Problem Solving in Hypertension

This work is dedicated to my daughter Rhona on her university graduation. I would like to extend my thanks also to all my family for their forbearance while I was engaged on this work.

Problem Solving in
Hypertension

LEE KENNEDY BSc, MB ChB, MD, PhD, FRCP, FRCPE, FRACP
Professor of Medicine, School of Medicine and Dentistry, Department of Medicine,
James Cook University, Queensland, Australia

CLINICAL PUBLISHING

OXFORD

CLINICAL PUBLISHING
an imprint of Atlas Medical Publishing Ltd
Oxford Centre for Innovation
Mill Street, Oxford OX2 0JX, UK

tel: +44 1865 811116
fax: +44 1865 251550

email: info@clinicalpublishing.co.uk
web: www.clinicalpublishing.co.uk

Distributed in USA and Canada by:
Clinical Publishing
30 Amberwood Parkway
Ashland OH 44805 USA
tel: 800-247-6553 (toll free within US and Canada)
fax: 419-281-6883
email: order@bookmasters.com

Distributed in UK and Rest of World by:
Marston Book Services Ltd
PO Box 269
Abingdon
Oxon OX14 4YN
UK
tel: +44 1235 465500
fax: +44 1235 465555
email: trade.orders@marston.co.uk

A catalogue record for this book is available from the British Library.

ISBN-13 978 1 84692 022 6
ISBN e-book 978 1 84692 617 4

The publisher makes no representation, express or implied, that the
dosages in this book are correct. Readers must therefore always check
the product information and clinical procedures with the most up-to-
date published product information and data sheets provided by the
manufacturers and the most recent codes of conduct and safety
regulations. The authors and the publisher do not accept any liability
for any errors in the text or for the misuse or misapplication of
material in this work.

Project manager: Gavin Smith, GPS Publishing Solutions, Herts, UK
Typeset by Phoenix Photosetting, Chatham, UK
Printed by Marston Book Services Ltd, Abingdon, Oxon, UK

Contents

SECTION 6   Complications and Emergencies

SECTION 7   Co-morbidities and Associated Disorders

SECTION 8   Secondary Causes of Hypertension

SECTION 9   Drugs to Treat Hypertension

Abbreviations

AASK	African American Study of Kidney disease and Hypertension	BMI	body mass index (kg/m^2)
		BNP	B-type natriuretic peptide
ABCD	Appropriate Blood pressure Control in Diabetes Study	BP	blood pressure
		CABG	coronary artery bypass grafting
ABPM	ambulatory blood pressure monitoring	CAD	coronary artery disease
ACE	angiotensin-converting enzyme	CAMELOT	Comparison of Amlodipine Versus Enalapril to Limit Occurrences of Thrombosis
ACE-I	angiotensin-converting enzyme inhibitor		
ACR	albumin/creatinine ratio	CAPP	CAptopril Prevention Project study
ACS	acute coronary syndrome	CB-1	cannabinoid-1
ACTH	adrenocorticotrophic hormone	CCB	calcium channel blocker
ADVANCE	Action in Diabetes and Vascular Disease: Preterax and Diamicron and MR Controlled Evaluation	CCF	congestive cardiac failure
		CD	collecting duct
		CgA	chromogranin A
AER	albumin excretion rate	CHARM	Candesartan in Heart failure – Assessment of Reduction in mortality and morbidity study
AF	atrial fibrillation		
AGE(s)	Advanced Glycation End Product(s)		
AHI	apnoea-hypopnoea index	CHD	coronary heart disease
ALLHAT	Antihypertensive and Lipid-Lowering Treatment to prevent Heart Attack Trial	CI	confidence interval
		CKD	chronic kidney disease
AME	apparent mineralocorticoid excess	CNS	central nervous system
cAMP	cyclic adenosine monophosphate	CO	cardiac output
ANBP-2	Australian National Blood Pressure Study-2	COC	combined oral contraceptive
		COMET	Carvedilol Or Metoprolol European study
ANF	antinuclear factor		
Ang I	angiotensin I	CONSENSUS	Cooperative North Scandinavian Enalapril Survival Study
Ang II	angiotensin II		
ANP	atrial natriuretic peptide	COPD	chronic obstructive pulmonary disease
APA	aldosterone producing adenoma	COMT	catechol O-methyltransferase
ARB	angiotensin receptor blocker	CPAP	continuous positive airways pressure
ARIC	Atherosclerosis Risk In Communities Study	CRH	corticotrophin-releasing hormone
		CROSS	Candesartan Role on Obesity and on Sympathetic System
ARR	aldosterone/renin ratio		
ASCOT	Anglo-SCandinavian Outcomes Trial	CT	computed tomography
ASCOT-BPLA	Anglo-Scandinavian Cardiac Outcomes Trial – Blood Pressure Lowering Arm	CURES	Chennai Urban Rural Epidemiology Study
ATP III	Cholesterol Education Program Adult Treatment Panel III	CV	cardiovascular
		CVD	cardiovascular disease
A-V	arteriovenous	DALY	disability-adjusted life-year
AVOID	Aliskiren in the Evaluation of Proteinuria in Diabetes	DASH	Dietary Approaches to Stop Hypertension
		DBP	diastolic blood pressure
BAH	bilateral adrenal hyperplasia	DCCB	dihydropyridine calcium channel blocker
BD	twice daily		
BENEDICT	BErgamo NEphrologic DIabetes Complications Trial	DCCT	Diabetes Control and Complications Trial
BEST	Beta-blocker Evaluation of Survival		
BK channel	large- (or big-)conductance calcium-activated potassium channel	DCT	distal convoluted tubule
		DHEA	dehydroepiandosterone

DHP	dihydropiridine	HOMA	homeostatic model assessment for insulin sensitivity/resistance
DM	diabetes mellitus		
DMSA	dimercaptosuccinic acid	HOPE	Heart Outcomes Prevention Evaluation Study
DOPA	dihydroxyphenylalanine		
DOPS	dihydroxyphenylserine	HOS	Hypertension-Obesity-Sibutramine study
DPP	dipeptidyl peptidase		
DREAM	Diabetes REduction Assessment with ramipril and rosiglitazone Medication study	HOT	Hypertension Optimal Treatment Study
		HR	heart rate
		HRs	hazard ratios
DRI	direct renin inhibitor	HRT	hormone replacement therapy
DVT	deep vein thrombosis	11β-HSD	11β-hydroxysteroid dehydrogenase
ECG	electrocardiogram	5-HT	5-hydroxytryptamine, serotonin
ED	erectile dysfunction	HTN	hypertension
EDC	Epidemiology of Diabetes Complications study	HyperGEN	Hypertension Genetic Epidemiology Network
EEG	electroencephalogram	HYVET	HYpertension in the Very Elderly Trial
EF	ejection fraction	IC	intermittent claudication
eGFR	estimated glomerular filtration rate	ICP	intracranial pressure
ELSA	European Lacidipine Study on Atherosclerosis	I/D	insertion/deletion
		IDF	International Diabetes Federation
EMEA	European Medicines Agency	IDNT	Irbesartan in Diabetic Nephropathy Trial
EPIC	European Prospective Investigation into Cancer		
		IFG	impaired fasting glucose
ESRD	end-stage renal disease	IGT	impaired glucose tolerance
EUROPA	EUropean trial on Reduction Of cardiac events with Perindopril	IHD	ischaemic heart disease
		IMPPACT	Investigation of Medical Professionals and Patients Achieving Control Together
FACET	Fosinopril versus Amlodipine Cardiovascular Events Trial		
		IMPROVE	Irbesartan in the Management of PROteinuric patients at high risk of Vascular Events
FBC	full blood count		
FDA	Food and Drug Administration		
FEVER	Felodipine Event Reduction	IMT	intima-media thickness
FFA	free fatty acids	INVEST	International VErapamil SR-Trandolapril study
FMD	fibromuscular dysplasia		
FPG	fasting plasma glucose	IP$_3$	inositol triphosphate
FPGL	functioning paraganglionoma	IRMA	Irbesartan in Diabetes with Microalbuminuria
GEMINI	Glycemic Effects in Diabetes Mellitus: Carvedilol-Metoprolol Comparison in Hypertensives		
		IRMA-2	IRbesartan MicroAlbuminuria type 2 diabetes in hypertension patients trial
GFR	glomerular filtration rate	i-SEARCH	International Survey Evaluating Microalbuminuria Routinely by Cardiologists in Patients with Hypertension
GI	gastrointestinal		
cGMP	cyclic guanosine monophosphate		
GP	general practitioner		
GRA	glucocorticoid-remediable aldosteronism		
		ISH	isolated systolic hypertension
GTN	glyceryl trinitrate	IUGR	intrauterine growth retardation
HBPM	home blood pressure monitoring	IV	intravenous
HCT	hydrochlorthiazide	JG	juxtaglomerular
HDFP	Hypertension Detection and Follow-up Programme	JNC7	US Joint National Committee
		JVP	jugular venous pressure
HELLP	Haemolytic anaemia, Elevated Liver enzymes and Low Platelets	LFT	liver function test
		LIFE	Losartan Intervention For Endpoint reduction Study
HERS	Heart and Estrogen Progestin Replacement Study		
		LV	left ventricular
HF	heart failure	LVA	low voltage activated
HOCM	hypertrophic obstructive cardiomyopathy	LVF	left ventricular failure
		LVH	left ventricular hypertrophy

LVMI	Left Ventricular Mass Index	PH	phaeochromocytoma
MA	microalbuminuria	PREVEND IT	Prevention of Renal and Vascular End
MAP	mean arterial pressure		Stage Disease Interventional Trial
MAG 3	mercaptoacetyltriglycine	PROactive	Prospective Pioglitazone Clinical Trial
MAO	monoamine oxidase		in Macrovascular Events
MARPLE	MicroAlbuminuria as Risk Predictor in	PROGRESS	Perindopril Protection against
	patients with arterial hypertension – a		Recurrent Stroke Study
	Long-time Evaluation with ramipril	PUFA	polyunsaturated fatty acid(s)
MEN	multiple endocrine neoplasia	PVD	peripheral vascular disease
MESA	Multi-Ethnic Study of Atherosclerosis	RAS	renin–angiotensin system
MetS	metabolic syndrome	RCT	randomized controlled trial
MHTN	masked hypertension	RENAAL	Reduction of Endpoints in NIDDM
MI	myocardial infarction		with the Angiotensin II Antagonist
MIBG	meta-iodobenzylguanidine		Losartan Trial
MMSE	Mini Mental State Examination	RR	relative risk
MONICA	MONitoring trends and determinants in	RRT	renal replacement therapy
	CArdiovascular disease	RUTH	Raloxifene Use for The Heart
MOXCON	Moxonidine Congestive Heart Failure	RVH	renovascular hypertension
	study	SAH	subarachnoid haemorrhage
MPA	medroxyprogesterone acetate	SAVE	Survival and Ventricular Enlargement
MRFIT	Multiple Risk Factor Intervention Trial	SBP	systolic blood pressure
MTHFR	methylenetetrahydrofolate	SCOPE	Study on COgnition and Prognosis in
	reductase		the Elderly
MUFA	monounsaturated fatty acid(s)	SCORE	Systemic Coronary Risk Evaluation
NA	noradrenaline	SCOUT	Sibutramine Cardiovascular OUTcomes
NAFLD	non-alcoholic fatty liver disease		Trial
NDCCB	non-dihydropyridine calcium channel	SDH	succinate dehydrogenase
	blocker	SENIORS	Study of the Effects of Nebivolol
NHANES	National Health And Nutrition		Intervention on Outcomes and
	Examination Survey		Rehospitalizations in Seniors with heart
NO	nitric oxide		failure
NOS	nitric oxide synthase	sFlt1	soluble fms-like tyrosine kinase 1
NSAID	non-steroidal anti-inflammatory drug	SHEP	Systolic Hypertension in the Elderly
NT-proBNP	N-terminal prohormone BNP		Program
NYHA	New York Heart Association	SNS	sympathetic nervous system
OA	osteoarthritis	SOLVD	Studies of Left Ventricular Dysfunction
OCP	oral contraceptive pill (combined)	SSRI	selective serotonin reputake inhibitor
OD	once daily	STEMI	ST elevation myocardial infarction
oGTT	oral glucose tolerance test	STOP	Swedish Trial in Old People with
OH	orthostatic hypertension		hypertension
OHTN	office (white coat) hypertension	SVT	supraventricular tachycardia
ONTARGET	Ongoing Telmisartan Alone and in	SWAN	Study of Women's health Across the
	Combination with Ramipril Global		Nation
	Endpoint Trial	Syst-Eur	Systolic Hypertension in Europe Study
OR	odds ratio	T2D	type 2 diabetes
OSAHS	obstructive sleep apnoea/hypopnoea	TG	triglycerides
	syndrome	TGF-β	transforming growth factor-β
PA	primary (hyper)aldosteronism	TIA	transient ischaemic attack
PAI-1	Plasminogen Activator Inhibitor-1	TNF-α	tumour necrosis factor-α
PAPY	Primary Aldosterone Prevalence in Italy	TPR	total peripheral resistance
PCKD	polycystic kidney disease	TOPH	Trials of Hypertension Prevention
PCOS	polycystic ovary syndrome	TROPHY	TRial Of Preventing HYpertension
PCT	proximal convoluted tubule	UAE	urinary albumin excretion
PDE5	phosphodiesterase type 5	U/E	urea and electrolytes
PEACE	Prevention of Events with ACE	UKPDS	United Kingdom Prospective Diabetes
	inhibition		Study

US	ultrasound
UTI	urinary tract infection
VALIANT	Valsartan in Acute Myocardial Infarction study
VALUE	Valsartan Antihypertensive Long-term Use Evaluation
VEGF	vascular endothelial growth factor
VSM	vascular smooth muscle
VTE	venous thromboembolism
WC	waist circumference
WCE	white coat effect
WHO	World Health Organization
WHR	waist-hip ratio

Hypertension – general

PROBLEM

01 Hypertension: When to Treat

Case History

Mrs LG is a 44-year-old mother of two. At a routine medical, her blood pressure (BP) is 140/92. She is rested, and when her BP is checked a week later a similar value is obtained. She was hypertensive in both her pregnancies, although did not require treatment. She is a non-smoker, does not drink alcohol, and has no regular medications. She is concerned about her BP as her father died in his 60s from heart disease and her mother had a stroke at a young age.

Does she have hypertension?

Does she require drug treatment for her BP?

Outline the general approach to her management

Background

Hypertension is a major risk factor for stroke, ischaemic heart disease, peripheral vascular disease, heart failure and chronic kidney disease. It is very common and can now be effectively treated. Starting at 115/75 mmHg, the risk of cardiovascular disease doubles for every 20/10 mmHg increase in BP. Individuals who are normotensive at age 55 have a lifetime risk of developing hypertension of 90%. Given its frequency and the fact that treatment is inevitably virtually life-long once started, it is critical to involve patients in

Table 1.1 Classification of hypertension (for adults)			
	Systolic mmHg		Diastolic mmHg
Normal	<120	and	<80
Prehypertension	120–139	or	80–89
Stage 1	140–159	or	90–99
Stage 2	160–179	or	100–109
Stage 3	≥180	or	≥110
Isolated systolic hypertension	≥140	and	<90

decisions regarding treatment. They should understand the potential benefits, and also possible side effects. See Table 1.1 for the classification of BP.

There are numerous local, national and international guidelines for managing hypertension. Many are based on the approach outlined in the report of the US Joint National Committee (JNC7).[1] BP should be measured using a suitable cuff, the bladder of which encircles at least 80% of the arm. The bladder should be centred over the brachial artery (located by palpation). A large cuff should be used for large individuals – if the cuff is too small an undue amount of pressure is required to compress the artery, yielding a falsely high reading.

Generally, BP should be recorded with the patient sitting, feet resting on the floor, with the arm supported at the level of the heart. When measured by auscultation, systolic is the pressure at which the first two or more sounds are heard (phase 1) and corresponds to ventricular contraction. Diastolic pressure corresponds to the ventricular filling phase and corresponds to the point at which sounds disappear (phase 5).

The patient should be rested for at least 5 minutes before measurement is made. The recording should be made on two separate occasions where important diagnostic or treatment decisions need to be made. The pressure should be recorded to the nearest 2 mmHg and the site of the recording (right or left arm) should be noted. Where there is doubt about accuracy of the measurement, pressure should be recorded in both arms. If there is a disparity, the arm with the higher pressure most accurately reflects BP.

The following may be helpful in making treatment decisions:

● Check systolic BP (SBP) by palpation: inflate cuff to above systolic and gradually deflate. SBP is that at which pulsation is first felt over the brachial or radial artery.

● Lying and standing BP: if postural symptoms are present or postural hypertension is suspected.

● Home BP monitoring (HBPM): this helps by excluding possible office or 'white coat' hypertension. Values above 135/85 are hypertensive. HBPM helps improve compliance with treatment.

● Ambulatory BP monitoring (ABPM): values are generally lower than office measurements and lower during the night. Hypertension is present when daytime values average >135/85 and sleeping values are >120/75.

The aims of assessment of patients with high BP are to:

- identify modifiable factors that may lower BP;
- assess overall risk of cardiovascular and renal complications;
- identify underlying causes;
- screen for end-organ damage, and
- plan treatment and follow-up.

Clinical examination should include pulse rate, jugular venous pressure, cardiac auscultation, and search for vascular bruits, oedema and palpation of peripheral pulses (dorsalis pedis and posterior tibial). Fundoscopy should be carried out to inspect for retinopathy. Patients with diabetes routinely have their fundi examined through dilated pupils. This is frequently omitted in patients with hypertension, although it is often difficult to obtain adequate views through undilated pupils. Weight and height, body mass index (kg/m^2) and waist circumference should be recorded. Urinalysis is essential. Plasma electrolytes and creatinine ($\pm$ estimated glomerular filtration rate), full blood count and fasting lipid profile (total, low-density lipoprotein and high-density lipoprotein cholesterol, and triglycerides) should always be requested. Electrocardiogram (ECG) is often omitted but useful to identify left ventricular hypertrophy. A spot check for albumin/creatinine ratio or timed collection for urinary protein output is also helpful.

The goals of treatment are summarized in Box 1.1.

Box 1.1 Aims of BP management

- Uncomplicated hypertension: 140/90
- Diabetes or chronic kidney disease: 130/80

Lifestyle modification should be incorporated into all regimens and may be sufficient alone in patients with prehypertension and in stage 1 hypertension. Average decreases in SBP with lifestyle modifications are as follows:

- Weight reduction to body mass index <25 kg/m^2: 5–20 mmHg
- Healthy eating plan: 8–14 mmHg
- Regular physical activity: 4–9 mmHg
- Restrict dietary salt: 2–8 mmHg
- Lower alcohol consumption: 2–4 mmHg

Thiazides are generally the first-line treatment in uncomplicated hypertension. Most patients require two agents to achieve targets. The most commonly used second-line agents are β-blockers, calcium channel blockers and angiotensin-converting enzyme inhibitors. Combination agents (e.g. diuretic + angiotensin-converting enzyme inhibitor) are very useful and improve compliance.

Recent Developments

1   Hypertension is becoming commoner in children and adolescents, but is frequently overlooked in this age group.[2] With rising prevalence of obesity, hypertension is more likely to develop in younger people. Early lifestyle interventions will prevent the progress of hypertension and may retard the onset of complications.

2   Self-monitoring of BP not only improves concordance with treatment but also improves the BP achieved during treatment.[3] Recent data[4] also demonstrate improvement in surrogate markers for complications – B-type natriuretic peptide (BNP) and urinary albumin excretion (UAE) – in patients who are self-monitoring. While there is acceptance among health professionals that HBPM is useful, many still rely more on office values when making diagnostic or treatment decisions.[5]

3   A recent study from the USA[6] examined the factors associated with poor awareness and control of hypertension. Women and non-Hispanic black patients were less likely to have well-controlled BP. Hypertension awareness was particularly poor among younger subjects. Poverty and lack of health insurance were particularly associated with ineffective treatment.

4   BP is labile and careful assessment of patients is necessary if they are not to be placed on unnecessary treatment. Marshall *et al.*[7] estimated the pretreatment BP in 'hypertensive' young people. It appeared that a large proportion might not actually require treatment. Obesity and the presence of renal abnormalities are strong correlates for the need for antihypertensive treatment.

5   Guidelines focus on fixed cut-off points for diagnosis and classification. These are artificial – risk with increasing BP is a continuous function and also related to other factors. There are arguments for the classification of hypertension based on overall cardiovascular risk assessment.[8] This would help us to target education and intervention to those most in need.[9]

6   Many practitioners record BP measurements rounded off to the nearest zero. This can result in many patients being misclassified in risk calculators[10] and may thus lead to inappropriate treatment. Automated BP measuring devices do not have rounding off errors.

Conclusions

By definition, the above patient is hypertensive. Given her history of gestational hypertension and her family history, she will almost certainly ultimately require drug treatment. However, as outlined in Figure 1.1, the first step is lifestyle management. She does not have a markedly elevated BP and attention to lifestyle factors may delay the need for drug treatment. Accurate assessment of BP and overall assessment of the patient's risk are critical when making treatment decisions. Involvement of the patient in decision-making is crucial to the success of hypertension management.

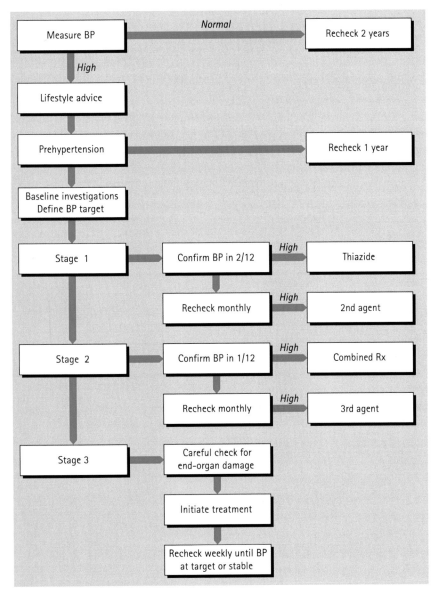

Figure 1.1 Management of hypertension.

References

1   Chobanian AV, Bakris GL, Black HR, Cushman WC, Green LA, Izzo JL, *et al.* The Seventh Report of the Joint National Committee on Prevention, Detection, Evaluation, and Treatment of High Blood Pressure. The JNC7 Report. *JAMA* 2003; **289**: 2560–72.

2   Hansen ML, Gunn PW, Kaelber DC. Underdiagnosis of hypertension in children and adolescents. *JAMA* 2007; **298**: 874–9.

3   Cappuccio FP, Kerry SM, Forbes L, Donald A. Blood pressure control by home monitoring: meta-analysis of randomised trials. *BMJ* 2004; **329**: 145–51.

4   Eguchi K, Matsui Y, Shibasaki S, Ishikawa J, Hoshide S, Ishikawa S, *et al.* Changes in self-monitored pulse pressure correlate with improvements in B-type natriuretic peptide and urinary albumin in treated hypertensive patients. *Am J Hypertens* 2007; **20**: 1268–75.

5   Logan AG, Dunai A, McIsaac WJ, Irvine MJ, Tisler A. Attitudes of primary care physicians and their patients about home blood pressure monitoring in Ontario. *J Hypertens* 2008; **26**: 446–52.

6   Ostchega Y, Hughes JP, Wright JD, McDowell MA, Louis T. Are demographic characteristics, health care access and utilization, and comorbid conditions associated with hypertension among US adults? *Am J Hypertens* 2008; **21**: 159–65.

7   Marshall T, Tennant R, Harrison WN. Estimating the proportion of young adults on antihypertensive treatment that have been correctly diagnosed. *J Hum Hypertens* 2008; **22**: 96–101.

8   Scheltens T, Bots ML, Numans ME, Grobbee DE, Hoes AW. Awareness, treatment and control of hypertension: the 'rule of halves' in an era of risk–based treatment of hypertension. *J Hum Hypertens* 2007; **21**: 99–106.

9   Weir MR. Risk-based classification of hypertension and the role of combination therapy. *J Clin Hypertens* 2008; **10** (Suppl 1): 4–12.

10   Broad J, Wells S, Marshall R, Jackson R. Zero end-digit preference in recorded blood pressure and its impact on classification of patients for pharmacologic management in primary care – PREDICT-CVD-6. *Br J Gen Pract* 2007; **57**: 897–903.

PROBLEM

02 Sphygmomanometers

Case History

Peter is a 58-year-old former policeman who gets frustrated with his blood pressure (BP). He has been treated for 8 years, complies with medication and does not mind taking treatment (amlodipine and bendrofluazide). He recently attended clinic as a prelude to day surgery for his hernia, and was told that his BP was not controlled. At his last visit to his general practice he was assured that the BP was controlled. He recently had it measured at his pharmacy where a value of 152/88 was recorded. He is considering buying a machine to monitor his BP.

Why is it so difficult to get a consistent measure of BP?

Is one type of BP measurement device better than others?

How should we ensure that a sphygmomanometer is functioning?

How helpful is home BP monitoring (HBPM)?

Background

The BP measured is an estimate of the pressure exerted against the vessel wall by the column of blood. It can be measured directly by arterial cannulation with a pressure transducer (only practical in intensive care settings). The earliest direct measurement of arterial pressure in animals was by Reverend Stephen Hales in 1733. Human arterial pressure was first measured directly by Karl Ludwig in 1847. Invention of the indirect method for measuring BP is credited to the Austrian-Jewish physician Samuel Siegfried Karl Ritter von Basch (1837–1905) in 1881, who used a water-filled bag connected to a manometer to occlude the arterial pulse. The mercury sphygmomanometer (Greek: sphygmós = pulse, manometer = pressure measuring device) was invented by the Italian paediatrician Scipione Riva-Rocci (1863–1937) in 1896. It was further developed by the neurosurgeon Harvey Cushing (1869–1939). Nikolai Sergeievich Korotkoff (1874–1920) described the measurement of BP using sounds heard over the partly occluded artery in 1903.

Although a variety of methods have been developed for BP measurement, use of a mercury device with auscultation is still the gold standard.[1] The artery is occluded by inflating the suitably placed cuff above systolic BP (SBP), and the cuff is gradually deflated. Korotkoff sounds (Box 2.1) are used to measure SBP and diastolic BP (DBP). These arise because of a combination of turbulent flow and oscillation in the arterial wall

> **Box 2.1 Korotkoff sounds**
>
> Phase 1: appearance of clear tapping sounds = systolic pressure
>
> Phase 2: sounds become softer and longer
>
> Phase 3: sounds become crisper and louder
>
> Phase 4: sounds become muffled and softer
>
> Phase 5: disappearance of sounds = diastolic pressure

while the vessel is partially obstructed – there are no sounds when the cuff is inflated above SBP and flow is completely obstructed, or when the cuff is below DBP and flow is unimpeded. The BP measured by this method is generally lower than that with direct intra-arterial measurement. There has been debate about whether phase 4 or 5 should be used for DBP, but there is now agreement that phase 5 should be used. Sometimes the sounds persist in spite of deflation of the cuff – pregnancy, arteriovenous fistula and aortic regurgitation. In this case, phase 4 should be used. The sounds may disappear and reappear between SBP and DBP in older patients with increased pulse pressure (the auscultatory gap). Mercury sphygmomanometers are now less widely used because of safety concerns with mercury.

Aneroid sphygmomanometers are now widely used. Here the column of mercury is replaced by a series of bellows and levers that allow an estimate of the pressure to be read on a circular dial. These devices tend to become inaccurate with time, particularly if they are moved around frequently. They need to be calibrated regularly. Hybrid devices use a pressure transducer to measure pressure. This can be linked to a digital readout or other display, but auscultation is still used to estimate the points at which SBP and DBP are reached. A 3 mmHg difference in readings between aneroid and mercury devices is considered acceptable.

Semi-automatic and automatic oscillometric devices are now widely used. These devices do not require the brachial artery to be located as they do not use pressure transducers. As with auscultatory determination, a cuff is placed around the arm and inflated above SBP. As it is deflated, oscillations are detected when flow is partially obstructed. Maximum oscillation is at mean arterial pressure. The devices use an algorithm to estimate SBP and DBP. The algorithms used vary between devices and are not disclosed by the manufacturers. There is a variation in performance between devices, and a variable relationship between pressure measured by mercury or aneroid devices. A list of machines that have been validated can be found at the British Hypertension Society website (http://www.bhsoc.org). Because of ease of use and safety, devices that use the oscillometric technique are suitable for HBPM and ambulatory BP monitoring. The recommended site for monitoring is the upper arm. Wrist devices can yield accurate readings but care has to be taken that the wrist is located at the level of the heart. Finger devices are also available but not currently recommended for routine use. Oscillometric devices tend to overestimate SBP and underestimate DBP. They should be validated for use in pregnancy, and may be inaccurate with increased arterial stiffness, e.g. diabetes and in older people. They are also often inaccurate when cardiac rhythm is irregular. Atrial fibrillation is the commonest arrhythmia and is associated with beat-to-beat varia-

Box 2.2 Non-representative blood pressure measurements

Too high

- Recorded by doctor or nurse
- Stress or anxiety
- Following physical exertion
- Smoking or caffeine intake
- Recent alcohol ingestion
- After meals
- Patient has a full bladder
- Early morning

Too low

- Recently taken medication
- During or after rest

tion in stroke volume, and therefore BP. Accurate BP measurements can be obtained with oscillometric devices in patients with atrial fibrillation.[2] However, the machine must be validated for use in atrial fibrillation and for the individual patient (variations in vascular compliance may affect performance).

Apart from variables related to the device used, a number of patient variables should be taken into account (Box 2.2). If a mercury device is used, calibration can be checked by establishing that the meniscus of the mercury column is at the zero level. The column should be free of dirt or debris and should rise and fall freely with cuff inflation and deflation. The bladder and tubing should be in good condition. The device should be calibrated every 2–5 years in a recognized laboratory against a reference mercury column or a non-mercury calibration device. In scientific studies, the random zero sphygmomanometer has been widely used to eliminate observer bias. Here, a variable baseline (hidden to the observer) is added to the measurement obtained. Once BP has been measured, the observer can subtract the baseline from the figures measured. Aneroid devices are mechanical devices and, particularly if they have been moved around a lot during usage, can yield inaccurate results. They should be calibrated every 6 months.

Given the vagaries of office BP measurement, it is not surprising that HBPM is finding wider usage. HBPM eliminates the white coat effect, is as predicative of end-organ damage as ambulatory BP monitoring, and helps to improve BP control by increasing patient awareness and their engagement with lifestyle and pharmacological management.[3] A list of validated devices can be found at http://www.bhsoc.org or http://dableducation.org. Note that measurement of BP at home is subject to many of the confounding factors that influence office measurements (Box 2.2). It is not always easy to translate HBPM measurements into office values and vice versa, and those using HBPM tend to have lower office values. However, consensus is being reached as to how HBPM should be carried out and what constitutes normal values.[1] Overuse of HBPM measurements may increase anxiety. Measurement of two morning and two evening (before dinner) values on three consecutive days each month is reasonable. SBP of less than 137 and DBP of 66–83 mmHg are considered normal for home values, and it is probably reasonable that these values are also used as targets for successful treatment.

Recent Developments

1   HBPM eliminates the white coat effect, but this is of independent prognostic significance. Stergiou *et al.*[4] did not find any superiority of HBPM over office or ambulatory measures in predicting cardiovascular end-points. By contrast, Shimbo *et al.*[5] found HBPM to be superior to office measurements in predicting cardiovascular end-points including increased Left Ventricular Mass Index.

2   The recent IMPPACT (Investigation of Medical Professionals and Patients Achieving Control Together) study[6] compared patients randomized to usual treatment with those randomized to use HBPM and participate in protocol-driven titration. The HBPM approach led to improvements in both SBP and DBP. This was confirmed by the J-HOME study,[7] involving nearly 2400 patients. Again, HBPM improved not only home but also office BP measures.

3   A morning BP surge is a marker for risk of renal end-points and left ventricular hypertrophy.[8] It is more likely to occur in older patients and those with a longer duration of hypertension. It also occurs in those who regularly drink alcohol in the evening.[9] This effect of alcohol may be missed when only office measurements are used. HBPM provides valuable feedback to the patients on what influences their BP and helps them make favourable lifestyle changes.

4   HBPM is useful in pregnant women,[10] although there are no agreed criteria for SBP and DBP in relation to hypertension diagnosis. SBP is more likely to show a disparity between home and office measures in pregnancy. There is an increasing interest in the use of telemedicine for those who live remotely or who otherwise might find it difficult to attend regular office appointments. In these circumstances, HBPM could prove a valuable asset in achieving safe BP control.[11]

Conclusions

The use of mercury sphygmomanometers has decreased recently because of concerns over safety and the high cost of cleaning up mercury spills. Whichever device is used they should be validated, well maintained and have been recently calibrated. In practice, surprisingly little attention is paid to the validity of the measuring device used. Up to 9% of consultations and 8% of prescriptions in general practice are for hypertension. On a population basis, even a relatively small error in BP measurement could greatly influence the number of patients diagnosed with, and treated for, hypertension. An office measurement of BP using an auscultatory technique and a suitably maintained and calibrated mercury or aneroid device is still the gold standard, and should be the ultimate arbitrator in major treatment decisions (Figure 2.1). Automated oscillometric devices are very useful and form the basis of ambulatory and other home monitoring devices. HBPM is finding increasing usage. It should not be used alone to diagnose hypertension but certainly improves engagement with management and allows for the monitoring of treatment response.

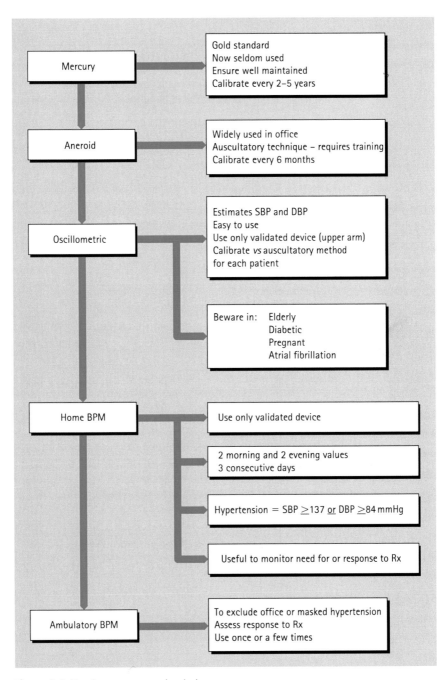

Figure 2.1 Blood pressure measuring devices.

References

1 Pickering TG, Hall JE, Appel LJ, Falkner BE, Graves J, Hill MN, *et al.* Recommendations for blood pressure measurement in humans and experimental animals. *Hypertension* 2005; **45**: 142–61.

2 Jani B, Bulpitt CJ, Rajkumar C. The accuracy of blood pressure measurement in atrial fibrillation. *J Hum Hypertens* 2006; **20**: 543–5.

3 Verberk WJ, Kroon AA, Jongen-Vancraybex HA, de Leeuw PW. The applicability of home blood pressure measurement in clinical practice: a review of literature. *Vasc Health Risk Manage* 2007; **3**: 959–66.

4 Stergiou GS, Baibas NM, Kalogeropoulos PG. Cardiovascular risk prediction based on home blood pressure measurement: the Didima study. *J Hypertens* 2007; **25**: 1590–6.

5 Shimbo D, Pickering TG, Spruill TM, Abraham D, Schwartz JE, Gerin W. Relative utility of home, ambulatory, and office blood pressures in the prediction of end-organ damage. *Am J Hypertens* 2007; **20**: 476–82.

6 Tobe SW, Hunter K, Geerts R, Raymond N, Pylypchuk G, Canadian Hypertension Society. IMPPACT: Investigation of Medical Professionals and Patients Achieving Control Together. *Can J Cardiol* 2008; **24**: 205–8.

7 Obara T, Ohkubo T, Asayama K, Metoki H, Inoue R, Kikuya M, *et al.* Home blood pressure measurements associated with better blood pressure control: the J-HOME study. *J Hum Hypertens* 2008; **22**: 197–204.

8 Ishikawa J, Hoshide S, Shibasaki S, Matsui Y, Kabutoya T, Eguchi K, *et al.* Relationship between morning hypertension identified by home blood pressure monitoring and brain natriuretic peptide and estimated glomerular filtration rate: the Japan Morning Surge 1 (JMS-1) Study. *J Clin Hypertens* 2008; **10**: 34–42.

9 Ishikawa J, Kario K, Eguchi K, Morinari M, Hoshide S, Ishikawa S, *et al.* Regular alcohol drinking is a determinant of masked morning hypertension detected by home blood pressure monitoring in medicated hypertensive patients with well-controlled clinic blood pressure: the Jichi Morning Hypertension Research (J-MORE) study. *Hypertens Res Clin Exp* 2006; **29**: 679–86.

10 Rey E, Pilon F, Boudreault J. Home blood pressure levels in pregnant women with chronic hypertension. *Hypertens Pregnancy* 2007; **26**: 403–14.

11 Palmas W, Pickering TG, Teresi J, Schwartz JE, Field L, Weinstock RS, *et al.* Telemedicine home blood pressure measurements and progression of albuminuria in elderly people with diabetes. *Hypertension* 2008; **51**: 1282–8.

PROBLEM

03 Ambulatory Blood Pressure Monitoring

Case History

Andrea is a 42-year-old woman. She had hypertension in both her pregnancies and has been attending regularly to have her blood pressure (BP) checked. Office measurements are usually high. Her neighbour has a home BP device and Andrea has noted that her home measurements are usually in the recommended range. She does get nervous at clinic visits, and would prefer not to take BP medications unless they are really necessary.

When should ambulatory blood pressure monitoring (ABPM) be used?

How are values obtained with ABPM interpreted relative to clinic measurements?

Does high BP on ABPM predict risk of cardiovascular (CV) events?

Background

ABPM is a non-invasive, automated technique where a series of BP recordings is made over a defined time – usually every 15–30 min for 24 h, yielding a total of 50–100 recordings. Most devices use an oscillometric technique, and only fully validated devices should be used (see http://www.bhsoc.org or http://www.dableducational.org). Office BP measurements are a useful surrogate marker for risk of end organ damage and for risk of CV events, including stroke and myocardial infarction. Studies in recent years have confirmed that averaged BP measurements are even more useful as a marker.[1]

The cut-off values for ABPM have been redefined using data from 5682 participants in different countries (Table 3.1)[2] – they are rounded up for convenience and compared with the equivalent values for office measurement. These thresholds were set taking into account a 10-year follow-up, during which there were 814 CV events including 377 strokes and 435 cardiac events. Not surprisingly, the average daytime thresholds do not differ from those for office BPs. The addition of night-time measurements adds an additional dimension. Mild, moderate and severe hypertension is present at systolic pressures of 141–155, 156–170 and >170 mmHg, respectively, for daytime. The corresponding diastolic ranges are 91–100, 101–110 and >110 mmHg. For night-time pressures 126–135, 136–150 and >150 mmHg systolic define mild, moderate and severe hypertension respectively. The corresponding figures for diastolic BP are 76–85, 86–100 and >100 mmHg.

Indications for ABPM are as follows:

Table 3.1 Threshold values (mmHg)			
	Optimal	Normal	High
Office			
SBP	120	130	140
DBP	80	85	90
ABPM, 24 h			
SBP	115	125	130
DBP	75	75	80
ABPM, day			
SBP	120	130	140
DBP	80	85	85
ABPM, night			
SBP	100	110	120
DBP	65	75	75

DBP, diastolic blood pressure; SBP, systolic blood pressure.

- *Suspected office or white coat hypertension.* This is present when office BP is consistently >140/90 and daytime ambulatory average is <135/85 or 24-h average is <125/80. The white coat effect is seen in patients who are normotensive or hypertensive and implies an increase of 20 mmHg systolic and/or 10 mmHg diastolic when BP is measured in the clinical setting. Office hypertension is hard to predict from clinical variables.

- *Masked hypertension.* Up to 1:3 patients with hypertension have higher measurements outside the clinic setting. Masked or reverse white coat hypertension should be suspected where there is an inappropriate amount of end organ damage (e.g. left ventricular hypertrophy, microalbuminuria or renal impairment) for the degree of BP elevation. It is commoner in men and risk increases with stress, smoking and high intake of alcohol or caffeine.

- *Nocturnal hypertension.* This is an important risk factor for CV disease with each 5% increase in either systolic or diastolic BP associated with a 20% increase in CV risk. Antihypertensive drugs are most frequently taken in the morning, often leaving the night time and early morning not covered. Non-dipping may account for some of the increased risk of African American subjects.

- *Nocturnal non-dippers.* Some people do not experience the normal decrease in BP overnight (non-dippers). They are at increased risk of CV disease and more likely to have a secondary cause for hypertension.

- *Variable BP measurements.* These can indicate variable compliance with medication. For untreated patients, episodic hypertension is a feature of phaeochromocytoma. It can also indicate a wide variation in exposure to stressful stimuli.

● *Planning antihypertensive treatment.* If ABPM yields a better measure of CV risk than office BP measures, then aiming for satisfactory control on ABPM should afford better CV protection. ABPM or home BP monitoring is also useful in assessing the impact of lifestyle interventions.

● *Hypotension.* BP is more variable in the elderly and isolated systolic hypertension (ISH) is frequently found on office BP measurements, which are not uncommonly 20 mmHg or more than those found with out of office measures. The elderly are more likely to have baroreceptor or autonomic failure. Signs of the latter may be episodic or sustained low BP during the day, with relatively high BP at night and decreases in BP after meals. If a Holter monitor is used simultaneously, the episodes of hypotension will be seen not to be accompanied by an appropriate increase in pulse rate.

● *Where control of BP is particularly important.* These are patients with diabetes or chronic kidney disease. There is very good evidence that tight BP control protects the kidneys. The degree of albuminuria can be used to monitor response. Patients with chronic kidney disease from non-diabetic causes also require tight BP control.

● *Pregnancy.* Treatment decisions are important but unnecessary drugs should be avoided. Tight control of BP in those with chronic or gestational hypertension will lessen the risk of hypertensive complications and operative delivery.

● *Children and adolescents.* Again, office measures of BP are frequently non-representative. Secondary causes are more common. Treatment decisions are difficult, particularly as the patient may require life-long treatment.

Potential problems with ABPM may be noted when the machine is being fitted to the patient. The most common problem is with arrhythmias – atrial fibrillation, frequent ectopics, episodic supraventricular tachycardia (SVT) – all of which may cause variable and spurious results. Elderly or diabetic patients with stiff arteries may have inaccurate measurements. ABPM is not currently recommended for those with very high BP. In this case, initial treatment to decrease BP should be instituted and ABPM used to titrate treatment. Some bruising or swelling round the cuff site may occur. Pressure effects on the ulnar nerve have been reported.

ABPM can give important information about the duration of effect of BP-lowering regimens. The majority of trials have been based on office BP measurements under defined and closely controlled conditions. There is a cost and inconvenience associated with ABPM but this must be weighed against the potential disadvantages of medication.

Recent Developments

1 With ABPM there is still scope for error in hypertension diagnosis with use of only a single recording.[3] The prevailing BP may be either over- or underestimated. When BP is elevated on ABPM and home BP monitoring, there is a greater correlation with end-points such as increased Left Ventricular Mass Index.[4] This relationship becomes more apparent with increased number of measurements. Hansen *et al.*[5] confirmed the superiority of ABPM over office measurements for predicating CV events. Compared with normotension the

relative risk of CV events with ABPM was 1.22 (95% CI: 0.96 to 1.53) for office hypertension (OHTN), 1.62 (95% CI: 1.35 to 1.96) for masked hypertension (MHTN), and 1.80 (95% CI: 1.59 to 2.03) for sustained hypertension.

2   A study of 3957 patients followed for over 27 000 person-years,[6] confirmed a relationship between increased nocturnal BP and mortality risk. A meta-analysis of four studies involving a total of 3468 patients has confirmed that the relationship between nocturnal BP abnormalities and CV mortality is stronger than that for daytime BP. There is a gradual shift in emphasis from daytime to night-time BP for predicting adverse prognosis.

3   In a recent large cohort study following patients over 5.8 years,[7] stroke risk was higher with nocturnal non-dipping, while increased daytime BP was a greater risk for cardiac events. Wider use of ABPM has been recommended on the basis of a national study in Spain involving about 20 000 patients.[8] While there is a correlation between office and ambulatory measures of BP, discrepancies are frequently found. In those with suspected hypertension, 60% will exhibit a non-dipping pattern and this is emerging as a major risk factor for CV disease.

4   Hyperaldosteronism is an under-recognized contributor to hypertension risk and aldosterone antagonists are finding increasing use, particularly in resistant hypertension. Office BP measurements may not be different in patients with high and normal aldosterone levels.[9] By contrast, average 24-h BP levels, daytime and night-time averages are all higher in patients with evidence of mineralocorticoid excess.

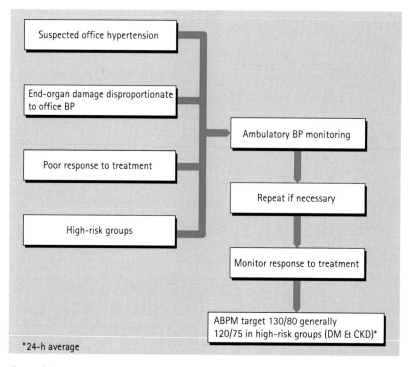

Figure 3.1 Use of ambulatory blood pressure monitoring. CKD, chronic kidney disease; DM, diabetes mellitus.

Conclusions

Out of office BPs are most useful when clinic BPs appear to be at variance with the clinical picture, and to give an indication of BP variability, including diurnal rhythm (Figure 3.1). The daytime average with ABPM is typically lower than clinic measures and 135/85 on ABPM daytime average corresponds generally to 140/90 – the cut-off for diagnosing hypertension. Diagnosis of OHTN is the most common use of ABPM. This is important as OHTN is hard to predict clinically and is relatively innocent as far as CV risk is concerned. MHTN is increasingly recognized as a CV risk factor with a relative risk for CV events of about 2.3 compared with normotensive subjects. With increasing evidence that ABPM gives a more reliable indication of underlying BP status than office BP and is more predictive of CV events, it is certain that this technique will find increasing usage in clinical practice within a relatively short space of time.

References

1   Pickering TG, Shimbo D, Haas D. Ambulatory blood-pressure monitoring. *N Engl J Med* 2006; **354**: 2368–74.

2   Kikuya M, Hansen TW, Thijs L, Bjorklund-Bodegard K, Kuznetsova T, Ohkubo T, *et al.* Diagnostic thresholds for ambulatory blood pressure monitoring based on 10-year cardiovascular risk. *Circulation* 2007; **115**: 2145–52.

3   Cuspidi C, Meani S, Sala C, Valerio C, Fusi V, Zanchetti A, *et al.* How reliable is isolated clinical hypertension defined by a single 24-h ambulatory blood pressure monitoring? *J Hypertens* 2007; **25**: 315–20.

4   Shimbo D, Pickering TG, Spruill TM, Abraham D, Schwartz JE, Gerin W. Relative utility of home, ambulatory, and office blood pressures in the prediction of end-organ damage. *Am J Hypertens* 2007; **20**: 476–82.

5   Hansen TW, Kikuya M, Thijs L, Bjorklund-Bodegard K, Kuznetsova T, Ohkubo T, *et al.* Prognostic superiority of daytime ambulatory over conventional blood pressure in four populations: a meta-analysis of 7,030 individuals. *J Hypertens* 2007; **25**: 1554–64.

6   Ben-Dov IZ, Kark JD, Ben-Ishay D, Mekler J, Ben-Arie L, Bursztyn M. Predictors of all-cause mortality in clinical ambulatory monitoring: unique aspects of blood pressure during sleep. *Hypertension* 2007; **49**: 1235–41.

7   Pickering T, Schwartz J, Verdecchia P, Imai Y, Kario K, Eguchi K, *et al.* Prediction of strokes versus cardiac events by ambulatory monitoring of blood pressure: results from an international database. *Blood Press Monit* 2007; **12**: 397–9.

8   Gorostidi M, Sobrino J, Segura J, Sierra C, de la Sierra A, Hernandez del Rey R, *et al.* Ambulatory blood pressure monitoring in hypertensive patients with high cardiovascular risk: a cross-sectional analysis of a 20,000-patient database in Spain. *J Hypertens* 2007; **25**: 977–84.

9   Pimenta E, Gaddam KK, Pratt-Ubunama MN, Nishizaka MK, Cofield SS, Oparil S, *et al.* Aldosterone excess and resistance to 24-h blood pressure control. *J Hypertens* 2007; **25**: 2131–7.

PROBLEM

04 Office and Masked Hypertension

Case History

Robert is a fit 36-year-old man. He has a strong family history of hypertension. He recently had an insurance medical at home and was noted to have blood pressure (BP) of 146/92. As suggested, he saw his general practitioner and was found to have normal BP (<140/90 on two occasions). His electrocardiogram (ECG) was normal, as was the fundoscopy, and he had no microalbuminuria. He would like to be sure that he does not need treatment for BP.

How often is there a difference between office BP and that measured at home?

Does masked hypertension (MHTN) need to be treated?

Does office hypertension (OHTN) need to be treated?

What factors contribute to variance between office and home BP measurements?

Background

OHTN and MHTN (defined in Box 4.1 and Figure 4.1) are very common, and although the presence of either diagnosis suggests that hypertension is not sustained they carry a worse prognosis than that for subjects who are normotensive. The terms 'white coat hypertension' and 'reverse white coat hypertension' are also used for these conditions. Office and home measurements are easy to deal with when they agree but harder when there is disagreement.

Clinic BP measurements have been the mainstay of diagnosis and management for many years. MHTN is present in up to 10% of the general population. It is easy to understand that the anxiety of having BP measured by a doctor or nurse increases the BP. However, this is a short-term phenomenon that indicates the individual's response to stressful events. However, those with MHTN have increased pressure for a larger part of

---

Box 4.1 Masked and office hypertension

- *Masked hypertension*: office or clinic BP is normal (<140/90) but out of clinic BP is elevated (>135/85) on daytime or home BP monitoring.

- *Office hypertension*: increased BP (>140/90) in the office or clinic setting but normal BP (<135/85) with ambulatory or home BP monitoring.

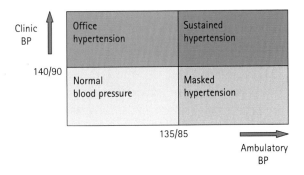

Figure 4.1 Classification of BP status. Adapted from Pickering *et al.* 2007.[1]

the day and are therefore at increased risk. Patients with MHTN are more likely to be young, male and subject to chronic stress. Smokers have higher than average BP but may have relatively low office BP measurements compared with their prevailing BP status. Alcohol is another confounding influence with higher alcohol consumption being associated with higher home BP (especially in the morning). MHTN is generally present in daytime hours and strongly linked with increased physical activity and stress levels, including occupational stress. Ambulatory BP monitoring (ABPM) tends to increase less with age than do clinic measures. Several studies[1] have confirmed a population prevalence of at least 10%, and a link with chronic stress. It is also documented to occur in children. Clearly, MHTN may be a precursor for sustained hypertension. MHTN is a marker for adverse end-points and increases risk of intermediate markers such as increased left ventricular (LV) mass and carotid intima-media thickness (IMT). The fact that it appears to be at least as important a risk factor as sustained hypertension suggests that aspects other than simply BP elevation may contribute to risk in patients susceptible to MHTN.

A substantial proportion of the population carries hypertensive risk that is not reflected in clinic BP measurements. Most intervention trials are based on clinic BP measures. It is not known whether treatment of patients with MHTN lowers their risk. Office BP measurements may reassure us that the patient is at low risk from hypertensive complications. Improved knowledge and measures of risk should help to identify those at risk of out of office hypertension and who may therefore benefit from either home BP monitoring (HBPM) or ABPM. Increased out of office hypertension may mask risk of renal complications, LV and other end-points. Clinic measurements of BP are fickle and only partly reflect risk. Some individuals at high risk from increased BP may not be identified by clinic BP measurements. Morning hypertension is the commonest form and, apart from normal diurnal variation, evening alcohol consumption and use of short-acting hypotensive agents, which only give partial 24-hour cover may contribute to this. Causes of increased night-time BP include high salt intake, renal impairment and sleep apnoea. It is intrinsically harder to identify hypertensive individuals whose predominant rise in BP is in out-of-clinic situations, but because of collateral risk and the proportion of their time that these individuals are hypertensive it is important to identify those with MHTN.

BP is often elevated when measured in the clinic setting, but may decrease by as much as 30 mmHg when the patient relaxes. The difference between the initial office measure and the measure taken with the subject fully relaxed is the 'white coat effect'. Both OHTN and MHTN are cardiovascular (CV) risk factors in their own right and are precursors to established hypertension. Patients with OHTN should be assessed for overall CV risk and for end-organ damage. While individuals with OHTN are at increased risk, antihypertensive treatment is less beneficial than in those with sustained hypertension. OHTN is defined as BP of 140/90 or above in the clinic and less than 135/85 in ABPM or HBPM. Office hypertension, unlike masked hypertension, is more common in women.

OHTN may be present in up to 25% of patients who fulfil diagnostic criteria for hypertension in an office BP measurement. ABPM is valuable in diagnosis but a single measurement is not necessarily sufficient to make a diagnosis – the first ABPM may be subject to similar influences that increase BP in office measurements. A suitably validated and calibrated machine must be used. OHTN appears to be commoner in women, in those with a family history of hypertension, with a faster pulse rate, and with a relatively small BP elevation (especially diastolic blood pressure [DBP]). Patients with OHTN do not have an increase in LV mass, alterations in carotid IMT, or retinal vascular changes. Their prognosis is better than that of patients with sustained hypertension. Patients with OHTN are more likely to have dyslipidaemia and elevated plasma glucose. There is also an increased risk of non-classical risk factors, including endothelial dysfunction and clotting disorders (increased fibrinogen and D-dimer). It is not entirely benign, but does not warrant routine prescription of antihypertensive drugs. Treatment should be considered if overall CV risk is 20% or more in 10 years. Otherwise the patient should be advised on lifestyle measures, and followed-up.

Recent Developments

1   There is a correlation between OHTN and metabolic CV risk factors. For example, Bo et al.[2] reported OHTN in 60% of patients attending a lipid clinic – careful evaluation of these patients revealed that the majority did not have worrying elevations in their BP outside the clinic. OHTN is also common among patients with diabetes. Prognosis in these patients is not as poor as those with sustained hypertension and probably differs very little to that of normotensive diabetic individuals.[3]

2   MHTN is much more difficult as we largely rely on clinic BP measurements, and may thus falsely reassure a patient. MHTN is common among patients with diabetes (up to 30%) and associated with increased albuminuria, increased LV mass and a higher prevalence of silent cerebral infarcts.[4] Other studies confirm that MHTN is an independent risk factor for increased urinary albumin excretion (UAE),[5] and the development of concentric LV hypertrophy.[6] These studies suggest that high-risk groups should be investigated for increased daytime BP and treated accordingly. Patients with OHTN do not carry a similar risk.

3   Data from the Ohasama Study[7] suggest that carotid IMT is increased in MHTN to a similar degree to that found in those with sustained hypertension. However, those with OHTN did not differ from normotensive subjects. These conclusions are at variance with the findings of two other recent studies. Investigating 2778 Italian hypertensives, de Simone et al.[8] documented that increased arterial stiffness was strongly correlated with the magnitude of the white coat effect. Puato et al.[9] carried out a 5-year follow-up study of carotid IMT in patients with

stage 1 hypertension. They demonstrated that IMT was greater and increased more rapidly in those with OHTN.

4   It has been suggested that any increased risk with OHTN may be related to associated features of metabolic syndrome (MetS), rather than to transient increases in BP. Mule et al.[10] confirmed that MetS variables were more likely to be associated with increased Left Ventricular Mass Index, but OHTN alone also correlated with LV structural abnormalities.

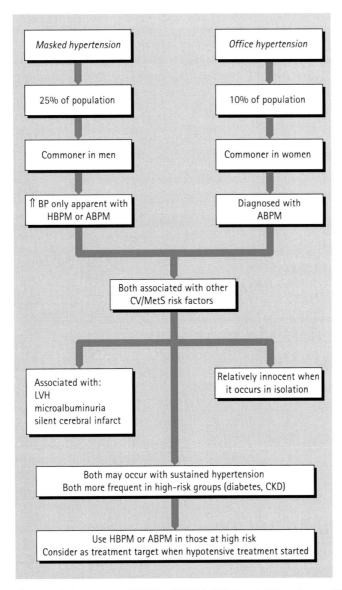

Figure 4.2 Comparison of OHTN and MHTN. CKD, chronic kidney disease; LVH, left ventricular hypertrophy; MetS, metabolic syndrome.

Conclusions

OHTN occurs in up to 25% of the population. It is due to sympathetic overactivity in the anxiety-provoking clinical situation and, when it occurs in isolation does not require treatment. It is frequently associated with other CV risk factors. Management of BP and other factors should be considered in the light of an overall CV risk assessment. When OHTN occurs alone, it is relatively benign but when superimposed upon other risk factors, it should be considered in the patient's management (Figure 4.2).

MHTN occurs in up to 10% of the population. It is associated with increased CV risk, particularly in high-risk groups, including those with diabetes or chronic kidney disease. Treatment is warranted if the patient's global CV risk is high (>20% event risk in 10 years). If daytime BPs are higher than office measurements in a patient treated for hypertension, consider irregular compliance with medications as a cause of the variation. The high frequency of differences in office and out of office BPs argues strongly for the increased use of HBPM and ABPM. MHTN is a particular problem as a normal office measurement of BP may be falsely reassuring.

References

1   Pickering TG, Eguchi K, Kario K. Masked hypertension: a review. *Hypertens Res* 2007; **30**: 479–88.

2   Bo M, Comba M, Canade A, Brescianini A, Corsinovi L, Astengo MA, *et al.* Clinical implications of white-coat effect among patients attending at a lipid clinic. *Atherosclerosis* 2008; **197**: 904–9.

3   Eguchi K, Hoshide S, Ishikawa J, Ishikawa S, Pickering TG, Gerin W, *et al.* Cardiovascular prognosis of sustained and white-coat hypertension in patients with type 2 diabetes mellitus. *Blood Press Monit* 2008; **13**: 15–20.

4   Leitao CB, Canani LH, Kramer CK, Boza JC, Pinotti AF, Gross JL. Masked hypertension, urinary albumin excretion rate, and echocardiographic parameters in putatively normotensive type 2 diabetic patients. *Diabetes Care* 2007; **30**: 1255–60.

5   Kato T, Horio T, Tomiyama M, Kamide K, Nakamura S, Yoshihara F, *et al.* Reverse white-coat effect as an independent risk for microalbuminuria in treated hypertensive patients. *Nephrol Dialysis Transplant* 2007; **22**: 911–16.

6   Tomiyama M, Horio T, Kamide K, Nakamura S, Yoshihara F, Nakata H, *et al.* Reverse white-coat effect as an independent risk for left ventricular concentric hypertrophy in patients with treated essential hypertension. *J Hum Hypertens* 2007; **21**: 212–19.

7   Hara A, Ohkubo T, Kikuya M, Shintani Y, Obara T, Metoki H, *et al.* Detection of carotid atherosclerosis in individuals with masked hypertension and white-coat hypertension by self-measured blood pressure at home: the Ohasama study.[See comment.] *J Hypertens* 2007; **25**: 321–7.

8   de Simone G, Schillaci G, Chinali M, Angeli F, Reboldi GP, Verdecchia P. Estimate of white-coat effect and arterial stiffness. *J Hypertens* 2007; **25**: 827–31.

9   Puato M, Palatini P, Zanardo M, Dorigatti F, Tirrito C, Rattazzi M, *et al.* Increase in carotid intima-media thickness in grade I hypertensive subjects: white-coat versus sustained hypertension. *Hypertension* 2008; **51**: 1300–5.

10 Mule G, Nardi E, Cottone S, Cusimano P, Incalcaterra F, Palermo A, *et al.* Metabolic syndrome in subjects with white-coat hypertension: impact on left ventricular structure and function. *J Hum Hypertens* 2007; **21**: 854–60.

Types of Hypertension and Hypotension

PROBLEM

05   Prehypertension

Case History

John is 44 years old. His blood pressure (BP) is 134/82, and has been at this level on his last three visits to his general practitioner over the past 6 months. His past medical history is unremarkable. He is a non-smoker but drinks a little too much alcohol (40+ units per week). He is also mildly overweight (body mass index 28 kg/m²). There is no family history of note and he is not taking any medication.

Does this level of BP place him at any risk in the future?

Does his BP need treatment?

How should he be investigated and followed up?

Background

The term prehypertension has been used over the past 5 years to replace what was called borderline hypertension, above optimal blood BP or high normal BP. It is a level of BP (see Box 5.1) that is associated with an increased risk of developing clinical hypertension. As the risk of complications increases linearly with BP and there are no threshold values,

Box 5.1 **Definition of prehypertension**

Systolic BP: 120–139 mmHg

or

Diastolic BP: 80–89 mmHg

- BP should be confirmed on at least two separate occasions
- If systolic BP and diastolic BP belong to different categories, the BP is classified according to the highest BP

prehypertension carries an increased risk of vascular and kidney diseases compared with normotension.

As BP tends to increase with age, patients with prehypertension are at risk for the development of hypertension. This occurs at a rate of 5–10% per year, but is greater in older subjects. Elderly subjects are more likely to have established hypertension at diagnosis than prehypertension. Men are more likely to have prehypertension, and there is a strong correlation with being overweight or obese. It clusters with other cardiovascular (CV) risk factors, 60–90% of patients having at least one other risk factor. All patients with prehypertension should be given healthy lifestyle advice:

- Healthy eating plan (high intake of fruit, vegetables, fibre and wholegrains, and lower intake of red meat and saturated fat)

- Manage body weight: as near ideal range as possible

- Regular exercise: 30 min most days

- Lower salt intake

- Moderate alcohol intake

Drug treatment is not routinely recommended. This would greatly increase the cost and burden of BP treatment and would expose a large number of relatively low-risk individuals to the disadvantages of drug treatment. The target BP for patients with diabetes or chronic kidney disease is 130/80. It follows that BP in the range that would normally be considered prehypertension is an indication for drug treatment in these high-risk groups.

The TROPHY Study[1] included 772 subjects with systolic BP of 130–139 mmHg and diastolic BP of 85–89 mmHg or with diastolic BP of 85–89 mmHg and systolic BP ≤139. They were randomized to either placebo or to candesartan for 2 years during which time hypertension developed in 154 in the placebo group compared with 53 in the candesartan group – a relative risk (RR) reduction of 66.3%. After 2 years medication was ceased, and BP rose more rapidly in the candesartan group. After 4 years (2 years on medication), 53% of the candesartan group had developed hypertension compared with 63% of the placebo group. This was a feasibility study and confirmed that while on BP-lowering medication, fewer patients crossed the threshold for hypertension. However, there was no suggestion that there was any lasting benefit of treatment in terms of long-term prevention of hypertension after medication was stopped.

There is no reason to suspect that the benefit of using medication to lower BP in those at risk of hypertension does not extend to other classes of drug. From a patient's perspective, the diagnosis of hypertension equates to starting drug treatment, and bringing forward the time when medication is required might not seem an advantage. There is also a chance of deflecting the patient from lifestyle interventions. By analogy with diabetes, it is possible that controlling the BP tightly from an earlier stage might prevent later deterioration of control to a degree where it is harder to get back to target values.

To date, there is no intervention study showing that aggressive treatment of prehypertension protects against adverse CV outcomes. It is, however, clear from a number of studies that prehypertension is associated with increased risk of ischaemic heart disease and myocardial infarction with conflicting results reported for stroke. For example, in the Women's Health Initiative cohort,[2] prehypertension was associated with a hazard ratio of 1.58 for CV death, 1.76 for myocardial infarction, 1.93 for stroke and 1.66 for any CV event. Prehypertension is associated with an increased prevalence of microalbuminuria, increased uric acid and increased inflammatory markers, all of which indicate increased vascular risk. An association with microcirculatory abnormalities has also been documented.

Recent Developments

1   Many of the major hypertension studies come from the USA. Recent national surveys from other countries have shown a rise in hypertension and prehypertension from previous levels. A Korean survey[3] found 22.9% (26.9% men, 20.5% women) of the population had hypertension, while prehypertension was present in 31.6% (41.9% men, 25.9% women). Only 30% of people surveyed were aware of their BP status. A survey of nearly 40 000 people in Thailand[4] revealed hypertension in 22% and prehypertension in 32.8%. Nearly 70% of subjects with increased BP were unaware of their condition. These studies highlight an important gender issue: women are more likely to have their BP checked and to seek advice for it while men are more likely to have high BP.

2   The prevalence of metabolic syndrome (MetS) increases with age. It is clear that prehypertension frequently coexists with insulin resistance and prediabetic states.[5,6] In the study by Cordero et al.,[5] prehypertension was related to the presence of MetS variables much more strongly than to abnormalities in renal function. Their study of over 19 000 subjects revealed MetS in only 0.9% of normotensives, but in 9.6% of those with prehypertension and in 30% of those with hypertension. Using the HOMA-R model, Player et al.[7] reported that insulin resistance was 60% more likely to occur in prehypertensive individuals compared with those who were normotensive. The association was only significant in men, confirming a need to target middle-aged men with multiple CV risk factors.

3   In the Strong Heart Study,[8] a large cohort of young people (14–39 years) were studied with echocardiography. Hypertension was present in 15% and prehypertension in 35%. Both were more prevalent in men, with increasing age, and in those with diabetes. Both were associated with increased left ventricular wall thickness and mass, as well as increased mean pulse pressure/stroke volume index. Total peripheral resistance (arterial stiffness was increased).

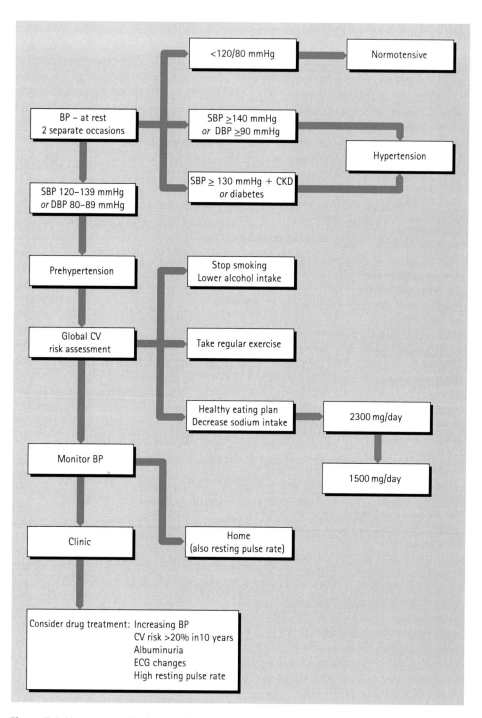

Figure 5.1 Management of prehypertension.

Prehypertension is common in young people, and arises because of increased carbon monoxide coupled with higher peripheral resistance.

4 Sironi *et al.*[9] confirmed that prehypertensive individuals had decreased left ventricular function and that this was associated with insulin resistance and ectopic fat accumulation in both the visceral and epicardial depots (assessed using magnetic resonance imaging). Ectopic fat contributes to local metabolic and inflammatory changes.

5 Means of identifying prehypertensive individuals at high risk would be useful. Data from the ARIC (Atherosclerosis Risk in Communities) study,[10] in which a large cohort was followed for 10 years, show the importance of resting heart rate in those with prehypertension. Those with increased resting heart rate and prehypertension were at increased risk of death. Both prehypertensive and prediabetic states are associated with subtle changes in retinal blood vessels.[11] These could assist in identifying those who are developing vascular complications and might help us to target treatment.

Conclusions

Prehypertension is even more common than hypertension. It is amenable to lifestyle intervention but should not, for now, be routinely treated with drugs. The above patient has up to 40% chance of developing hypertension within the next 4 years, and a greater than 90% lifetime chance of developing hypertension. He should be counselled on lifestyle factors to lower his BP and decrease his overall CV risk. The approach to prehypertension is summarized in Figure 5.1. In advising the patient with mildly elevated BP, it is important to encourage a positive outlook and not to regard the patient as having a disease state. Men are more likely to have prehypertension and are less likely to be aware of it.

References

1 Julius S, Nesbitt SD, Egan BM, Weber MA, Michelson EL, Kaciroti N, *et al.* Feasibility of treating prehypertension with an angiotensin-receptor blocker. *N Engl J Med* 2006; **354**: 1685–97.

2 Hsia J, Margolis KL, Eaton CB, Wenger NK, Allison M, Wu L, *et al.* Prehypertension and cardiovascular disease risk in the Women's Health Initiative. *Circulation* 2007; **115**: 855–60.

3 Choi KM, Park HS, Han JH, Lee JS, Lee J, Ryu OH, *et al.* Prevalence of prehypertension in a Korean population: Korean National Health and Nutrition Survey 2001. *J Hypertens* 2006; **24**: 1515–21.

4 Aekplakorn W, Abbott–Klafter J, Khonputsa P, Tatsanavivat P, Chongsuvivatwong V, Chariyalertsak S, *et al.* Prevalence and management of prehypertension and hypertension by geographic regions of Thailand: the Third National Health Examination Survey, 2004. *J Hypertens* 2008; **26**: 191–8.

5 Cordero A, Laclaustra M, Leon M, Grima A, Casasnovas JA, Luengo E, *et al.* Prehypertension is associated with insulin resistance state and not with an initial renal function impairment. A Metabolic Syndrome in Active Subjects in Spain (MESYAS) Registry substudy. *Am J Hypertens* 2006; **19**: 189–96.

6 Kanauchi M, Kanauchi K, Inoue T, Kimura K, Saito Y. Surrogate markers of insulin resistance in assessing individuals with new categories 'prehypertension' and 'prediabetes'. *Clin Chem Lab Med* 2007; **45**: 35–9.

7 Player MS, Mainous AG, 3rd, Diaz VA, Everett CJ. Prehypertension and insulin resistance in a nationally representative adult population. *J Clin Hypertens* 2007; **9**: 424–9.

8 Drukteinis JS, Roman MJ, Fabsitz RR, Lee ET, Best LG, Russell M, *et al.* Cardiac and systemic hemodynamic characteristics of hypertension and prehypertension in adolescents and young adults: the Strong Heart Study. *Circulation* 2007; **115**: 221–7.

9 Sironi AM, Pingitore A, Ghione S, De Marchi D, Scattini B, Positano V, *et al.* Early hypertension is associated with reduced regional cardiac function, insulin resistance, epicardial, and visceral fat. *Hypertension* 2008; **51**: 282–8.

10 King DE, Everett CJ, Mainous AG, 3rd, Liszka HA. Long-term prognostic value of resting heart rate in subjects with prehypertension. *Am J Hypertens* 2006; **19**: 796–800.

11 Nguyen TT, Wang JJ, Wong TY. Retinal vascular changes in pre-diabetes and prehypertension: new findings and their research and clinical implications. *Diabetes Care* 2007; **30**: 2708–15.

06 Resistant Hypertension

Case History

Mr TO is a 62-year-old man and has been treated for hypertension over the past 10 years. His blood pressure (BP) has never been well controlled. Currently, he takes lisinopril 10 mg OD, atenolol 50 mg OD, amlodipine 10 mg OD and prazosin 2 mg BD. He attends for review and his BP is once more elevated at 165/90, but has been much higher than this previously. He may have had a transient ischaemic attack 6 months ago when he lost speech for 2 hours. An electrocardiogram (ECG) shows borderline left ventricular hypertrophy. His body mass index is 30 kg/m².

Can we label him as having resistant hypertension?

Why is his drug therapy not working?

What is the best approach to managing resistant hypertension?

Should we accept that, while not ideal, his hypertension is improved?

Background

Only about 25% of patients with diagnosed hypertension are effectively treated with medications to render BP in the target range. Fifty per cent of patients taking medications remain poorly controlled with BPs in excess of 140/90. The majority of patients with hypertension require more than one agent to control their BP. Resistant hypertension occurs in up to 10% of patients with hypertension (Box 6.1).[1,2]

Causes of treatment failure (Box 6.2)

Poor patient compliance is common. Reasons for this include cost of the treatment, complexity of the regimen, and side effects from drugs. The patient often does not understand, or agree with, the reason for the prescription. The drug regimen should be kept as

---

Box 6.1 Resistant hypertension

Failure to control BP (>140/90) in a patient who has been taking an optimal combination of at least three medications for at least 1 month. A cut-off point of 130/80 is more appropriate for patients with diabetes or chronic kidney disease.

> **Box 6.2 Causes of resistant hypertension**
>
> | **Apparent resistance** | **True resistance to treatment** |
> |---|---|
> | ● Poor patient compliance | ● Secondary hypertension |
> | ● Inadequate dosing of drugs | ● Renal |
> | ● Poor choice of drug combinations | ● Endocrine |
> | ● Drugs – see text | ● Obesity |
> | ● Excessive alcohol intake | ● Sleep apnoea |
> | ● Cocaine use | ● Volume/salt overload |
> | ● Pseudohypertension | |
> | ● Office hypertension | |

simple (and inexpensive) as possible with both the number of preparations and the number of doses being kept to a minimum. Short-acting preparations are generally best avoided, as they need to be taken two to three times per day. This includes captopril, clonidine, hydralazine and short-acting nifedipine preparations. Combination preparations are very useful – particularly those that combine a diuretic with either angiotensin-converting enzyme inhibitors or angiotensin receptor blockers. Patients who have poor memory are also less likely to comply.

Treatment regimens are often inadequate in either not using sufficient doses of drugs or using combinations that are not fully synergistic. Drugs prescribed for other indications can increase BP. These include oral contraceptives, corticosteroids, cyclosporine, erythropoietin, non-steroidal anti-inflammatory drugs and appetite suppressants. Alcohol intake above 30 g (three standard drinks) per day is likely to increase BP. The alcohol history is often neglected when planning treatment and follow-up of hypertensive patients. Cocaine use also commonly increases BP, sometimes to a dangerous level.

Pseudohypertension describes the situation where sclerosis in the large arteries renders them less compressible meaning that higher pressure has to be applied to occlude the artery leading to a falsely high blood BP reading. It may be present in up to 7% of elderly people. The Osler manoeuvre (**not** described by Sir William Osler, 1849–1919) has been suggested as a test – the BP cuff is inflated to in excess of the auscultated BP, and in Osler-positive patients the radial or brachial artery remains palpably pulsatile. Intra-arterial BP measurement is required to definitively confirm pseudohypertension (not routinely indicated). Office hypertension is very common and can be diagnosed by asking the patient to self-monitor BP or by use of ambulatory BP monitoring.

True resistant hypertension

Secondary renal causes include renal artery stenosis, polycystic kidney disease, chronic nephritis, diabetic nephropathy, hydronephrosis and acute glomerulonephritis. The most common endocrine cause for resistant hypertension is primary hyperaldosteronism (Table 6.1). Patients with atherosclerotic renal artery stenosis may only be partially

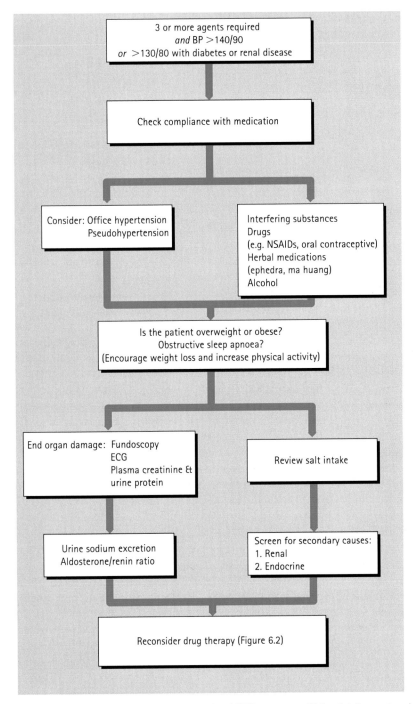

Figure 6.1 Evaluation of resistant hypertension; NSAIDs, non-steroidal anti-inflammatory drugs.

Table 6.1 Prevalence of secondary causes	
	Prevalence (%)
Hyperaldosteronism	1.5–15
Renal parenchymal disease	1.0–8.0
Renal artery disease	3.0–4.0
Thyroid disorders	1.0–3.0
Coarctation of the aorta	<1.0
Cushing's syndrome	<0.5
Phaeochromocytoma	<0.5

Prevalence quoted is percentage of total hypertensive patients.
Adapted from Moser and Setaro.[1]

improved by intervention. Other causes include Cushing's syndrome, congenital adrenal hyperplasia, acromegaly and thyrotoxicosis. Underlying secondary disease states are found in 10% of patients with resistant hypertension overall, but in a greater percentage of the elderly. Coarctation of the aorta should be considered, though rare, and excluded initially clinically by looking for radiofemoral delay and for rib notching on chest X-ray.

Obese subjects tend to be hypertensive and antihypertensive drugs tend not to be as effective. Even lean people with insulin resistance or metabolic syndrome (MetS) are more resistant to the effects of antihypertensives. Sleep apnoea is associated with resistant hypertension, an effect that is independent of obesity. Patients should be asked about interrupted sleep, snoring and daytime somnolence. Evidence of polycythaemia or carbon dioxide retention should be sought and, if necessary, a sleep study carried out.

Volume overload arises from excessive salt intake or inadequate use of diuretics. All patients with hypertension should be advised to limit salt intake. Daily sodium excretion >150 mmol/l (in the absence of diuretic therapy) suggests that sodium intake is excessive. As more antihypertensive drugs have become available, there has been a tendency to underuse diuretics. Patients with low glomerular filtration rate (<35 ml/min) usually require loop diuretics to control BP. Investigation and non-pharmacological management of a patient with resistant hypertension are summarized in Figure 6.1. Before considering the most appropriate drug regimen, confounding factors such as compliance, office hypertension, and use of drugs that elevate BP should be considered. Also, lifestyle factors should be attended to. At least 50% of patients will respond to initiating or increasing diuretic. Initially 12.5–25 mg hydrochlorthiazide (maximum dose 50 mg/day) is suitable for patients with normal renal function. Frusemide or bumetanide (loop diuretics) are necessary for those with renal impairment (estimated glomerular filtration rate <35 ml/min, plasma creatinine >120 µmol/l). Twice daily dosing should be used to avoid compensatory sodium retention offsetting any BP-reducing effect. Diuretic treatment may lead to stimulation of the renin–angiotensin system (RAS), an effect counteracted by use of a β-blocker, angiotensin-converting enzyme inhibitor or angiotensin receptor blocker. Combined α- and β-blocking agents may be useful in some cases.

Despite the fact that resistant hypertension is common, there are limited trial data on combinations of three or more medications. Treatment needs to be tailored to the

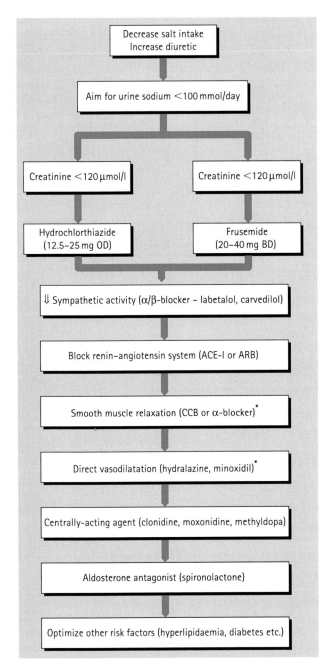

Figure 6.2 Pharmacological treatment. *Use with β-blocker and diuretic to minimise reflex tachycardia and oedema. ACE-I, angiotensin converting enzyme inhibitor; ARB, angiotensin receptor blocker; CCB, calcium channel blocker.

patient's needs (e.g. using β-blockers in patients with concurrent angina), and adjusted according to response and the presence of side effects. Hyperaldosteronism is common in resistant hypertension and addition of spironolactone (12.5–50 mg per day) should be considered. Combination medications and once daily preparations are useful to minimize the treatment burden to patients and to maximize compliance. Drug treatment is considered in Figure 6.2 – this is not a fixed flow of treatment, but a general consideration of available agents.

Recent Developments

1 Mineralocorticoid receptors are expressed in the brain, heart and blood vessels. Some of the effects of activation of the RAS on increasing BP are mediated by aldosterone (which may be locally generated) rather than by angiotensin II.[3] These include resetting the baroreflex arc, local electrolyte fluxes, vascular remodelling and response to pressor substances. In ASCOT (Anglo-Scandinavian Cardiac Outcomes Trial),[4] spironolactone along with three other agents decreased BP from 157/85 at baseline to 135/76.

2 Obstructive sleep apnoea/hypopnoea syndrome (OSAHS) is very common in patients with resistant hypertension. Hypoxia and increased upper airways pressure leads to sympathetic activation and thus increased BP. In a recent case–control study,[5] OSAHS was present in 71% with resistant hypertension compared with only 38% of matched controls with well-controlled hypertension. Patients with OSAHS have increased plasma aldosterone, the concentration of which correlates with symptom severity.[6]

3 Carotid sinus baroreceptors (innervated through the glossopharyngeal nerve) respond to increased BP by activating neurones in the caudal ventrolateral medulla. These, in turn, inhibit neurones in the rostral ventrolateral medulla leading to decreased sympathetic activation. Electrical stimulation of the carotid sinus is a novel method for controlling resistant hypertension. An implantable pulse generator is connected to bilateral perivascular leads located at the carotid sinuses. The method appears to be safe with no side effects such as bradycardia. Initial studies suggest that systolic BP reductions of between 28 and 41 mmHg can be achieved.[7,8]

4 Many patients with resistant hypertension do not have the normal nocturnal dip in their BP, and this constitutes a significant cardiovascular risk factor. Use of ambulatory monitoring and timing of drug doses to achieve a night-time dip could increase the protective effect of drug regimens.[9]

Conclusions

All patients with hypertension, but particularly those with resistant hypertension, should be screened for end-organ damage. Before diagnosing resistant hypertension, compliance should be checked. Also, it is striking that the above patient is not using a diuretic. The patient is obese and may require higher doses of antihypertensive drugs. Attempts should be made to help him lose weight. Resistant hypertension is often associated with relatively higher systolic than diastolic BP, an effect that is exaggerated with age and increased body weight. The approach to a patient with resistant hypertension is summarized in Figures 6.1 and 6.2. Salt and water overload is a common cause of treatment failure. We often have to accept that patients do not reach treatment targets. However, we should try hard to identify reasons why this happens in each patient. With a rational approach to treatment, control of even resistant hypertension can be achieved in many cases.

References

1   Moser M, Setaro JF. Resistant or difficult-to-control hypertension. *N Engl J Med* 2006; **355**: 385–92.

2   Calhoun DA, Jones D, Textor S, Goff DC, Murphy TP, *et al.* Resistant hypertension: diagnosis, evaluation and treatment. A scientific statement from the American Heart Association Professional Education Committee of the Council for High Blood Pressure Research. *Hypertension* 2008 (published online 7 April 2008).

3   Duprez DA. Aldosterone and the vasculature: mechanisms mediating resistant hypertension. *J Clin Hypertens* 2007; **9** (Suppl 1): 13–18.

4   Chapman N, Dobson J, Wilson S, Dahlof B, Sever PS, Wedel H, *et al.* Effect of spironolactone on blood pressure in subjects with resistant hypertension. *Hypertension* 2007; **49**: 839–45.

5   Goncalves SC, Martinez D, Gus M, de Abreu-Silva EO, Bertoluci C, Dutra I, *et al.* Obstructive sleep apnea and resistant hypertension: a case–control study. *Chest* 2007; **132**: 1858–62.

6   Pratt-Ubunama MN, Nishizaka MK, Boedefeld RL, Cofield SS, Harding SM, Calhoun DA. Plasma aldosterone is related to severity of obstructive sleep apnea in subjects with resistant hypertension. *Chest* 2007; **131**: 453–9.

7   Illig KA, Levy M, Sanchez L, Trachiotis GD, Shanley C, Irwin E, *et al.* An implantable carotid sinus stimulator for drug-resistant hypertension: surgical technique and short-term outcome from the multicenter phase II Rheos feasibility trial. *J Vasc Surg* 2006; **44**: 1213–18.

8   Tordoir JHM, Scheffers I, Schmidli J, Savolainen H, Liebeskind U, Hansky B, *et al.* An implantable carotid sinus baroreflex activating system: surgical technique and short-term outcome from a multi-center feasibility trial for the treatment of resistant hypertension. *Eur J Vasc Endovasc Surg* 2007; **33**: 414–21.

9   Hermida RC, Ayala DE, Fernandez JR, Calvo C. Chronotherapy improves blood pressure control and reverts the nondipper pattern in patients with resistant hypertension. *Hypertension* 2008; **51**: 69–76.

07 Isolated Systolic Hypertension

Case History

John is a 75-year-old man who is a carer for his disabled wife. He is quite active and copes well with household chores. He has high cholesterol and takes a statin as well as aspirin. Blood pressure (BP) has been high for some time, and at this visit is 168/82. The time has come to start treatment, and you wish to discuss this with him. Renal function and creatinine are both normal. Urine is negative on stick testing but he has microalbuminuria on laboratory testing.

Is isolated systolic hypertension (ISH) common, and is it important?

Why does systolic BP (SBP) selectively increase in the elderly?

What is the optimal approach to management?

Background

SBP rises progressively with age, while after about the age of 65 there is a modest decline. ISH with increased pulse pressure (Figure 7.1) is the commonest form of hypertension in the elderly and is a major risk factor for cardiovascular (CV) disease.[1–3] ISH is defined as SBP >140 mmHg and diastolic BP (DBP) <90 mmHg. It should probably be distinguished from essential hypertension (where SBP and DBP are both increased). Pathogenesis of the two conditions overlaps, but is not identical. There are subtle differences in the approach to treatment. ISH and essential hypertension are not entirely distinct – a patient with essential hypertension may later present with ISH as the DBP decreases with age. However, over 60% of patients with ISH have no preceding hypertension. ISH affects two-thirds of patients over 65 years and three-quarters of patients over 75. It is by far the most common form of hypertension in later life (Figure 7.2). With the ageing population, this is clearly a very major public health problem.

The relative increase in SBP, compared with DBP, relates to decreased vascular compliance with ageing. The latter arises from atherosclerosis, collagen cross-linking and glycosylation, vascular calcification and elastin fragmentation. The aorta and larger vessels lose the ability to expand to accommodate the pulse wave during systole and there is decreased recoil during diastole. Decreased baroreceptor responses and increased salt sensitivity contribute to hypertension in the elderly. Although plasma catecholamines are relatively increased, sensitivity of adrenoreceptors is decreased. Increased sympathetic drive is, therefore, a less important mechanism and because of this as well as often

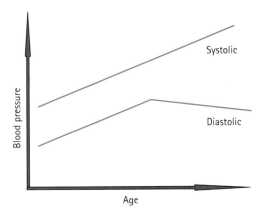

Figure 7.1 Change in blood pressure with age.

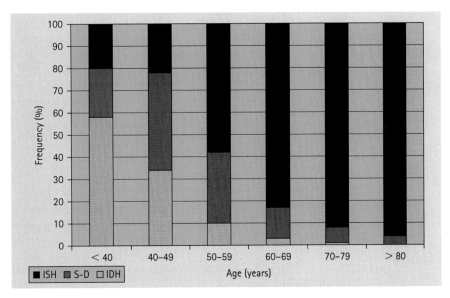

Figure 7.2 Presentation of untreated hypertension. IDH, isolated diastolic hypertension; ISH, isolated systolic hypertension; S-D, systolic-diastolic (essential) hypertension. Adapted from Chobanian.[1]

decreased myocardial function, increased cardiac output is less important than in younger subjects. Activation of the renal artery stenosis is also relatively less important in ISH, explaining why angiotensin-converting enzyme inhibitors and angiotensin receptor blockers are often not the most effective drugs. The addition of angiotensin-converting enzyme inhibitors and angiotensin receptor blockers to treatment is logical where ISH is placing the patient in danger of end-organ damage. There is particularly strong evidence that these agents may bring about regression of left ventricular hypertrophy and retard

Table 7.1 ISH and essential hypertension		
	Essential	ISH
Increased cardiac output	+	–
Arterial compliance	+	–
Peripheral resistance	++	+
Left ventricular mass	+	++
Baroreceptor sensitivity	--	–
Plasma catecholamines	+	++
Plasma renin	+	–
Salt sensitivity	+	++

Adapted from Pannarale.[3]

the development of nephropathy. Salt sensitivity is increased in older subjects, and this contributes to increased arterial stiffness. Thus, lower salt intake and diuretic therapy are central in management. ISH and essential hypertension are compared in Table 7.1.

Even a modest decrease in SBP of <5 mmHg reduces cardiac mortality by 7% and stroke mortality by 10%. A target BP of 140/90 seems reasonable for the elderly, but is often not achievable, let alone the tighter target of 130/80, which is recommended for those at higher risk (e.g. those with diabetes and chronic kidney disease). Effective treatment of ISH decreases the risk of CV events by 23%.[2] The landmark trials in this area (see Duprez for a review[2]) were:

● SHEP (1991) followed 4736 patients with ISH for 4.5 years. In treated patients, the rate of non-fatal stroke was decreased by 36%, cardiac disease by 25%, and heart failure by 53%. A more recent (2005) extension of this study following patients for up to 14.3 years showed continuing benefit in terms of event rate reduction. Benefit extended to those with pre-existing diabetes, while those who developed diabetes during the follow-up period but had their BP treated had no different risk to patients without diabetes. This study was based on the use of chlorthalidone with other agents added as needed.

● Syst-Eur (1997) and Syst-China (1998) followed 4695 and 2394 patients respectively for 2–3 years, with initial therapy based on calcium channel blockers (CCB). These studies showed a reduction in stroke of about 40% and of total CV outcomes of 31–39% for treated patients.

More recent studies have included: LIFE (2002) in which losartan decreased CV outcomes compared with an atenolol-based regimen in 1326 patients with ISH and left ventricular hypertrophy followed for 4.7 years; the Systolic Hypertension in the Elderly Long-term Lacidipine study (SHELL, 2003) in which 1882 patients with ISH were followed for 32 months, showed a 9.3% reduction in event rate with the CCB; the International Nifedipine GITS Study; the Intervention as a Goal in Hypertension Treatment study (INSIGHT, 2004) which included 1498 patients with ISH followed for 3 years, and showed a 6% decrease in the CV event rate. These, and a number of other shorter-term studies have, in recent years, highlighted ISH as a clinical problem in the elderly. They have also shown that decreasing BP leads to lower CV risk. Although the various classes of agent are similar in BP-decreasing potency, renin-angiotensin system blocking drugs and CCBs have the most trial evidence. The former may be slightly superior in preventing stroke and are slightly better tolerated because of the relatively high incidence of peripheral oedema seen with CCBs.

As with all patients with hypertension, the elderly with ISH should have an overall assessment of CV risk, secondary causes of hypertension should be considered (particularly renovascular), and they should be screened for end-organ damage (eyes, heart and kidneys). Consider also conditions that increase cardiac output and may selectively increase SBP. These include anaemia, thyrotoxicosis, Paget's disease and aortic regurgitation. Lifestyle modifications should be instituted where possible – maintain or decrease body weight, regular exercise, balanced diet, lower salt intake and avoid excess alcohol. It is assumed that the major advantage of drug treatment is through lowering BP, and none of the major classes has a specific action in ISH. In the elderly, it is important to start with low doses of drugs where possible, and to titrate gradually with careful monitoring of BP response, renal function and electrolytes. Over-vigorous reduction in DBP should be avoided as this may decrease myocardial perfusion.

The first choice of treatment for ISH is low-dose thiazide. The greatest evidence is with hydrochlorthiazide and chlorthalidone. Bendrofluazide is also widely used. The latter is more potent on a milligram for milligram basis and also has a longer half-life (48–72 h vs 16–24 h). The disadvantages of thiazides are hypokalaemia, increased uric acid, dyslipidaemia, hyperglycaemia, and erectile dysfunction in men. All of these are commoner in the elderly but less likely to occur with low doses – 12.5 mg of hydrochlorthiazide is a suitable starting dose. Long-acting CCBs should also be considered early in the treatment. These are of proven efficacy and have beneficial effects on vascular remodelling. β-blockers are no longer considered first-line for the elderly patient with ISH, but should certainly be used in those with angina or previous myocardial infarction, and considered in those with heart failure (Figure 7.3).

Recent Developments

1 High SBP is very variable in older subjects with reduced vascular compliance. There is an argument for confirming ISH on at least three occasions before the diagnostic label is assigned.[4] A recent large Portuguese study confirmed that ISH was common, particularly after the age of 70.[5] It was not, however, particularly associated with premature mortality, and CV complications often developed very late in life.

2 In a follow-up of participants in the SHEP trial at 14.3 years,[6] a chlorthalidone-based antihypertensive regimen decreased CV mortality – RR 0.86 (95% CI: 0.76 to 0.98). Patients who had sustained stroke experienced a particularly poor mortality experience. We should not be over-pessimistic about the dangers of ISH, or over-optimistic about the benefits of treatment. For population-based risk reduction, many patients would have to be treated for many years to appreciably impact on mortality.

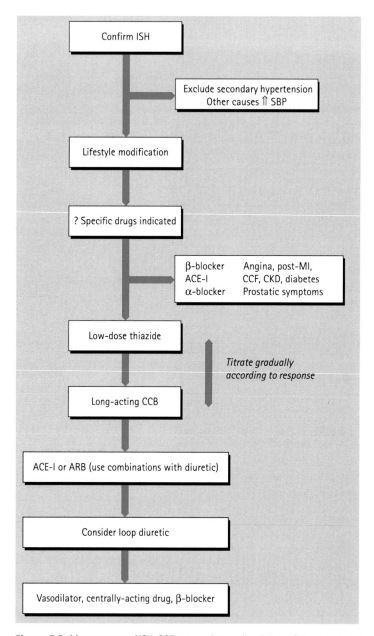

Figure 7.3 Management of ISH. CCF, congestive cardiac failure; CKD, chronic kidney disease.

3 Over-aggressive treatment of systolic hypertension may lead to an unwanted decrease in DBP. In the elderly, DBP <60 mmHg has been associated with poor prognosis independent of large artery stiffness and left ventricular function.[7] Elderly people taking antihypertensives should be carefully monitored. DBP decreases with age and may warrant altering treatment for ISH.

4 Long-acting CCBs are a very useful adjunct to thiazides as first-line treatment. A recent trial compared amlodipine with a newer CCB manidipine.[8] Chlorthalidone was added where needed. Both CCBs effectively decreased BP. Manidipine had the advantage of a lower incidence of peripheral oedema.

5 The importance of exercise as an intervention for the elderly is often forgotten. Apart from general well-being, exercise has tangible benefits including reducing SBP.[9] Given the now proven benefits of exercise in elderly patients with chronic disease, including diabetes and pulmonary disease, we need to examine how to actively engage elderly people in exercise programmes.

Conclusions

The vast majority of us will develop hypertension as we age, and ISH is by far the commonest form in older people. Subtly, the pathogenesis is different to that of essential hypertension, which is a disease of younger people. Decreased vascular compliance is the hallmark. The underlying cause of hypertension shifts from more humoral mechanisms in younger subjects to more mechanical causes in the elderly. This explains why some drugs are less effective in ISH. The condition is important, being strongly linked with adverse CV outcomes, particularly stroke. Treatment with two or more drugs is often needed. Over-vigorous treatment may control ISH but at the expense of undue lowering of DBP, which may reduce coronary perfusion. Low-dose thiazides and long-acting CCBs are the cornerstone of treatment. These should be initiated cautiously and titrated gradually, especially in very aged or frail patients.

References

1 Chobanian AV. Clinical practice. Isolated systolic hypertension in the elderly. *N Engl J Med* 2007; **357**: 789–96.

2 Duprez DA. Systolic hypertension in the elderly: addressing an unmet need. *Am J Med* 2008; **121**: 179–84.e3.

3 Pannarale G. Optimal drug treatment of systolic hypertension in the elderly. *Drugs Aging* 2008; **25**: 1–8.

4 Talleruphuus U, Bang LE, Wiinberg N, Mehlsen J, Svendsen TL, Bentzon MW. Isolated systolic hypertension in an elderly Danish population. Prevalence and daytime ambulatory blood pressure. *Blood Press* 2006; **15**: 347–53.

5 Seto S, Soda M, Nakashima E, Yano K, Akahoshi M. Longitudinal analysis of blood pressure trends and prognosis in isolated systolic hypertension in elderly individuals. *Am J Hypertens* 2007; **20**: 134–9.

6 Patel AB, Kostis JB, Wilson AC, Shea ML, Pressel SL, Davis BR. Long-term fatal outcomes in subjects with stroke or transient ischemic attack: fourteen-year follow-up of the systolic hypertension in the elderly program. *Stroke* 2008; **39**: 1084–9.

7 Protogerou AD, Safar ME, Iaria P, Safar H, Le Dudal K, Filipovsky J, *et al.* Diastolic blood pressure and mortality in the elderly with cardiovascular disease. *Hypertension* 2007; **50**: 172–80.

8   Payeras AC, Sladek K, Lembo G, Alberici M. Antihypertensive efficacy and safety of manidipine versus amlodipine in elderly subjects with isolated systolic hypertension: MAISH study. *Clin Drug Invest* 2007; **27**: 623–32.

9   Westhoff TH, Franke N, Schmidt S, Vallbracht-Israng K, Meissner R, Yildirim H, *et al.* Too old to benefit from sports? The cardiovascular effects of exercise training in elderly subjects treated for isolated systolic hypertension. *Kidney Blood Press Res* 2007; **30**: 240–7.

08 Orthostatic Hypotension

Case History

HT is a 72-year-old man who is complaining of increasing dizziness. He is light-headed if he stands up quickly or when he gets up at night to pass urine. He has actually lost consciousness during these episodes on at least three occasions over the past 6 months. His frail elderly wife is concerned that he will fall and injure himself. His general health is reasonable. He takes metformin 500 mg BD, aspirin 100 mg OD, and tamsulosin 400 µg OD for prostatic symptoms. His recumbent blood pressure (BP) is 160/98 and this falls to 134/80 when he stands up.

What are the common causes of orthostatic hypotension (OH)?

How should the patient be evaluated?

What treatment options are available?

Background

Orthostatic (or postural) hypotension is defined as a decrease in systolic BP of 20 mmHg or diastolic BP of 10 mmHg within 3 minutes of assuming upright posture. OH often occurs in the elderly and may occur alongside hypertension, and is commonly precipitated or exacerbated by antihypertensive medications – particularly those that cause either volume depletion or vasodilatation (dihydropyridine calcium channel blockers). Some of the older vasodilators are less likely to cause OH because they cause sodium and water retention in addition to vasodilatation. OH is not always symptomatic. Symptoms include light-headedness, dizziness, nausea, blurred vision, paraesthesiae, tremor, fatigue, impaired cognitive function and syncope. Causes of OH are divided into non-neurogenic, neurogenic and iatrogenic (drugs – Box 8.1). OH is present in up to 20% of 65-year-olds, 30% of 75-year-olds, and up to 50% of nursing home residents. It is associated with general frailty, risk of falls and fractures, and risk of cardiovascular events (particularly transient ischaemic attack and stroke).[1]

On standing, up to 800 ml of blood is pooled in the peripheries. Muscle contraction along with competent venous valves normally ensure the cardiac return is maintained. Baroreceptors in the aorta and carotid artery sense the drop in BP and mediate an increased sympathetic output, which, in turn, increases venous and arterial tone. Also, there is a reflex increase in heart rate and contractility so that increased cardiac output helps to maintain systemic BP. Factors that predispose the elderly include decreased baroreceptor sensitivity, decreased α_1-adrenergic vasoconstrictor response, diminished

Box 8.1 **Drugs that cause orthostatic hypotension**

- Diuretics
- Tricyclic antidepressants
- Vasodilators
- Phenothiazines
- Dihydropyridine calcium channel blockers
- MAO inhibitors
- α-blockers
- Marijuana
- β-blockers
- Narcotics
- Nitrates
- Dopamine agonists (bromocriptine)
- PDE5 inhibitors (sildenafil etc.)
- Vincristine

MAO, monoamine oxidase; PDE5, phosphodiesterase-5.

parasympathetic responsiveness, decreased renal artery sympathetic activity and increased natriuretic peptides leading to a tendency for renal sodium loss, arterial stiffness and decreased left ventricular diastolic filling.

In evaluating the patient, a careful history should be taken, including severity of symptoms, timing, aggravating and relieving factors, and drug history. BP should be measured after at least 5 minutes lying and at 1 and 3 minutes after standing. Passive head up tilt-table testing is recommended if the standing test is negative or if the patient has motor impairment.[2] If there is a diurnal variation, e.g. symptoms in early morning or after meals, then home or ambulatory BP monitoring may be required. Volume status should be assessed. Peripheral oedema may suggest heart failure or venous obstruction. If postural BP drop is not accompanied by increased heart rate (at least 10 beats per minute), autonomic failure should be suspected and autonomic function tests considered. Other features of autonomic neuropathy include dry feet, bowel and bladder dysfunction, unexplained vomiting (gastroparesis), gustatory sweating and erectile dysfunction in men. Neurological examination should aim to identify possible underlying causes including Parkinson's disease, multiple sclerosis and cardiovascular disease. Causes are summarized in Table 8.1.

Simple measures can go a long way to alleviating symptoms. Below are some simple 'dos' and 'don'ts':

Table 8.1 Non-iatrogenic causes of OH

Non-neurological	Neurological
Cardiac pump failure	*Primary autonomic disorders*
Coronary heart disease	Multiple system atrophy*
Aortic stenosis	Parkinson's disease
Arrhythmias	Lewy-body dementia
Carditis	Pure autonomic failure
Decreased intravascular volume	*Peripheral neuropathies*
Vomiting, diarrhoea, dehydration	Alcohol
Burns	Diabetes
Haemorrhage	B_{12} deficiency
Adrenal insufficiency	Amyloidosis
Salt-losing nephropathy	HIV/AIDS
	Guillain–Barré syndrome
Venous pooling	Paraneoplastic
Postprandial	HSAN type III**
Fever	
Sepsis	*Spinal cord disorders*
Heat	Syringomyelia
Venous obstruction	Tumours
	Syphilis (tabes dorsalis)
	Transverse myelitis
	Brain disorders
	Cerebrovascular disease
	Multiple sclerosis
	Brainstem lesions
	Carotid sinus hypersensitivity

*Also known as Shy–Drager syndrome.
**Hereditary sensory and autonomic neuropathy (familial dysautonomia).

Dos:

- Stand up slowly and avoid sudden posture changes
- Dorsiflex and plantarflex feet several times before standing
- Maintain salt intake (up to 10 g per day)
- Drink plenty of fluids
- Elevate head of bed 5–20 degrees
- Eat small, frequent meals (eating lowers BP)
- Wear compression stockings
- Stooping or squatting may alleviate symptoms

Don'ts:

- Do not stand motionless for prolonged periods

- Avoid straining at toilet if possible

- Avoid large meals

- Restrict alcohol intake

- Beware of vigorous exercise

- Hot environments, hot baths or showers may precipitate symptoms

- Hyperventilation

Drugs that precipitate orthostatic symptoms should be withdrawn if possible, or their dose reduced. Postural symptoms with antihypertensives sometimes improve with continuing treatment. The following can be considered for the symptomatic patient:

- Fludrocortisone: a mineralocorticoid, initially at a dose of 0.1 mg/day. Side effects include oedema, headache, hypertension and hypokalaemia.

- Midodrine: an α-agonist with selective vasopressor properties. Start at 2.5 mg TDS. Side effects include hypertension, pruritis, piloerection and paraesthesiae. It is not available in all countries, and is contraindicated with cardiac or renal failure, urinary retention or thyrotoxicosis.

- Non-steroidal anti-inflammatory drugs: e.g. ibuprofen 400–800 mg TDS interferes with vasodilatory responses and retention of sodium.

- Caffeine: 100–250 mg daily, by tablet or as two to three cups of strong brewed coffee.

- Erythropoietin: used in patients with OH and anaemia.

Other drugs that have been used include octreotide (inhibits release of some vasodilatory peptides), ephedrine (adrenoreceptors agonist), yohimbine (α_2-adreno-receptor antagonist, desmopressin (to decrease nocturnal polyuria).

Recent Developments

1 Arterial stiffness, a determinant of systolic hypertension in the elderly, also places patients at risk of OH. In the Rotterdam Study,[4] 3362 patients were divided into quartiles according to arterial stiffness as measured by carotid–femoral wave velocity. OH prevalence increased with increasing arterial stiffness.

2 It has been estimated[5] that OH accounts for over 80 000 hospital admissions per year in the USA – a rate of 36 per 100 000 adults. In the over-75s, the admission rate was 233 per 100 000 and was particularly high in Caucasian males. Data from the ARIC (Atherosclerosis Risk in Communities) study[6] confirm that patients with OH are at increased risk of premature death, an association that is not completely explained by the association of hypotensive symptoms with traditional cardiovascular risk factors.

3   Dihydroxyphenylserine (DOPS, Droxidopa) is an amino acid that is converted by dihydroxyphenylalanine (DOPA) decarboxylase to noradrenaline. Administration of 200–400 mg daily can improve symptoms of OH. The effect of this drug has now been confirmed in a number of controlled trials.[7] Another novel treatment is the acetylcholinesterase inhibitor pyridostigmine, which increases baroreceptor sensitivity. Although not recommended currently for routine use, there are consistent data from trials to support its safety and efficacy.[8]

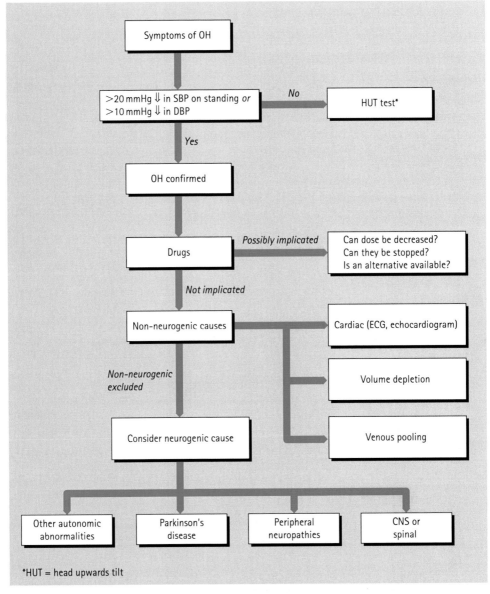

*HUT = head upwards tilt

Figure 8.1 Assessment of the patient with orthostatic hypotension.

4   There is also a novel surgical treatment, use of which has been studied in a small-scale trial.[9] Electrical stimulation of the midbrain in the region of the periventricular/periaqueductal grey areas is known to affect BP in animals. In the study, symptoms of OH were reversed – this was presumed to be through increased sympathetic activity and improved baroreflex sensitivity.

5   OH can occur early in Parkinson's disease, and symptoms from this may initially be more prominent than those of movement disorder. It is not only associated with disease progression, but also with cognitive decline. Parkinson's patients with OH are more likely to be older, male and to be using dopaminergic agents.[10]

Conclusions

OH is common, prevalence increases with age, and it correlates with increased risk of morbidity and mortality. Causes are divided into iatrogenic, non-neurological and neurological. Management is summarized in Figure 8.1. Drugs are a very common cause, but it is not always possible to withdraw offending agents. For the above patient, it is highly likely that the α-blocker is contributing to his symptoms, but it may not be the sole cause. The non-pharmacological management options should be extensively explored before resorting to drug treatment unless symptoms are severe and the cause is clear. Fludrocortisone is the most widely used drug but the range of treatment options for this, sometimes difficult, clinical problem is increasing.

References

1   Gupta V, Lipsitz LA. Orthostatic hypotension in the elderly: diagnosis and treatment. *Am J Med* 2007; **120**: 841–7.

2   Lahrmann H, Cortelli P, Hilz CJ, Mathias CJ, Struhal W, Tassinari M. EFNS guidelines on the diagnosis and management of orthostatic hypotension. *Eur J Neurol* 2006; **13**: 930–6.

3   Freeman R. Neurogenic orthostatic hypotension. *N Engl J Med* 2008; **358**: 615–24.

4   Mattace-Raso FUS, van der Cammen TJM, Knetsch AM, van den Meiracker AH, Schalekamp MADH, Hofman A, *et al.* Arterial stiffness as the candidate underlying mechanism for postural blood pressure changes and orthostatic hypotension in older adults: the Rotterdam Study. *J Hypertens* 2006; **24**: 339–44.

5   Shibao C, Grijalva CG, Raj SR, Biaggioni I, Griffin MR. Orthostatic hypotension-related hospitalizations in the United States. *Am J Med* 2007; **120**: 975–80.

6   Rose KM, Eigenbrodt ML, Biga RL, Couper DJ, Light KC, Sharrett AR, *et al.* Orthostatic hypotension predicts mortality in middle-aged adults: the Atherosclerosis Risk In Communities (ARIC) Study. *Circulation* 2006; **114**: 630–6.

7   Mathias CJ. L-dihydroxyphenylserine (Droxidopa) in the treatment of orthostatic hypotension: the European experience. *Clin Auton Res* 2008; **18** (Suppl 1): 25–9.

8   Gales BJ, Gales MA. Pyridostigmine in the treatment of orthostatic intolerance. *Ann Pharmacother* 2007; **41**: 314–18.

9   Green AL, Wang S, Owen SLF, Paterson DJ, Stein JF, Aziz TZ. Controlling the heart via the brain: a potential new therapy for orthostatic hypotension. *Neurosurgery* 2006; **58**: 1176–83.

10 Allcock LM, Kenny RA, Burn DJ. Clinical phenotype of subjects with Parkinson's disease and orthostatic hypotension: autonomic symptom and demographic comparison. *Mov Disord* 2006; **21**: 1851–5.

Lifestyle Factors

PROBLEM

09 Dietary Salt

Case History

James is a 46-year-old man who was noted to be hypertensive – blood pressure (BP) 142/90 – at an insurance medical. He attends asking for advice on this. His general health is very good and he takes no medications. He would be reluctant to start medication. However, his mother had high BP and suffered a stroke at age 65, and he is aware that hypertension runs in families and that it is important to control. He confesses to a liking for salt, and would like to know if cutting down would reduce his BP.

What are the current recommendations for salt intake?

Does high salt intake cause hypertension?

Does restricting salt intake improve BP control?

Background

The use of salt dates back to at least 6000 BC, and the increasing use of salt as a seasoning and food preservative has paralleled the development of human civilization. Throughout the world, daily sodium intake is remarkably consistent at between 100 and 200 mmol/day. Those at the higher end of this range may be consuming up to 10-fold more salt than was the norm in primitive societies. It is common knowledge that eating too much salt (sodium chloride) is bad for your BP. However, this has been a controversial area in the medical literature. It is inherently difficult to accurately estimate the salt intake of individuals or populations; salt is only one of a number of factors that influence BP; and the population is heterogeneous with respect to salt sensitivity.

Sodium is an essential element, necessary to maintain plasma volume and thus tissue perfusion. The recommended dietary intake is 1500 mg per day. Without added salt, a diet consisting only of vegetables provides only 200 mg, while a mixed diet provides 600 mg and a diet consisting largely of meat provides up to 1000 mg. We rely on added salt to maintain our daily requirement (Box 9.1).

Box 9.1 Dietary salt intake

- 100 mmol salt = 6 g = 1 teaspoonful = 2300 mg sodium*
- Recommended dietary intake: 1500 mg sodium per day
- Low salt diet: 1500–2300 mg sodium per day
- Average dietary intake: 2300–4600 mg sodium per day
- High salt diet: >4600 mg sodium per day

*There is potential for confusion as most food labels show sodium content, whereas dietary guidelines stipulate salt (sodium chloride) levels.

There is a wealth of data from animal studies that increasing salt intake increases BP while decreasing intake has the reverse effect. The controversy around dietary salt that existed 10 years ago partly arose from the variable design and quality of studies. These suggested that, at best, salt restriction would modestly lower BP but the effect was not consistent between individuals. The INTERSALT Study,[1] published in 1988, investigated the relationship between salt intake and BP in 10 079 subjects in 52 locations in 32 countries. There was a clear linear relationship between sodium intake and BP: a 100 mmol/day higher salt intake was estimated to increase systolic BP by 3–5 mmHg while diastolic BP increased by up to 3 mmHg. BP rises with age. Changes in renal haemodynamics dictate that a higher perfusion pressure is required to achieve natriuresis, water and other metabolite excretion as the subject ages. In the INTERSALT Study, a 100 mmol/day increase in salt intake equated to 11 mmHg systolic and 6 mmHg diastolic rise between the ages of 25 and 55.

Animal studies, observational human studies and randomized trials now overwhelmingly confirm the importance of dietary salt intake as a determinant of BP. In the DASH (Dietary Approaches to Stop Hypertension) Sodium Trial,[2] individuals were randomized to one of three levels of salt intake (140, 104 and 62 mmol/day), each for 30 days. While the response to salt restriction was highly variable, more than one-third of subjects decreased systolic BP by more than 10 mmHg when salt was restricted. It is now recognized that the population can be divided into individuals who are salt-sensitive and those who are not. Patients with hypertension are more likely to be salt-sensitive. The phenomenon is partly genetic but increases with age: 50% of hypertensives under the age of 40 are salt-sensitive, compared with 80% of those over 60 years old. Salt sensitivity is defined as a mean rise in arterial pressure of 10 mmHg when the individual consumes a high salt diet. Obese or diabetic subjects are more likely to be salt sensitive.

The volume expansion that follows increased salt intake raises BP, leading to pressure natriuresis, an important mechanism in regulating sodium balance. Reflex vasoconstriction in the preglomerular capillaries can lead to focal ischaemia. The resulting tubulo-interstitial injury provides a stimulus for lymphocyte and macrophage infiltration. These cells secrete a variety of mediators including chemokines and angiotensin II, and also contribute to oxidative stress. The ability to excrete a salt load is genetically determined. Some 20–30 genes have been documented to participate. Individuals who are more able to secrete salt from the kidneys rely less on pressure natriuresis to excrete a sodium load, and are therefore less likely to develop hypertension in response to increased dietary salt. Genes involved include the epithelial sodium channel, activating mutations of which cause Liddle's syndrome – an autosomal dominant condition where increased sodium retention leads to hypertension, which responds to potassium-sparing diuretics. Other genes include the cytoskeletal protein adducing and the Na^+-H^+ exchanger-3. Volume expansion also increases the secretion of endogenous digitalis-like substances, which contribute to hypertension by inhibiting membrane Na^+-K^+-ATPase. Increased digitalis-like substances are found in patients with high volume, low renin hypertension and, in animal models, administration of polyclonal antibody to digoxin (Digibind) lowers BP.

Some of the controversy that arose over dietary salt came from the publication of data from the National Health and Nutrition Examination Survey (NHANES) I and II.[3] These studies reported that lower salt intake was associated with increased mortality. One of the proposed mechanisms was that decreasing salt, as with using diuretics, activates the renin–angiostensin system and may thus cause insulin resistance and worsen overall cardiovascular profile. These studies have been criticized as salt intake was estimated using a single 24-h dietary recall, which is unreliable and does not necessarily take into account discretionary salt (i.e. added at the table). It is vastly preferable to assess salt intake by measuring 24-h urine sodium excretion. An important intervention study was published in 2007[4] – the Trials of Hypertension Prevention (TOHP) study randomized patients to low sodium intake for 18 months (TOHP1) or for 36–48 months (TOHP2). The 2007 study reported follow-up of the patients over 10–15 years. Those randomized to a lower salt diet achieved a reduction in urinary sodium of 44 and 33 mmol/day, respectively, in TOHP1 and TOHP2. The RR of a coronary event was 0.75 (95% CI: 0.57 to 0.99; $P < 0.04$). The RR was lower when data were adjusted for body weight and baseline sodium excretion.

Dietary sodium restriction is important on a population basis to decrease the prevalence of hypertension and thus minimize the burden of cardiovascular disease. For the individual, it may prevent hypertension developing or delay the need for medication. There is a dose-dependent decrease in BP with salt restriction with no threshold effect. Changes in BP with salt restriction are independent of baseline BP, body mass index, gender, ethnicity and age. High salt diet may also predispose to bone demineralization and carcinoma of the stomach. It is important to recognize that salt is not the only important dietary factor, and salt intake should be considered in the context of an overall dietary review in the patient with hypertension.

Generally, when a patient starts taking antihypertensive drugs, they remain on them for life. It seems reasonable to assess the need for drugs at the outset. The most reliable way to assess excessive sodium intake is to measure the amount in a 24-h urine collection. It is reasonable for a patient who has a high salt intake to decrease their intake (confirmed on a second urine collection) and to see whether BP is decreased. High sodium intake leads to increased urinary potassium loss. Furthermore, potassium intake is frequently less than the recommended level. Low potassium status is associated with increased BP, and increasing potassium status can lower BP. Finally, for some patients, a diuretic is needed. Thiazide diuretics can increase urinary sodium loss up to 1000 mmol/day.

Recent Developments

1   A simple questionnaire may assist in assessing an individual's sodium intake.[5] Much of the salt ingested actually comes from relatively few food types. The effect of discretionary salt, which typically accounts for 20% or more of the daily total, is often underestimated. This may be one reason why dietary questionnaires have been found to be much less reliable than measuring the sodium content of urine samples.[6] The sodium content of common classes of foodstuffs is shown in Table 9.1.

2   Salt intake is a major determinant of fluid intake. In children, higher salt intake is associated with increased intake of sugar-sweetened drinks.[7] Decreased salt intake could thus contribute to lower calorie intake and therefore decreased risk of obesity.

3   Activation of the renin–angiostensin system and sympathetic nervous system both result from salt restriction. Because of this, β-blockers and angiotensin-converting enzyme inhibitors or angiotensin receptor blockers are the logical choice of treatment for hypertension following salt restriction or diuretic therapy. Activation of the renin–angiotensin system following salt restriction may decrease insulin sensitivity and predispose to the development of type 2 diabetes.[8]

4   Not only is there genetic variability in the ability to excrete a salt load but individuals who are salt-sensitive may also be more susceptible to hypertension with other predisposing genetic polymorphisms.[9] This includes the I polymorphism of the angiotensin-converting enzyme gene.[10] Independent of genetic influences on salt sensitivity, salt restriction may also be important in patients who have other genetic predispositions to hypertension.

5   The effects of changes in sodium and potassium balance are mediated not only through changes in plasma volume but also through direct alterations in vascular physiology. Salt loading increases vascular tone by decreasing endothelial nitric oxide generation.[11] Also, the protective effect of increased potassium intake may operate through increased nitric oxide generation in the vascular wall, and protect from the effect of a relatively high sodium intake.[12]

Conclusions

Obesity is the most important nutritional factor associated with high BP. Salt intake is the next most important and can account for up to one-fifth of the variation in BP in the population. The management of salt status is summarized in Figure 9.1. Susceptibility to increased BP is variable within populations and is a complex trait that is partly inherited but also relates to obesity, insulin resistance and age. In many individuals, high salt intake predisposes to hypertension, exacerbates any underlying tendency towards hypertension,

Table 9.1 Sodium content of common foodstuffs

Food	Portion size	Salt/portion (mg)
Bread	100 g (2 slices)	425
Processed cereals (cornflakes etc.)	30 g	140–210
Less processed cereals (whole grain cereals, etc.)	50 g	80
Baked snacks, biscuits	20–30 g	120–230 mg
Potato crisps	50 g	600
Pizza	170 g	800–1000
Pastry	40–50 g	85–280
Pasta (uncooked)	70 g	20
Pasta ready meal	250–340 g	600–900
Commercial pie	140 g	650
Commercial stock		
not salt reduced	250 ml	1370
salt reduced	250 ml	1020
Tinned soup	300 ml	1000
Baked beans	210 g	630
Tinned beans (kidney, butter)		
salt added	120 g	320
no salt	120 g	15
Tinned tomatoes		
with salt	125 g	450
no salt added	125 g	8
Tinned fish (salmon, tuna)	80 g	200–350
Corned or other processed beef	80 g	400–500
Cheese	40 g	200–400
Milk	250 ml	115
Ice cream	100 g	50–60
Fruit juice	200 ml	10
Beer	375 ml	30
Ketchup	15 ml	180
Soy sauce	15 ml	1210

and can decrease the response to treatment. Lowering sodium intake has the potential to prevent hypertension, lower BP in the early stages, and to increase the effect of drug treatments. All too often, we neglect salt intake and other lifestyle factors before resorting to pharmacological treatment of high BP.

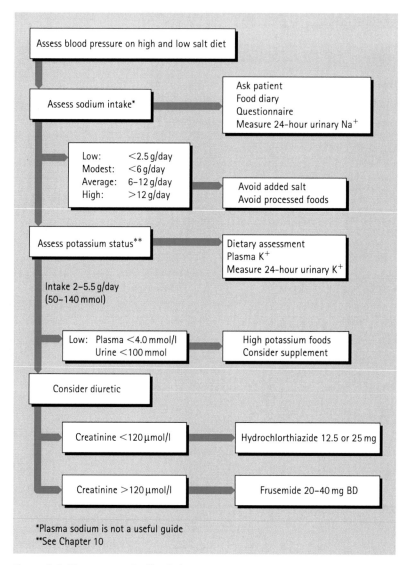

Figure 9.1 Management of sodium balance.

References

1 Stamler J. The INTERSALT Study: background, method, findings, and implications. *Am J Clin Nutr* 1997; **65** (Suppl): 626–42S.

2 Oberzanek E, Proschan MA, Vollmer WM, Moore TJ, Sacks FM, Appel LJ, *et al.* Individual blood pressure response to changes in salt intake. Results from the DASH–sodium trial. *Hypertension* 2003; **42**: 459–67.

3 Cohen HW, Hailpern SM, Fang J, Alderman MH. Sodium intake and mortality in the NHANES II follow-up study. *Am J Med* 2006; **119**: e7–e14.

4   Cook NR, Cutler JA, Oberzanek E, Buring JE, Kumanyika SK, Appel LJ, Whelton PK. Long term effects of dietary sodium reduction on cardiovascular disease outcomes: observational follow-up of the trials of hypertension outcome (TOHP). *BMJ* 2007; **334**: 885–93.

5   Charlton KE, Steyn K, Levitt NS, Jonathan D, Zulu JW, Nel JH. Development and validation of a short questionnaire to assess sodium intake. *Public Health Nutr* 2007; **11**: 83–94.

6   Hashimoto T, Yagami F, Owada M, Sugawara T, Kawamura M. Salt preference according to a questionnaire vs dietary salt intake estimated by a spot urine method in participants at a health check-up center. *Intern Med* 2008; **47**: 399–403.

7   He FJ, Marrero NM, MacGregor GA. Salt intake is related to soft drink consumption in children and adolescents; a link to obesity. *Hypertension* 2008; **51**: 629–34.

8   Townsend RR, Kapoor S, McFadden C. Salt intake and insulin sensitivity in healthy human volunteers. *Clin Sci* 2007; **113**: 141–8.

9   Gu D, Rice T, Wang S, Yang W, Yang W, Gu C, Chen C-S, *et al*. Heritability of blood pressure responses to dietary sodium and potassium intake in a Chinese population. *Hypertension* 2007; **50**: 116–22.

10   Yamagishi K, Tanigawa T, Cui R, Tabata M, Ikeda A, Yao M, *et al*. High sodium intake strengthens the association of ACE I/D polymorphism with blood pressure in a community. *Am J Hypertens* 2007; **20**: 751–7.

11   Oberleithner H, Riethmüller C, Schillers H, MacGregor GA, de Wardnere HE, Hausberg M. Plasma sodium stiffens vascular endothelium and reduces nitric oxide release. *Proceedings of the National Academy of Sciences USA* 2007; **104**: 16281–6.

12   Fang Y, Mu J-J, He L-C, Wang S-C, Liu Z-Q. Salt loading on plasma asymmetrical dimethylarginine and the protective role of potassium supplement in normotensive salt-sensitive Asians. *Hypertension* 2006; **48**: 724–9.

10 Other Dietary Factors

Case History

Mr TW is 49 years old and generally fit. He was recently found to be hypertensive – blood pressure (BP) at his last clinic visit was 146/92. His parents were both hypertensive and required BP-lowering medications. He is anxious to avoid medications for as long as possible. He attends with his wife who is an aromatherapist. They would like to know what he could do to lower his BP. He has decreased his alcohol intake and is trying to decrease his weight (body mass index 27.5 kg/m²).

Is lifestyle management effective in lowering BP?

What lifestyle factors should he focus on?

Would drug treatment be more effective and desirable at this stage?

Background

Hypertension affects one in three adults in the USA, i.e. a total of 65 million people. While many require drug treatment, many could achieve better BP control and minimize reliance on medications by following current nutritional recommendations:

- Maintain a healthy body weight.
- Maintain physical activity: 30 min moderate exercise most days.
- An eating plan that incorporates a low salt intake.
- Drink alcohol in moderation.

The US government initiative Dietary Approaches to Stop Hypertension (DASH)[1] provides an excellent framework for lifestyle management to prevent and manage hypertension (Box 10.1). The DASH diet is based on a decreased sodium intake along with a higher intake of electrolytes that protect against hypertension (potassium, calcium and magnesium). The diet is high in fruit, vegetables and fibre while relative restriction in the intake of meat is encouraged.

The typical BP response with a DASH diet is a reduction of 5.5/3.0 mmHg.[2] Greater effects are seen in patients with hypertension. Also, black subjects respond better (reduction of 7.0/4.0 on average). Diets higher in vegetable content and lower in meat are more effective – several studies have demonstrated that vegetarians tend to have lower BP. The OmniHeart trial[2] used the DASH approach, but demonstrated a further decrease in BP when some of the dietary carbohydrate was substituted either by protein or by monounsaturated fatty acid.

Box 10.1 Goals of the DASH Diet for Hypertension: 2100 calorie diet

- Total fat: 27% of calories
- Saturated fat: 6% of calories
- Protein: 18% of calories
- Carbohydrate: 55% of calories
- Cholesterol: 150 mg/day
- Sodium 2300 mg/day*
- Potassium 4700 mg/day
- Calcium 1250 mg/day
- Magnesium 500 mg/day
- Fibre 30 g/day

*BP is lower with a sodium intake of 1500 mg/day.

Finally, PREMIER is an approach where the DASH-based diet is combined with exercise and other lifestyle modifications. Use of this was associated with 14.2/7.4 reduction in the BP of hypertensives, and a 9.2/5.8 reduction in the BP of non-hypertensives.

Potassium

Only between 10% and 40% of adults consume the recommended intake, which is 4700 mg or 120 mmol/day. In the NHANES III study,[2] men consumed an average of 3000 mg/day compared with only about 2000 mg in women. There is now a general consensus that higher potassium intake is associated with better BP control. Numerous studies have now demonstrated an inverse relationship between potassium status and BP, both in hypertensives and in non-hypertensives. Increasing potassium intake (and therefore excretion) by 2000 mg (50 mmol)/day could decrease population average BP by about 4.5/2.5 mmHg. Tangible benefits in BP control are easily achievable through dietary change. These changes are generally more apparent in black subjects and in those with a relatively high salt intake. Potassium content is high in many fruits and vegetables, some dairy products, and in fish (Table 10.1).

Note that care has to be taken with potassium supplementation if renal function is compromised (estimated glomerular filtration rate <60 ml/min). Also, certain drug classes tend to increase plasma potassium levels: angiotensin-converting enzyme inhibitors, angiotensin receptor blockers, non-steroidal anti-inflammatory drugs and potassium-sparing diuretics. The benefits of a higher potassium intake have now been noted in studies with children. There appears to be a particularly high protective effect in relation to stroke. The benefits of potassium supplementation are irrespective of the salt (chloride or citrate), suggesting that dietary manoeuvres are as likely to be effective as potassium chloride tablets. Chang et al.[3] studied 1981 institutionalized elderly people randomized to use either potassium-enriched salt or regular salt. The risk per 1000 of cardiovascular (CV) death was 13.1 and 20.5 respectively. The heart rate was 0.59 (95% CI: 0.37 to 0.95) in favour of the potassium-enriched group, which also had lower in-patient costs for CV complications.

Table 10.1 Dietary sources of potassium	
Foodstuff	Potassium content (mg)
Potato (medium, with skin)	930
Sweet potato (medium)	540
Banana (medium)	420
Orange (medium)	240
Cantaloupe melon (half cup)	220
Lentils, kidney beans (cooked, half cup)	360
Milk (1 cup)	380
Fish (3 ounces)	200–400

Calcium supplementation

The benefits of this have been less certain than those for potassium. Forty per cent of the adult population do not consume the recommended dietary intake, and this has implication for risk of osteoporosis as well as for BP control. Increasing calcium intake has a modest effect on BP control, particularly where the diet is relatively high in sodium. In a recent meta-analysis of 40 published trials,[4] calcium decreased systolic BP by an average of 1.86 mmHg (95% CI: –2.91 to –0.81). Reduction in diastolic BP was 0.99 mmHg (–1.61 to –0.37).

Magnesium

To date, information about magnesium supplementation and BP have been inconsistent. A modest decrease of about 0.6/0.8 mmHg has been noted, and attributed to vasodilatation. At present, routine calcium or magnesium supplementation is not warranted but their intake levels should be considered in the overall design of a dietary strategy.

Alcohol

A modest intake of alcohol is protective against insulin resistance and CV disease. Men are recommended to consume no more than two standard drinks per day, while women and men of small stature are recommended to limit themselves to one drink per day (Box 10.2). For those who habitually consume moderate to high amounts of alcohol, limiting themselves to the above will modestly decrease BP (typically by 3–4 mmHg systolic and 2–3 mmHg diastolic). Also, the calorie content of alcoholic drinks should not be forgotten. Alcohol metabolism generates 7 kcal/g. For example, half a bottle of wine (12.5% alcohol) contains 40 ml alcohol or 280 kcal.

Box 10.2 Definition of a standard drink

- 285 ml of standard beer (4.9% alcohol)
- 375 ml of mid-strength beer (3.5% alcohol)
- 100 ml or one small glass wine (12% alcohol)
- 30 ml spirit ± mixer (40% alcohol)

Fish oil

Dietary supplementation with omega-3 polyunsaturated fatty acids (PUFA) has been considered to have modest effects in lowering BP, although effects may only be seen with higher doses (e.g. 3 g/day). Typically, lower by no more than 4/2.5 mmHg is seen. The effect varies between individuals and may depend on other dietary components, including other fats (omega-6 polyunsaturated, saturated and monounsaturated fatty acids).

Recent Developments

1 In a study of nearly 21 000 middle-aged women,[5] there was no relationship between adherence to a DASH-type diet and either hypertension or mortality from CV disease after adjusting for other risk factors. One of the possible factors was a less than perfect concordance with DASH nutrition goals by participating subjects. Increasing patient choice may improve concordance with the diet. A recent study by Swain et al.[6] has shown that there can be reasonable flexibility with respect to macronutrient components of the diet.

2 Recent work with Dahl salt-sensitive rats[7] has not only confirmed the protective effects of potassium against salt loading but shows that the mechanism may be through decreased generation of reactive oxygen species. While data are accumulating to support the protective role of higher potassium intake, there is still a degree of uncertainty: The Rotterdam study[8] followed individuals aged 55 years and older for 5 years. No relationship was demonstrated between sodium or potassium status and mortality.

3 A recent study[9] of nearly 29 000 women aged ≥45 has confirmed the protective role of calcium. There was a significant trend for lower incidence of hypertension with increasing intake of low-fat dairy products. While current data do not support routine calcium supplementation, we should encourage patients to maintain their intake as part of a balanced diet.

4 While the effects of dietary omega-3 PUFA on BP may be modest, they have now been confirmed in a variety of studies including the recent INTERMAP study.[10] In addition to their effect on BP, they protect against sudden death following coronary events, and data from the Atherosclerosis Risk In Communities (ARIC) study[11] suggest that they may protect against cognitive decline when administered to patients with hypertension. The protective effects almost certainly do not just relate to decreasing BP.

5 Dietary phosphorus intake levels correlate inversely with BP,[12] adding to the range of mineral micronutrients, which may have protective effects. Again, available data do not allow us to make firm recommendations about dietary change or supplementation for now.

Conclusions

An overview of the lifestyle management of hypertension is presented in Figure 10.1. Management of body weight is the single most important factor followed by salt intake. Overall management of lifestyle factors has considerable potential to lower BP in many

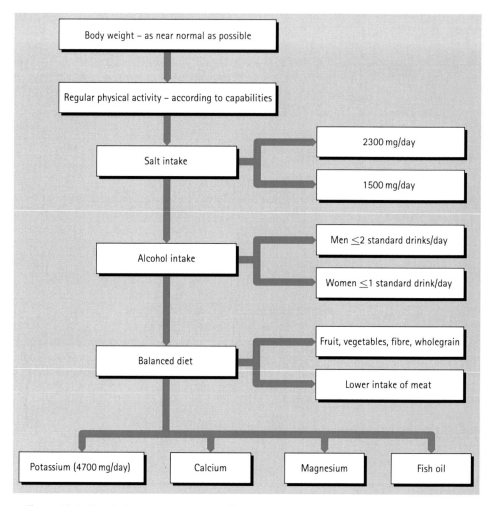

Figure 10.1 Lifestyle factors in management of hypertension.

patients, and also to favourably impact on other aspects of CV risk. Initial management of patients with prehypertension or stage I hypertension should generally be non-pharmacological. While some areas remain controversial (e.g. calcium supplementation), these should be viewed in the context of an overall balanced diet.

References

1   *Your guide to lowering your blood pressure with DASH*. US Department of Health and Human Services. NIH Publication No. 06-4082; Revised April 2006.

2   Appel LJ, Brands MW, Daniels SR, Karanja N, Elmer PJ, Sacks FM. Dietary approaches to prevent and treat hypertension: a scientific statement from the American Heart Association. *Hypertension* 2006; **47**: 296–308.

3   Chang H-Y, Hu Y-W, Yue C-SJ, Wen Y-W, Yeh W-T, Hsu L-S, *et al.* Effect of potassium-enriched salt on cardiovascular mortality and medical expenses of elderly men. *Am J Clin Nutr* 2006; **83**: 1289–96.

4   van Mierlo LAJ, Arends LR, Streppel MT, Zeegers MPA, Kok FJ, Grobbee DE, Geleinjnse JM. Blood pressure response to calcium supplementation: a meta-analysis of randomized controlled trials. *J Hum Hypertens* 2006; **20**: 571–80.

5   Folsom AR, Parker ED, Harnack LJ. Degree of concordance with DASH diet guidelines and incidence of hypertension and fatal cardiovascular disease. [See comment.] *Am J Hypertens* 2007; **20**: 225–32.

6   Swain JF, McCarron PB, Hamilton EF, Sacks FM, Appel LJ. Characteristics of the diet patterns tested in the optimal macronutrient intake trial to prevent heart disease (OmniHeart): options for a heart-healthy diet. *J Am Diet Assoc* 2008; **108**: 257–65.

7   Kido M, Ando K, Onozato ML, Tojo A, Yoshikawa M, Ogita T, *et al.* Protective effect of dietary potassium against vascular injury in salt-sensitive hypertension. *Hypertension* 2008; **51**: 225–31.

8   Geleijnse JM, Witteman JCM, Stijnen T, Kloos MW, Hofman A, Grobbee DE. Sodium and potassium intake and risk of cardiovascular events and all-cause mortality: the Rotterdam Study. *Eur J Epidemiol* 2007; **22**: 763–70.

9   Wang L, Manson JE, Buring JE, Lee IM, Sesso HD. Dietary intake of dairy products, calcium, and vitamin D and the risk of hypertension in middle-aged and older women. *Hypertension* 2008; **51**: 1073–9.

10 Ueshima H, Stamler J, Elliott P, Chan Q, Brown IJ, Carnethon MR, *et al.* Food omega-3 fatty acid intake of individuals (total, linolenic acid, long-chain) and their blood pressure: INTERMAP Study. *Hypertension* 2007; **50**: 313–19.

11 Beydoun MA, Kaufman JS, Sloane PD, Heiss G, Ibrahim J. n-3 fatty acids, hypertension and risk of cognitive decline among older adults in the Atherosclerosis Risk in Communities (ARIC) study. *Public Health Nutr* 2008; **11**: 17–29.

12 Elliott P, Kesteloot H, Appel LJ, Dyer AR, Ueshima H, Chan Q, *et al.* Dietary phosphorus and blood pressure: international study of macro- and micro-nutrients and blood pressure. *Hypertension* 2008; **51**: 669–75.

11 Stress and Blood Pressure

Case History

Paul is a successful 53-year-old businessman who has been noted to be hypertensive. He has a happy home life but has many business pressures. When he attends for routine review, his blood pressure (BP) is 160/96. He has it taken often when he is away on business and has a BP machine at home and says that his BP is often quite normal. He drinks alcohol regularly (30–40 units a week), is a non-smoker, and takes no medications apart from aspirin intermittently. His father had a stroke in his late 50s.

Does this man need treatment for his BP?

What is the optimal approach to managing stress-induced hypertension?

Do behavioural interventions to combat stress also lower BP?

Background

Psychological and physical stress is a component of how we react to demands placed upon us. It has a positive aspect, helping us cope with and deal with these demands. However, when stress is either severe and acute or chronic, it has the potential to impact negatively on mental and physical well-being. There is a huge variation between individuals in the reaction to stress. Because of this and the variety of stressful stimuli, it is hard to define stress scientifically. Common sources of stress are summarized in Box 11.1. Many patients complain of stress, and rating scores are available to help quantify the phenomenon. Stress is not always precipitated by a single factor or event, and the individual's response does not necessarily directly relate to the apparent severity of the stressor(s).

There is no question that stress can affect many aspects of health. Increase in BP in response to stress if it becomes chronic will contribute to increased cardiovascular (CV) risk. Some individuals, so-called type A personalities, are attracted to stressful situations and often thrive on them. Characteristics of this personality type include competitive and assertive behaviour, being generally less relaxed and more time-conscious. This character type may be associated with increased CV events. The stress consequences of earthquakes and other natural disasters have been extensively studied.[1] Acute responses include increased sympathetic nervous system activity and increased circulating catecholamines leading to increased heart rate. In those with pre-existing cardiac disease, these changes may provoke myocardial ischaemia, arrhythmia, give rise to cardiac wall motion abnormalities, and decrease ejection fraction. Acute stressful events may create life changes that

Box 11.1 Common causes of stress

- Ageing
- Decline in health
- Post-traumatic
- Care giving
- Life experiences
- Occupational
- Relationship breakdown
- Income/financial
- Social status
- Discrimination

cause chronic stress, or the individual may develop post-traumatic stress disorder. A number of studies have confirmed that chronic stress is associated with a more than doubling of CV events. In the INTERHEART study, the rate of myocardial infarction was 2.1-fold increased in those with stress.[1] The mechanisms through which chronic stress increases CV risk are multiple and some of them may operate through increasing BP. Increased sympathetic and decreased parasympathetic activity contribute to the blunting of baroreceptor reflexes so that increased BP is not accompanied by a compensatory decrease in heart rate. Endocrine changes include hypercortisolaemia and, in men, decreased testosterone. Both sympathetic overactivity and decreased insulin sensitivity contribute to sodium and water retention. Finally, there is a strong association with unhealthy lifestyle choices.

Exercise is an important component of stress management. Randomized trials, which have included BP reduction as an outcome, have yielded conflicting results. Typically, a 1–2% reduction in systolic BP (SBP) and diastolic BP (DBP) is reported. Exercise programmes are often disappointing in promoting weight loss but they certainly impact favourably on body composition and well-being. Dietary factors are also important – no single change will consistently control BP but collectively a healthy diet that is low in salt and high in potassium coupled with limited alcohol intake can make a difference. Other methods of controlling stress-induced hypertension include yoga, mediation, progressive relaxation programmes, biofeedback and cognitive-behavioural therapy approaches. Inconsistent trial design and small sample size have contributed to inconsistent conclusions in the literature.[2]

Several observational and cross-sectional studies have confirmed the association between chronic stress and hypertension, as well as end-organ damage (e.g. left ventricular hypertrophy). The latter may occur before hypertension is too advanced as multiple causative factors are involved. Stress-induced hypertension is more common in men and in postmenopausal women, in those with a family history of hypertension, and in certain racial groups including African Americans. Three main approaches have been studied.[2]

- *Biofeedback*: early studies in the 1980s were encouraging, and suggested that SBP and DBP might be decreased by up to 8 and 6 mmHg respectively. Unfortunately, subsequent studies have yielded inconsistent results.

- *Relaxation therapies*: again, preliminary studies in the 1980s suggested that modest reductions in both SBP and DBP were possible, alongside other benefits of the therapy in patients with stress.

- *Stress management programmes*: a number of studies have shown a modest reduction in both SBP and DBP but, once more, results are not consistent. A recent 1-year study employed a cognitive-behavioural intervention.[3] At the end of the study there was no difference in the BP between treated patients and controls.

There are considerable methodological difficulties with the type of study that is required: subjects get used to having their BP measured, and there is a tendency for values to drift downwards with time; there are confounding influences from drug treatments and life events during the study period; responses are heterogeneous. The approach needs to be tailored to the individual's needs and, as with drug treatment for hypertension, combination treatments may be required. Linden *et al.*[4] investigated the effect of an individualized programme on BP. During this programme, SBP decreased by 6.1 and DBP by 4.3 mmHg.

Medical practitioners are generally not skilled in identifying stress and, therefore, helping patients to cope with it. Some simple initial steps are to:

- help the patient to list factors that are causing stress;

- encourage them to make choices that minimize stress;

- develop coping strategies to deal with stressors that cannot be removed;

- help build relaxation and time to themselves into their routine (hobbies etc.);

- encourage a healthy lifestyle: diet and exercise, and

- identify possible support mechanisms.

It can be helpful to keep a journal, noting stressful events and how they reacted to them, and also identifying opportunities to use their coping strategies. Poor time management is often a feature of stress. Identifying this and using a structured approach can help. Signs of poor time management include always rushing, missing deadlines, trying to do several things at once, inability to find things and difficulty with prioritization.

Recent Developments

1   Recent data from the EPIC study[5] involved 20 627 subjects without stroke at baseline. Risk of stroke on follow-up was clearly related to symptoms of psychological distress and depression. Hypertension could be an important mediator of this effect. However, in the Whitehall II study,[6] where work-related stress increased risk of coronary events, hypertension was not thought to be a major factor in the increased risk of stressed workers. Linden *et al.*[7] conducted a meta-analysis of psychological interventions in patients who had suffered a coronary event. The interventions decreased risk of mortality and event recurrence, but did not produce major affects on measures of affective disorder.

2 Stress is an important predictor of depression in high-risk groups such as African American patients with hypertension.[8] The presence of depression is an important determinant of prognosis in patients with vascular disease. For example, after myocardial infarction, both early and late depression appears to increase mortality.[9] Stress obviously predisposes to depression. It is important to recognize when clinical depression has developed in a stressed patient as it may require specific treatment, including pharmacotherapy.

3 Edelman *et al.*[10] used an integrative approach with stress management combined with traditional risk factor treatments. Compared with a standard approach, the integrative approach showed a greater effect on the Framingham risk score. The intervention group experienced a decrease in 10-year risk from 9.3% at baseline to 7.8% at 10 months of follow-up. Drug treatments are very effective for BP and lipid control in high-risk populations, and should not be withheld. However, psychological interventions may provide additional benefits in terms of symptom relief, compliance with lifestyle and drug treatment, and the development of depression.[11]

4 A long-term follow-up of a large cohort of young Finns[12] provides strong evidence for a relationship between stress-related (type A) personality traits and risk of atherosclerosis. Increased carotid intima-media thickness was documented

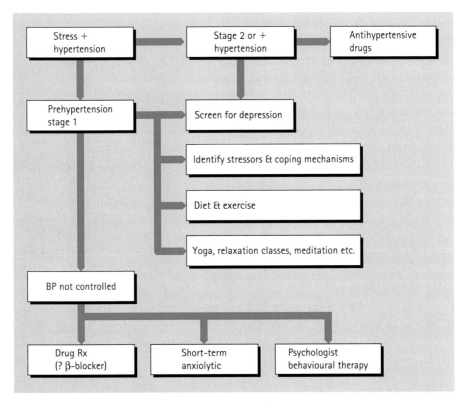

Figure 11.1 Management of stress and hypertension.

in those who scored highly for type A personality traits. Such traits may not only directly influence pathogenetic mechanisms, including those involved in BP control, but are also linked with unhealthy behaviour choices such as smoking, high alcohol intake and unhealthy diet choices.[13]

Conclusions

 Increased BP is part of the body's response to stress, and this contributes to the increased CV risk among those who suffer stress. Individual psychological or behavioural interventions may alleviate stress-related symptoms, but so far have proved limited in their impact on hypertension. Combinations of intervention treatments tailored to the patient's need, and used along with pharmacotherapy provide hope for the future. The above patient requires both stress and BP measurement. A treatment flow is suggested in Figure 11.1. It is reasonable to focus on the stress initially but not to withhold specific BP-lowering therapy for too long. In the individual patient, a stress management approach can be very effective if it meets the patient's requirements and this can certainly minimize the need for medication if not avoid the need for drugs.

References

1   Dimsdale JE. Psychological stress and cardiovascular disease. *J Am Coll Cardiol* 2008; **51**: 1237–46.

2   Blumenthal JA, Sherwood A, Gullette ECD, Georgiades A, Tweedy D. Biobehavioral approaches to the treatment of essential hypertension. *J Consult Clin Psychol* 2002; **70**: 569–89.

3   Claesson M, Birgander LS, Jansson JH, Lindahl B, Burell G, Asplund K, *et al.* Cognitive-behavioural stress management does not improve biological cardiovascular risk indicators in women with ischaemic heart disease: a randomized-controlled trial. *J Intern Med* 2006; **260**: 320–31.

4   Linden W, Lenz JW, Con AH. Individualized stress management for primary hypertension: a randomized trial. *Arch Intern Med* 2001; **161**: 1071–80.

5   Surtees PG, Wainwright NWJ, Luben RN, Wareham NJ, Bingham SA, Khaw KT. Psychological distress, major depressive disorder, and risk of stroke. *Neurology* 2008; **70**: 788–94.

6   Kivimaki M, Head J, Ferrie JE, Shipley MJ, Steptoe A, Vahtera J, *et al.* Hypertension is not the link between job strain and coronary heart disease in the Whitehall II study. *Am J Hypertens* 2007; **20**: 1146–53.

7   Linden W, Phillips MJ, Leclerc J. Psychological treatment of cardiac patients: a meta-analysis. *Eur Heart J* 2007; **28**: 2972–84.

8   Dennis JP, Markey MA, Johnston KA, Vander Wal JS, Artinian NT. The role of stress and social support in predicting depression among a hypertensive African American sample. *Heart Lung* 2008; **37**: 105–12.

9   Parakh K, Thombs BD, Fauerbach JA, Bush DE, Ziegelstein RC. Effect of depression on late (8 years) mortality after myocardial infarction. *Am J Cardiol* 2008; **101**: 602–6.

10 Edelman D, Oddone EZ, Liebowitz RS, Yancy WS, Jr, Olsen MK, Jeffreys AS, *et al.* A multidimensional integrative medicine intervention to improve cardiovascular risk. *J Gen Intern Med* 2006; **21**: 728–34.

11 Koertge J, Janszky I, Sundin O, Blom M, Georgiades A, Laszlo KD, *et al.* Effects of a stress management program on vital exhaustion and depression in women with coronary heart disease: a randomized controlled intervention study. *J Intern Med* 2008; **263**: 281–93.

12 Keltikangas-Jarvinen L, Hintsa T, Kivimaki M, Puttonen S, Juonala M, Viikari JSA, *et al.* Type A eagerness-energy across developmental periods predicts adulthood carotid intima-media thickness: the Cardiovascular Risk in Young Finns Study. *Arterioscler Thromb Vasc Biol* 2007; **27**: 1638–44.

13 Krueger PM, Chang VW. Being poor and coping with stress: health behaviors and the risk of death. *Am J Public Health* 2008; **98**: 889–96.

12 Obesity and Hypertension

Case History

TW is a 47-year-old woman with a body mass index (BMI) of 34 kg/m². She and her family are becomingly concerned that her weight is affecting her health. She has developed arthritis in her knees and has been diagnosed with sleep apnoea following complaints from her husband that she snores loudly. She has a persistently high BP with typical value of 164/96. There is a strong family history of weight problems, hypertension, and a number of family members have died prematurely from vascular problems.

How is the link between obesity and weight problems explained?

Will losing weight improve her BP?

How should her hypertension be managed?

Is there a role for pharmacological treatment to help weight loss?

Background

Prevalence of being overweight or obese has increased markedly in recent years: two-thirds of the population of developed countries is overweight and obesity affects one in five. Obesity decreases life expectancy with severely obese men living 13 years less, and severely obese women living 8 years less, than their lean counterparts. This decrease in life expectancy, and much of the morbidity that accompanies obesity, is due to cardiovascular (CV) disease. There is clear evidence that obesity increases risk of CV disease in young and middle-aged adults, reasonable evidence that it is linked to stroke and heart failure, and strong evidence for a link between visceral obesity and CV risk. At least 70% of obese adult males and 60% of obese females have a CV problem, including those with hypertension. The World Health Organization (WHO) defines obesity on the basis of BMI (Table 12.1). Visceral obesity is particularly associated with increased vascular risk (Table 12.2). Waist circumference is at the core of the International Diabetes Federation definition of the metabolic syndrome.

Increased body weight is an important risk factor for hypertension. This has been confirmed in a number of studies, including NHANES (National Health and Nutrition Examination Survey), INTERSALT and WHO Monica.[1] In NHANES, only 12% of those with normal body weight were hypertensive while hypertension increased steadily with increasing BMI to about 40% of those with BMI ≥30. In general, an increase in BMI of one unit equates to a systolic BP increase of 0.91 mmHg in men and 0.72 mmHg in

Table 12.1 Classification of BMI for adults

BMI (kg/m²)	Classification
<18.5	Underweight
18.5–24.9	Healthy body weight
25.0–29.9	Overweight or pre-obese
≥30.0	Obese
30.0–34.9	Class I
35.0–39.9	Class II
≥40	Class III

Table 12.2 Increased waist circumference and waist–hip ratio

	Men	Women
Waist circumference associated with higher cardiovascular risk	94 cm	80 cm
Waist–hip ratio		
Low risk	≤0.95	≤0.80
Medium risk	0.96–1.0	0.81–0.85
High risk	>1.0	>0.85

women. This holds well across different races, although the figures vary, e.g. in high-risk groups such as South Asians and African Americans, only modest weight increases may lead to major increases in BP. Only a minority of patients with hypertension are of normal body weight (Figure 12.1).

The reasons for the association between obesity and hypertension are complex (Figure 12.2). In obesity, there is increased carbon oxide, expanded plasma volume and increased total peripheral resistance – all of which contribute to hypertension. There is activation of the renin–angiotensin system (RAS), including within adipose tissue. Weight loss in subjects with obesity leads to decreased angiotensinogen, angiotensin-converting enzyme and aldosterone levels. Increased leptin (a product of adipose tissue) directly increases sympathetic nervous system (SNS) activity and contributes to sodium retention. Decreased atrial natriuretic peptide levels further contribute to sodium retention. Renal changes increase matrix deposition and endothelial cell proliferation. Haemodynamic changes cause hyperfiltration with consequent tubular damage and glomerulosclerosis. Increase expression of 11β-hydroxysteroid dehydrogenase type 1 (11β-HSD-1) in adipose tissue leads to increased conversion of inactive cortisone to active cortisol. Hypertension may predispose to obesity as well as vice versa: increased SNS in patients with hypertension leads to β-adrenergic receptor down-regulation with consequent decreased thermogenic responses. Similar changes are seen with β-blocker

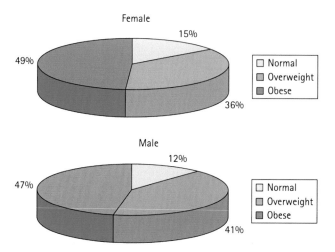

Figure 12.1 Increased body weight and hypertension.

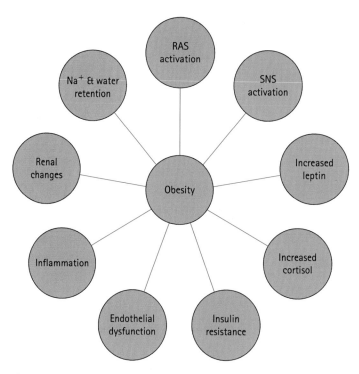

Figure 12.2 Pathogenesis of hypertension in obesity.

therapy. While not all patients with obstructive sleep apnoea/hypopnoea syndrome (OSAHS) are obese, most are. Sleep-disordered breathing has been reported in up to 30% of hypertensives, while more than 50% of those with OSAHS have increased BP. The

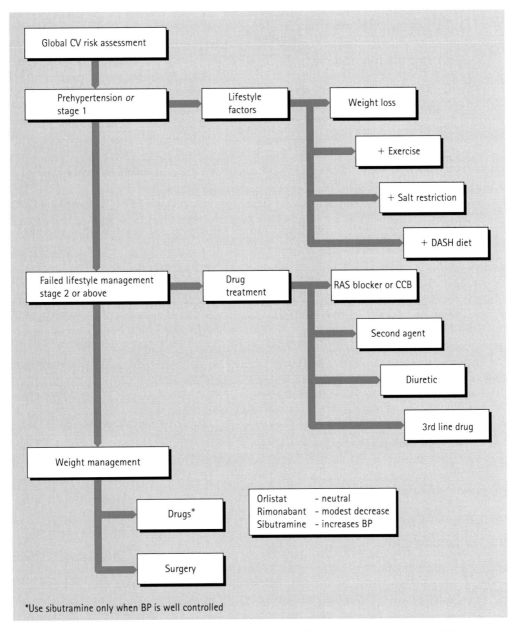

Figure 12.3 Management of hypertension with obesity. CCB, calcium channel blocker; DASH, dietary approaches to stop hypertension; RAS, renin–angiotensin system.

combination of hypertension and OSAHS has now been noted in 9% of US females and in up to 20% of US males.

There are no specific guidelines for managing hypertension in obesity. The accepted target BP is 140/90 unless there is diabetes or chronic kidney disease (130/80). Both diuretics and β-blockers increase the risk of diabetes, or may worsen glycaemic control in pre-existing diabetes. This adverse effect of diuretics may be offset by benefits in CV end-point reduction. β-blockers, in addition, can cause modest weight gain, or contribute to difficulty in losing weight. Several studies have demonstrated the efficacy of RAS-blocking drugs in obese subjects:[1] the TROPHY (Trial of Preventing Hypertension) study (1997) demonstrated the superiority of angiotensin-converting enzyme inhibitors over diuretics. In the CROSS (Candesartan Role on Obesity and on Sympathetic System) study (2003) candesartan proved superior to hydrochlorthiazide in obese subjects. The LIFE (Losartan Intervention For Endpoint Reduction) (2005) substudy reported that losartan was superior to atenolol. An algorithm is proposed in Figure 12.3.

There is considerable interest in drugs to assist with weight loss/maintenance. Two drugs are in common usage: Orlistat (Zenecal) is a gastrointestinal lipase inhibitor with an excellent evidence base supporting its use and safety. Given at a dose of 120 mg TDS (with each meal), it induces modest weight loss with a decrease in BP in proportion to the degree of weight loss. Sibutramine (Meridia, Reductil) is a centrally-acting noradrenaline and 5-hydroxytryptamine reuptake inhibitor, and is used at doses of 10 or 15 mg OD. While effective when used for up to 2 years with suitable diet and exercise, it increases heart rate and BP. It should not be used in patients with uncontrolled hypertension. It may be used along with antihypertensives and the recent Hypertension–Obesity–Sibutramine (HOS) Study[2] showed that a regimen based on angiotensin-converting enzyme inhibitors or calcium channel blockers was preferable to one based on β-blocker ± diuretic as the latter could decrease the beneficial effects of sibutramine. In the very large SCOUT (Sibutramine Cardiovascular OUTcomes) trial,[3] 88% of patients were hypertensive. Although a short-term study, sibutramine was effective when used alongside hypertension treatment. A third drug, rimonabant (Accomplia), is a selective cannabinoid-1 (CB-1) receptor antagonist. Studies in America and Europe have shown that this drug is effective in inducing weight loss and improving CV risk profile, although the reduction in systolic BP and diastolic BP is modest.[4] However, due to the potential side-effects caused by rimonabant acting on the central nervous system, this drug failed to gain approval by the FDA for use in the US. Subsequently, rimonabant was voluntarily withdrawn altogether by the manufacturer following advice by the EMEA for practitioners not to prescribe the drug due to adverse psychological effects.

Recent Developments

1   Increasing understanding of the biology of adipocytes is helping to explain the links between obesity and CV risk. Adiponectin levels decrease with increasing obesity and low adiponectin is a risk factor for diabetes and CV disease. Low adiponectin has been directly linked to hypertension,[5] although it is not clear whether this association is causal or coincidental. The RAS in adipose tissue contributes to adipocyte differentiation and may contribute to hypertension. In an obese mouse model, mineralocorticoid receptor blockade decreased the expression of inflammatory cytokines and increased adiponectin.[6]

2   COMT is an enzyme involved in the breakdown of catecholamines and oestrogens. It is a yet unexploited therapeutic target for hypertension associated with obesity. The val158-met polymorphism of the COMT gene determines

enzyme activity with the met allele having lower activity. Those with the met allele are predisposed to abdominal obesity and hypertension.[7]

3 In the MESA (Multi-Ethnic Study of Atherosclerosis) Study,[8] obesity was a powerful determinant of markers of evolving CV disease (coronary artery calcification and increased carotid intima-media thickness). There were important ethnic differences with those of Chinese descent having a lesser tendency to become obese. In all ethnic groups, development of severe obesity leads to the accumulation of CV risk factors. The proportion of US adults who are severely obese has increased steadily in recent years – now at least 1.5% of the population.[9]

Conclusions

Obesity has overtaken smoking as a modifiable risk factor. Recent evidence strengthens arguments for weight management as first-line treatment in obese and hypertensive individuals. Among the many factors linking obesity to high BP are activation of the SNS and RAS. Weight loss is an effective means of lowering BP, and will favourably impact on other CV risk factors. RAS-blocking drugs and calcium channel blockers are logical first-line treatments. Because of the association with salt and water retention, diuretics are also useful in many patients in spite of their metabolic disadvantages. Of those weight loss drugs currently in wide usage: (1) orlistat decreases BP in proportion to the amount of weight loss; (2) sibutramine increases BP but can be very useful where hypertension is either not present or is well controlled. For patients with severe obesity, bariatric surgery is increasingly used and leads to significant weight loss, although patients with well-established hypertension may not experience marked BP reductions after surgery.

References

1 Narkiewicz K. Diagnosis and management of hypertension in obesity. *Obes Rev* 2006; **7**: 155–62.

2 Scholze J, Grimm E, Hermann D, Unger T, Kintscher U. Optimum treatment of obesity-related hypertension: the Hypertension-Obesity-Sibutramine (HOS) study. *Circulation* 2007; **115**: 1991–8.

3 Torp-Pedersen C, Caterson I, Coutinho W, Finer N, Van Gaal L, Maggioni A, *et al.* Cardiovascular responses to weight management and sibutramine in high-risk subjects: an analysis from the SCOUT trial. *Eur Heart J* 2007; **28**: 2915–23.

4 Ruilope LM, Despres JP, Scheen A, Pi-Sunyer X, Mancia G, Zanchetti A, Van Gaal L. Effect of rimonabant on blood pressure in overweight/obese patients with/without co-morbidities: analysis of pooled RIO study results. *J Hypertens* 2008; **26**: 357–67.

5 Li HY, Chiu YF, Hwu CM, Sheu WHH, Hung YJ, *et al.* The negative correlation between plasma adiponectin and blood pressure depends on obesity: a family-based association study in SAPPHIRe. *Am J Hypertens* 2008; **21**: 471–6.

6 Guo C, Ricchiuti V, Lian BQ, Yao TM, Coutinho P, Romero JR, *et al.* Mineralocorticoid receptor blockade reverses obesity-related changes in expression of adiponectin, peroxisome

proliferator-activated receptor-gamma, and proinflammatory cytokines. *Circulation* 2008; **117**: 2253–61.

7   Annerbrink K, Westberg L, Nilsson S, Rosmond R, Holm G, Eriksson E. Catechol O-methyltransferase val158-met polymorphism is associated with abdominal obesity and blood pressure in men. *Metab Clin Exp* 2008; **57**: 708–11.

8   Burke GL, Bertoni AG, Shea S, Tracy R, Watson KE, Blumenthal RS, *et al.* The impact of obesity on cardiovascular disease risk factors and subclinical vascular disease: the Multi-Ethnic Study of Atherosclerosis. *Arch Intern Med* 2008; **168**: 928–35.

9   Mondolfi RN, Jones TM, Hyre AD, Raggi P, Muntner P. Comparison of percent of United States adults weighing > or = 300 pounds (136 kilograms) in three time periods and comparison of five atherosclerotic risk factors for those weighing > or = 300 pounds to those <300 pounds. *Am J Cardiol* 2007; **100**: 1651–3.

Hypertension at Different Ages

PROBLEM

13 Children and Adolescents

Case History

Kevin is 14 years old and attends with his mother. He has been feeling tired and not finding it easy to concentrate on schoolwork. He is generally fit and plays football regularly. He is, however, slightly overweight (body mass index 28 kg/m²). You note that his blood pressure (BP) is elevated (134/96). This has also been noted on previous visits and there is a strong family history of hypertension. He has had normal childhood illnesses, but nothing major. Growth and development have been normal and he is peri-pubertal. He is quite tall for his age (96th centile).

What are the common causes of increased BP in childhood and adolescence?

When should investigations for a secondary cause be undertaken?

How should high BP be managed in a young person?

Background

BP is lower in children than adults. It increases through the first two decades of life. Those with high BP at an early age have a tendency to maintain that position relative to their peers into adult life. BP measurement is now being undertaken more frequently in young people. BP is strongly related to height, weight and age (Table 13.1). It is slightly higher in boys than in girls, and this difference widens in the second decade. Gender and racial differences are not as marked as in adults. Black children tend to have higher BP than white and those of South Asian descent tend to show an increase in BP in adolescence. BP is higher in children who have a family history of hypertension. As in adults, BP should be measured under controlled conditions with the patient rested and abnormal results should be confirmed on several separate occasions. Auscultatory methods are more accurate. Measurement of BP in younger people requires a set of three paediatric cuffs: a normal adult cuff, a large adult cuff and a thigh cuff. Cuff size is important – too large and BP may be underestimated, too small and it may be overestimated. Err on the side of a larger cuff. Lower limb BP should be measured to exclude coarctation. Automated devices are used in very young patients where auscultatory methods are not possible, and are also useful where repeated measurements are needed and for home BP monitoring. Ambulatory BP monitoring is useful where office hypertension is suspected and when investigating for a possible secondary cause.

Table 13.1 95th centile blood pressures for adolescents

Age (years)	Boys height centile			Girls height centile		
	5th	50th	95th	5th	50th	95th
Systolic BP						
13	121	126	130	121	125	128
14	124	128	132	123	126	130
15	127	131	135	124	128	131
16	129	134	138	125	128	132
17	132	136	140	126	129	132
Diastolic BP						
13	79	82	84	80	82	84
14	80	82	85	81	83	85
15	81	83	86	82	83	86
16	83	85	87	83	84	86
17	85	87	89	83	84	86

Young patients with BP below the 90th centile are normotensive. Those between the 90th and 95th centile have been designated borderline, but this probably overestimates the true prevalence of hypertension in childhood (which is 1–2%). Those with BP greater than the 99th centile have severe hypertension. It is common to find a cause for hypertension in those less than 10 years of age, while essential hypertension is commoner in the teens, particularly with obesity. Relative prevalence of underlying causes by age is shown in Table 13.2. Renovascular (particularly fibromuscular dysplasia) and renal parenchymal causes are the commonest in those under 10 years. In the very young, other vascular abnormalities associated with hypertension include patent ductus arteriosus, bronchopulmonary

Table 13.2 Relative frequency of secondary causes

	Age (years)			
	Birth to 1	1–6	6–12	12–18
Vascular abnormalities	+	–	–	–
Coarctation	+	+	+	±
Renal vascular	++	++	++	+
Renal parenchymal	++	++	+	+
Iatrogenic	–	±	±	+
Endocrine	–	±	+	+
Essential hypertension	–	–	±	++

dysplasia and intraventricular haemorrhage. Metabolic and endocrine causes (Box 13.1) are rare individually but collectively account for a sizeable proportion of secondary hypertension. Neurofibromatosis (1 in 3000 children) should not be forgotten (autosomal dominant). Iatrogenic causes include steroids, non-steroidal anti-inflammatory drugs, erythropoietin, cocaine, amphetamines and the contraceptive pill.

In utero development has important influences on the development of hypertension and other CV risk factors later in life. Placental under-nutrition, which is associated with maternal insulin resistance and microvascular disease, leads to a low birth weight. This and the associated accelerated growth rate in early life have been strongly related to later risk of hypertension and diabetes. The prevalence of overweight and obese subjects more than doubled between the 1960s and the 1990s. Obese children are at least three times as likely to develop hypertension as their lean counterparts. Prevention of childhood obesity is currently a major public health focus and could decrease the incidence of hypertensive disorders in early life and beyond.

Clinical assessment should include pregnancy, birth, and developmental and family history. Examination should include assessment for end-organ damage – retinopathy, cardiomegaly and stick testing of urine.[1] Coarctation may be detected by radio-femoral delay in association with a systolic murmur. Renal bruit is present in 40% of patients with renal artery stenosis. Syndromes should be considered including Turner's (coarctation), neurofibromatosis and Cushing's. All patients should have measurement of electrolytes, creatinine, full blood count and thyroid function. Urine should be tested for blood and protein (microalbumin is useful), and examined for casts that suggest glomerular disease. If renal function is impaired, the cause should be determined. In younger people, renal ultrasound is indicated – scarring may reflect recurrent infections and a small kidney could suggest renal artery stenosis. Where indicated, more specialized investigations for secondary causes are required. For renal artery stenosis, ultrasound is a suitable screening test, and angiography remains the gold standard. An exaggerated decrease in BP and increase in renin after captopril is a useful test. Decreased renal function after captopril can also be documented using the radionuclides DMSA or MAG3. Magnetic resonance angiography is now widely used. Diagnosis of phaeochromocytoma may require adrenal vein sampling and MIBG. Cushing's syndrome is initially diagnosed by 24-hour urine free cortisol measurements and dexamethasone suppression test, with further investigations to determine whether it is of pituitary or adrenal origin.

The goal of treatment is to lower BP to below the 95th centile value for age and height. Trial data are lacking for the use of antihypertensive medications in children. Broadly speaking, the same drugs are used as in adults with doses adjusted for age and body weight. Secondary causes require tailored approaches, which are often influenced by age, level of maturity, family circumstances and other psychosocial factors. A conservative approach is often appropriate for essential hypertension in older children with a focus on lifestyle factors, including weight loss where indicated. Where drug treatments are needed, angiotensin-converting enzyme inhibitors and calcium channel blockers are good initial choices as there is extensive experience with their use and they are relatively free of side effects in young people. Diuretics, usually loop diuretics, are required for most patients with renal disease.

Box 13.1 Endocrine and metabolic causes of hypertension in children

- Hypercalcaemia
- Hyperthyroidism
- Corticosteroid excess (Cushing's syndrome)
- Mineralocorticoid excess:
  - Primary hyperaldosteronism (Conn's syndrome)
  - Congenital adrenal hyperplasia: 11β-hydroxylase deficiency; 17α-hydroxylase deficiency
  - Liddle's syndrome
  - Apparent mineralocorticoid excess
  - Glucocorticoid-remediable hyperaldosteronism
- Growth hormone excess

Recent Developments

1 Using the 90th and 95th centiles respectively as cut-offs for prehypertension and hypertension, a study of 6790 adolescents[2] reported that prehypertension was present in 9.5% and hypertension in 9.4% at initial screening. These figures changed to 15.7% and 3.2% respectively after repeated screening. This underlines the importance of multiple measurements, but also emphasizes that a high proportion of young population are at risk of hypertensive problems. In a large UK study,[3] about 1:5 boys and girls were overweight. The odds ratio (OR) for high systolic BP with overweight boys was 2.50 (95% CI: 1.73 to 3.60), and for a girl the OR was 3.39 (95% CI: 2.36 to 4.85).

2 A number of studies have now established a link between the amount of time spent watching television and the risk of obesity. A recent study[4] has confirmed that prolonged time spent watching television is also associated with hypertension in children. Obesity in young people is also related to the consumption of soft drinks, which in turn is associated with high salt intake from snack foods. Average salt intake increases with age in children, and there is a strong relationship with the risk of hypertension, as in adults.[5]

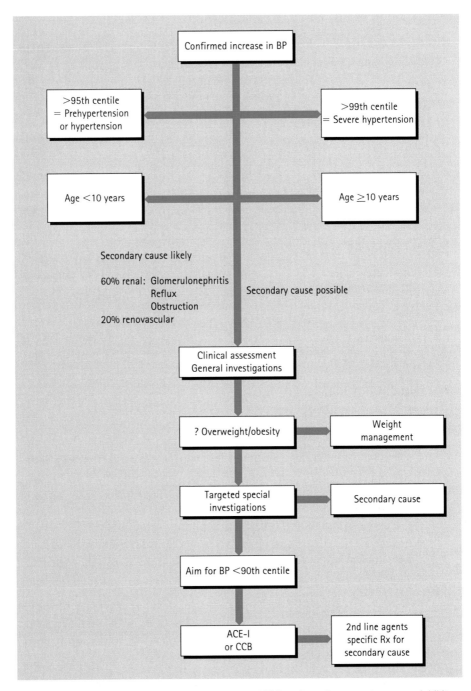

Figure 13.1 Hypertension in children and adolescents. ACE-I, angiotensin-converting enzyme inhibitor; CCB, calcium channel blocker.

3 Office hypertension is extremely common in children.[6] Its prevalence decreases with age and, in most adolescents, office and home BP measurements are broadly comparable. Ambulatory BP monitoring can be extremely useful in children and measures of systolic BP are highly indicative of risk of increased Left Ventricular Mass Index.[7] The nocturnal elevation of BP is much more common in overweight and insulin-resistant children,[8] and is a marker for risk of sustained hypertension in later life.

Conclusions

Hypertension is not rare in children or adolescents. An underlying cause should always be suspected, particularly before the age of 10. Essential hypertension is becoming commoner as overweight and obesity have increased in recent years. The common secondary causes of hypertension in younger people include renal, renovascular and endocrine. A secondary cause should be considered when the hypertension is of sudden onset, is severe or difficult to control, and in all children under 10 years. Lifestyle factors are always important, but particularly so in obesity-related hypertension. The principles of pharmacological management are similar to those in adults with hypertension. Angiotensin-converting enzyme inhibitors and calcium channel blockers are reasonable choices for first-line agents. Specific secondary causes will require treatment, according to the underlying condition. Hypertension in children and adolescents requires effective treatment to decrease the risk of vascular problems in later life (Figure 13.1).

References

1 Varda NM, Gregoric A. A diagnostic approach for the child with hypertension. *Pediatric Nephrol* 2005; **20**: 499–506.

2 McNiece KL, Poffenbarger TS, Turner JL, Franco KD, Sorof JM, Portman RJ. Prevalence of hypertension and pre-hypertension among adolescents. *J Pediatr* 2007; **150**: 640–4.

3 Harding S, Maynard MJ, Cruickshank K, Teyhan A. Overweight, obesity and high blood pressure in an ethnically diverse sample of adolescents in Britain: the Medical Research Council DASH study. *Int J Obes* 2008; **32**: 82–90.

4 Pardee PE, Norman GJ, Lustig RH, Preud'homme D, Schwimmer JB. Television viewing and hypertension in obese children. *Am J Prev Med* 2007; **33**: 439–43.

5 He FJ, Marrero NM, Macgregor GA. Salt and blood pressure in children and adolescents. *J Hum Hypertens* 2008; **22**: 4–11.

6 Stergiou GS, Rarra VC, Yiannes NG. Changing relationship between home and office blood pressure with increasing age in children: the Arsakeion School study. *Am J Hypertens* 2008; **21**: 41–6.

7 Richey PA, Disessa TG, Hastings MC, Somes GW, Alpert BS, Jones DP. Ambulatory blood pressure and increased left ventricular mass in children at risk for hypertension. *J Pediatr* 2008; **152**: 343–8.

8 Lurbe E, Torro I, Aguilar F, Alvarez J, Alcon J, Pascual JM, *et al.* Added impact of obesity and insulin resistance in nocturnal blood pressure elevation in children and adolescents. *Hypertension* 2008; **51**: 635–41.

14 Hypertension in a Young Man

Case History

James is 38 years old. His blood pressure (BP) has been high since he was 34. He had taken treatment (thiazide) for 6 months but developed erectile dysfunction (ED). He is reluctant to accept advice that his hypertension should be treated. There is a family history of hypertension, and he understands the risks associated with high BP. He is happily married and he and his wife have recently had their first child. There is no evidence of end-organ damage, and he is in excellent health overall although overweight (body mass index 27 kg/m²). He does not smoke but drinks about 40 units of alcohol per week. He is stressed by his job.

How common is ED among men with hypertension?

What causes this association?

Do antihypertensive drugs commonly cause ED?

What is the best approach to treating hypertension in a young man?

Background

ED is an inability to sustain an erection sufficiently for satisfactory sexual performance. It is common and prevalence increases with age (three-fold increase between the ages of 40 and 70). Numerous studies have documented an association between hypertension and ED (up to 65% of men with hypertension may have some degree of ED).[1,2] The association increases with age, is greater in those with multiple cardiovascular (CV) risk factors, and where there is established vascular disease. Common causes of ED are summarized in Box 14.1. These should be considered before accepting that the hypertension *per se* is the cause of ED. Most patients with ED have an underlying physical cause, although underlying or resulting psychological factors often worsen the situation.

The penis consists of two columns of spongy erectile tissue, the corpora cavernosa, separated by an incomplete septum that allows them to function as a single unit. Endothelial cells line the network of cavernous spaces. The ventrally placed corpus spongiosum surrounds the urethra and expands distally to form the glans penis. Blood flow is derived from the internal pudendal artery, and increased flow through the terminal branches of this artery leads to filling of the cavernous spaces. During erection, increased blood inflow leads to compression of the venous plexuses on the exterior of the corpora cavernosa, and thus decreased venous drainage. These venous plexuses normally drain into emissary veins that traverse the tunica albuginea and drain into the dorsal vein of the penis. Central sexual stimulation or tactile stimulation of the sensory nerves in the penis, or a combination of the two, leads to increased somatic and parasympathetic nerve discharge with production of nitric oxide and thence cyclic guanosine monophosphate. These mediators cause relaxation of the smooth muscle of the arteriolar blood vessels and the corpora cavernosa, thus increasing blood influx.

Box 14.1 Causes of erectile dysfunction

Demographic and lifestyle
- Ageing
- Smoking
- Heavy alcohol intake

Neurogenic
- Spinal cord injury
- Multiple sclerosis
- Lumbar disc herniation

Drugs
- See Table 14.1

Endocrine
- Hypogonadism
- Hyperprolactinaemia
- Thyroid disease

Systemic diseases
- Diabetes
- Atherosclerosis
- Hypertension
- Renal failure
- Hepatic failure

Penile pelvic
- Trauma
- Irradiation
- Peyronie's disease
- Anatomical developmental
- Prostatic disease

Psychological
- Depression
- Anxiety
- Stress

Assessment of the patient with ED should include full medical and drug history. Symptoms and signs of hypogonadism, vascular disease and neurological disease should be sought. Drugs contribute to at least a quarter of all cases (Figure 14.1). Antihypertensive drugs are the most common offenders. Enquiry should be made about other aspects of sexual function – libido and ejaculatory disorders. This may give a clue to aetiology. Endocrine and psychological problems usually cause decreased libido in addition to ED. Routine use of nocturnal tumescence, ultrasonography or penile injection trials is not warranted. Oral phosphodiesterase (PDE) 5 inhibitors are widely used as first-line treatment. Start with a middle dose – sildenafil (Viagra) 50 mg, tadalafil (Cialis) 10 mg, or vardenafil (Levitra) 10 mg. They should be taken within 1–2 h of anticipated sexual activity, preferably on an empty stomach. They should not be used more than once in 24 hours. Non-arteritic anterior ischaemic optic neuropathy is a rare side effect. There is a slight increase in risk of myocardial ischaemia with these drugs, and they should not be used concurrently with nitrates. Alprostadil is a stable form of prostaglandin E_1 and increases smooth muscle relaxation through increasing cyclic adenosine monophosphate. It may be given transurethrally or by intracavernous injection. Trimix is a combination of alprostadil, phentolamine (α_1-antagonist) and papaverine (non-specific PDE inhibitor), which is given by intracavernous injection. Penile tumescence device or prosthetic devices may be useful in those who do not respond to

Table 14.1 Drugs and male sexual function

	ED	Decreased libido	Ejaculatory dysfunction
Antihypertensives			
β-blockers	+	+	-
α-blockers	+	-	+
Sympatholytics	+	+	-
Thiazides	+	+	-
Spironolactone	+	+	-
Psychiatric medications			
Tricyclics	+	+	-
SSRIs	+	-	+
Benzodiazepines	-	+	-
Antipsychotic	+	+	+
Anti-androgenic drugs			
Digoxin	+	+	-
H_2 receptor blockers	+	+	-
Various			
Alcohol	+	+	-
Phenytoin	+	+	-
Ketoconazole	+	+	-

SSRIs, selective serotonin reuptake inhibitors.

pharmacotherapy. The role of psychological counselling should not be forgotten, and the partner should be involved in treatment decisions.

Sympatholytic agents were among the earliest drugs for hypertension. Guanethidine and reseprine were associated with a high incidence of male sexual problems. Methyldopa also has an appreciable incidence. Clonidine is associated with a high incidence of ED. Because the major trials of these drugs were carried out before ED was recognized as a clinical problem, the evidence base is not as strong as it might be. In the MRC Hypertension Trial,[1] follow-up for a total of 3582 patient-years was completed. After 2 years, the prevalence of ED was 10.1% in the placebo group, 13.2% in the β-blocker group, and 22.6% with bendrofluazide. Patients with severe ED are likely to withdraw from trials, thus introducing a selection bias. Thiazides induce ED by interfering with smooth muscle relaxation and also by partly blocking effects of catecholamines. While the trial data are perhaps not as extensive as would be desirable, there is no doubt that thiazides, and both non-selective and $β_1$-selective β-blockers increase risk of ED. Angiotensin-converting enzyme inhibitors and calcium channel blockers are neutral with respect to male sexual function, while angiotensin receptor blockers may actually improve ED.[1] Oral PDE5 inhibitors are suitable for hypertensive men with ED, including those in whom antihypertensive drugs are contributing to ED. Caution should be exercised in combining PDE5 inhibitors with an α-blocker because of risk of postural hypotension. Currently available PDE5 inhibitors have a small, probably not clinically significant, additive effect in lowering BP when used with hypotensive medications.

Recent Developments

1. Data from the 2001–2002 NHANES (National Health and Nutrition Examination Survey)[3] suggest that the prevalence of ED in men in the USA was 18.4%, amounting to a total of 18 million men. Prevalence increased with age and the number of CV risk factors or with CV disease. Prevalence in diabetes was greater than 50%. In another study of 11 252 men aged 25–40 years,[4] there was no apparent increase in ED among men with prehypertension or hypertension. It may be that young age is protective for ED in patients with high BP.

2. Increased catecholamines in response to stress lead to increased BP. Lack of exercise and the development of abdominal obesity often go hand in hand with stress and contribute to it. Another component is sleep disorders,[5] which are frequently neglected in clinical practice. These may contribute directly to ED but also indirectly through hypertension.

3. Increased arterial stiffness is a surrogate marker for hypertensive complications. Vasodilatation after exercise lowers BP. This is attenuated in young African American men, who are more susceptible to hypertension than Caucasians.[6] Arterial stiffness increases with increasing number of metabolic syndrome components, and is strongly linked with insulin resistance, low-grade inflammation and sympathetic activation.

4. Routine androgen replacement is not warranted for patients with ED. However, many patients with ED have low normal or borderline low testosterone and dehydroepiandrosterone levels.[7] Obesity and high alcohol consumption are associated with low bioavailable testosterone. Although these low androgen levels do not reflect underlying disease, a number of studies have suggested that androgen supplementation improves sexual performance and enhances well-being.

5. While the effect of PDE5 inhibitors on BP is modest, effective treatment of ED does improve BP control in hypertensive men.[8] The vasodilatory effect of PDE5 inhibitors, may synergize with antihypertensives. However, just as important may be increased health-seeking behaviour (including medication compliance). PDE5 inhibitors are already approved for the treatment of pulmonary hypertension. The fact that they are only used with sexual activity means that they do not contribute to BP control. With newer and longer-acting agents, PDE inhibition may contribute to hypertension treatment.[9]

Conclusions

Hypertension and ED are mutually associated. A number of antihypertensive medications increase the risk of ED, which is a major consideration when treating men, particularly younger men (Figure 14.1). If antihypertensive treatment is required, calcium channel blockers and renin–angiotensin system blocking drugs should be considered as first-line treatment. The latter may actually improve endothelial dysfunction and thus have a beneficial effect on ED. Thiazides and β-blockers should be avoided unless there are other reasons to prescribe them. Prescription of these drugs may lead to poor compliance because of their effect on sexual function. Sexual health and performance is a critical determinant of quality of life, particularly in younger subjects. Problems in this area

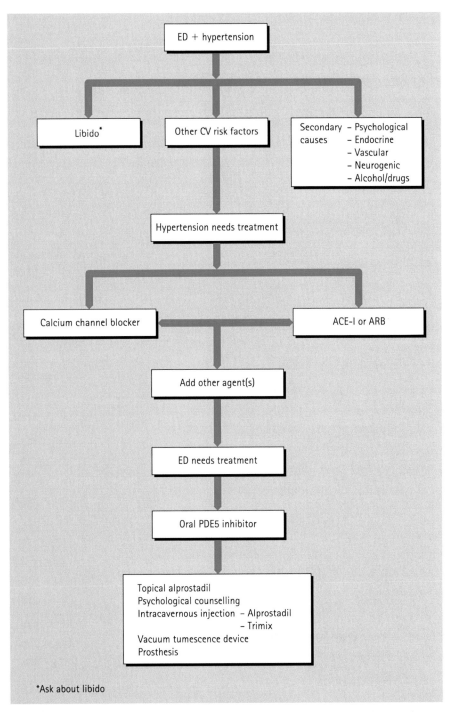

Figure 14.1 ED and hypertension. ACE-I, angiotensin-converting enzyme inhibitor; ARB, angiotensin receptor blocker; ED, erectile dysfunction; PDE5, phosphodiesterase 5.

merit effective investigation and management, and the association with increased CV risk should also be considered.

References

1   Dusing R. Sexual dysfunction in male patients with hypertension: influence of antihypertensive drugs. *Drugs* 2005; **65**: 773–86.

2   Kloner R. Erectile dysfunction and hypertension. *Int J Impot Res* 2007; **19**: 296–302.

3   Selvin E, Burnett AL, Platz EA. Prevalence and risk factors for erectile dysfunction in the US. *Am J Med* 2007; **120**: 151–7.

4   Heruti RJ, Sharabi Y, Arbel Y, Shochat T, Swartzon M, Brenner G, *et al.* The prevalence of erectile dysfunction among hypertensive and prehypertensive men aged 25–40 years. *J Sex Med* 2007; **4**: 596–601.

5   Jankowski JT, Seftel AD, Strohl KP. Erectile dysfunction and sleep related disorders. *J Urol* 2008; **179**: 837–41.

6   Heffernan KS, Jae SY, Fernhall B. Racial differences in arterial stiffness after exercise in young men. *Am J Hypertens* 2007; **20**: 840–5.

7   Ahn TY, Park JK, Lee SW, Hong JH, Park NC, Kim JJ, *et al.* Prevalence and risk factors for erectile dysfunction in Korean men: results of an epidemiological study. *J Sex Med* 2007; **4**: 1269–76.

8   Scranton RE, Lawler E, Botteman M, Chittamooru S, Gagnon D, Lew R, *et al.* Effect of treating erectile dysfunction on management of systolic hypertension. *Am J Cardiol* 2007; **100**: 459–63.

9   Ghiadoni L, Versari D, Taddei S. Phosphodiesterase 5 inhibition in essential hypertension. *Curr Hypertens Rep* 2008; **10**: 52–7.

15 Hypertension in a Young Woman

Case History

Sandra is a 28-year-old single mother. Her daughter by a previous relationship is 3 years old. She had difficulty conceiving, but her pregnancy was uncomplicated. She has recently entered into a new relationship. She and her new partner would like to have a child soon. For now, she has asked if she can start using a contraceptive pill. Her periods are irregular and infrequent and she has facial hirsutism. She is overweight at 92 kg, with a body mass index of 31 kg/m². Her blood pressure (BP) is elevated–142/96 at this visit.

What is the relationship between oral contraceptive pill (OCP) use and BP?

She probably has polycystic ovary syndrome (PCOS): how should this be managed?

Her BP is high: how should this be managed?

Background

Hypertension is not uncommon in young women, affecting 2–6%. The vast majority have essential hypertension but secondary causes should be considered, particularly where BP is difficult to control or there are electrolyte abnormalities. Where drug treatment is required (Figure 15.1), the woman's intention to become pregnant should be considered; If she is likely to conceive in the foreseeable future, it is best not to choose drugs that would need to be stopped in pregnancy (angiotensin-converting enzyme inhibitors, angiotensin receptor blockers and atenolol). If pregnancy could be imminent, choose drugs that would be used in pregnancy (labetalol, methyldopa). Young women are at relatively low cardiovascular (CV) risk, and thus benefit relatively less from BP-lowering than other groups. Black women are at higher risk, and thus benefit more. The risk of mortality from CV events is low in young women,[1] e.g. in women aged 35–44 years, mortality is as follows:

- Myocardial infarction (MI), 1–7 per 100 000 woman-years; men are at two- to three-fold higher risk

- Stroke, 4–12 per 100 000 woman-years; men have twice the risk

- Venous thromboembolism, <1 per 100 000 woman-years

While OCP do increase the risk of CV events, the absolute event rate is low. The combined OCP is the most widely used contraceptive in developed countries. Eighty per cent

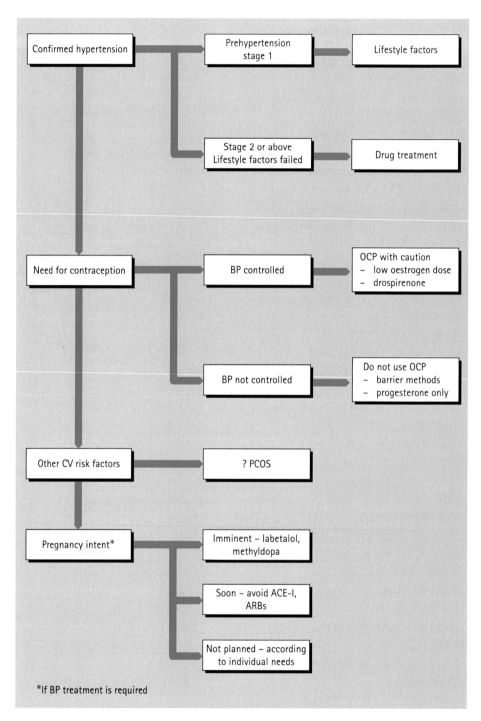

Figure 15.1 Hypertension in a young woman. ACE-I, angiotensin-converting enzyme inhibitor; ARB, angiotensin receptor blocker; OCP, oral contraceptive pill; PCOS, polycystic ovary syndrome.

of women will use OCP at some time, and they are used by over 18 million women in the USA, representing at least 30% of women of reproductive age. Up to half will switch brands because of perceived or actual side effects. These include mood changes, weight gain and fluid retention. Overall, up to 60% of women using OCP will discontinue because of concerns over adverse effects, and the average duration of usage is less than 5 years. OCPs contain an oestrogen and progestagen. Ethynyloestradiol is used at doses of 30–50 μg. For those at risk of hypertension, the lowest possible dose of oestrogen should be used. In pharmacological doses, oestrogen increases BP – mean daily systolic BP (SBP) increased by up to 8 mmHg and night-time SBP by up to 6 mmHg.[1] There is usually only a minimal effect on diastolic BP. Mechanisms by which oestrogen increase BP include activation of the renin–angiotensin system and altered expression of adrenoreceptors in vascular tissues. Choice of progestagen is also important (Table 15.1). Side effects often relate to androgenic activity. However, the effects of an agent with androgenic activity are preferred by some. Drospirenone, like native progesterone, has mineralocorticoid blocking activity and an OCP with this (Yasmin) is a logical choice in women with higher BP.

Table 15.1 Properties of commonly used progestagens

Agent	Prog	Mineralo block	Andro block	Andro neutral	Andro pro
Progesterone	+	+	±	–	–
Drospirenone	+	+	+	–	–
MPA	+	–	–	+	–
Dydrogesterone	+	–	–	+	–
Norgestrel	+	–	–	–	+
Levonorgestrel	+	–	–	–	+
Norethisterone	+	–	–	–	+
Cyproterone	+	–	+	–	–

Andro block, androgen blocking; Andro neutral, neither androgen blocking or androgenic; Andro pro, androgenic; Mineralo block, mineralocorticoid blocking; MPA, medroxyprogesterone acaetate; Prog, progestagenic.

Although oestrogen may be protective against atherosclerosis because of effects on lipid profile, event rate is increased in those with overall higher CV risk and in those with CV disease. This is because oestrogen may destabilize atherosclerotic plaques and also has a prothrombotic action. Risk is not increased with progestagen-only contraceptives. Increased risk with OCP has been confirmed in a number of studies, including the Nurses Health Study.[1] Compared with non-users, OCP users have an odds ratio (OR) for MI of 2.5 (95% CI: 1.9 to 3.2), an OR of 2.7 (95% CI: 2.2 to 3.3), and up to six-fold increased risk of venous thromboembolism (VTE) (particularly in the first year). Fatality rate from VTE is not markedly increased in OCP users. Risk of CV events is higher if the patient is obese, smokes, has diabetes, or is over 35. VTE risk with OCP is increased markedly if the patient has a prothrombotic state, the most common of which is factor V

Leiden, which occurs in up to 5% of Caucasians and up to 30% of patients with deep vein thrombosis (DVT). This variant factor V is not inactivated by activated protein C.

Risks during pregnancy should also be considered in women with hypertension. MI occurs in 1:10 000 pregnancies. Only about half have atherosclerosis with thrombotic occlusion. Coronary artery dissection accounts for about 15%. Stroke occurs in one pregnancy in every 5000–20 000. It is especially common in the third trimester and following delivery. VTE occurs in 15 per 10 000 pregnancies and in 1–2% of patients after Caesarean section; 85% are left sided (compared with 55% in non-pregnant patients). The majority of DVTs in pregnancy are ileofemoral (72%) compared with the minority in non-pregnant patients. Warfarin is contraindicated in pregnancy because of its teratogenicity. Low molecular weight heparin is preferred because of its low incidence of reactions compared with unfractionated heparin.

Although BP frequently increases with OCP use (Box 15.1), it usually returns to normal when OCP is stopped. The increased BP is accompanied by modest increases in urinary albumin excretion (UAE) and a slight decrease in glomerular filtration rate. There is a graded risk with hypertension and combined oral contraceptive (COC) use with no threshold for increased risk of CV events.[1] Hypertensive women using OCP are up to 60 times more likely to have an MI and 15 times more likely to have a stroke compared with normotensive non-users. Haemorrhagic stroke is 20 times more likely in those with severe and uncontrolled hypertension. The increased risk related to OCP use is only among current users. Higher lifetime exposure to oestrogen (duration rather than dose) appears to be protective, particularly for stroke. The absolute CV event rate in hypertensive young women is low:

- At age 24: 312 per million woman-years with COC; 134 per million woman-years without COC.

- At age 44: 1213 per million woman-years with COC; 529 per million woman-years without COC.

PCOS is a combination of oligomenorrhoea, hyperandrogenism, and multiple cysts or follicles on ovarian ultrasound. It commonly occurs with obesity and insulin resistance. PCOS patients have a high prevalence of metabolic syndrome (MetS) and its components, but the link between PCOS and future risk of CV events has not clearly been established. PCOS affects up to 10% of young women, accounting for more than 10 million cases in the USA. It is the commonest cause of menstrual irregularity and anovulatory subfertility. It is becoming commoner, partly because it is now more widely recognized. Hypertension is twice as common in women with irregular menses, and occurs in up to 40% of women with PCOS.

Obesity is the major determinant of increased BP in PCOS. This leads to endothelial dysfunction and to other vascular changes, including decreased vascular compliance. As a precursor to sustained increases in ambulatory BP, women with PCOS may have increased office hypertension or decreased nocturnal dipping. In a recent study of 11 035 women with PCOS,[2] the population prevalence was estimated at 2.6%. Women with PCOS were more likely to be obese (OR 4.21; 95% CI 3.96 to 4.47) and to have hypertension (OR 1.41; 95% CI 1.31 to 1.51). Hypertension was most common in black women and least common in Hispanic women. Chen et al.,[3] found a strong relationship between increased androgen status and hypertension. The OR for hypertension in

Box 15.1 Recommendations for oral contraceptive pill use

- Use with caution:

  Obesity   Obese   Age >35 years

  Smokers   Diabetes

- Relatively contraindicated:

  SBP 140–149 mmHg or diastolic BP 90–99 mmHg

  Past history of stage 2 hypertension or above (even if controlled)

- Absolutely contraindicated:

  SBP ≥160 mmHg or diastolic BP ≥100 mmHg

  End-organ damage from hypertension

  Any degree of hypertension with high overall CV risk

women with PCOS in this study was 3.8. There may be racial differences in susceptibility to hypertension among patients with PCOS.

Recent Developments

1 Girouard et al.[4] reported that hypertensive disorders of pregnancy were associated with an increased risk of development of insulin resistance in the future. It is not known whether prevention and effective treatment of pregnancy-related hypertension would decrease later prevalence of metabolic risk factors. Pregnancy itself appears to be a risk factor for future development of systolic hypertension, particularly with younger age at delivery.[5]

2 Drospirenone is a progestagen with anti-mineralocorticoid activity. Combined with ethynyloestradiol (Yasmin), it is an effective and well tolerated contraceptive. While there are no prolonged studies, available evidence[6] suggests that drospirenone at doses used in the OCP has a useful BP-lowering effect. Use of drospirenone has been associated with falsely positive increased aldosterone levels.[7] Where possible, antihypertensive drugs should be stopped before screening for secondary causes of hypertension. Verapamil and α-blockers are less likely than other agents to affect renin and aldosterone measurements.

3 Women should be screened for factors that increase risk with OCPs, and they should also be counselled about possible adverse effects. However, the health of women taking OCPs may be better than that of non-users.[8] This may be because women with poor health are excluded from using OCPs. Quality of life also seems to be enhanced in OCP users.[8]

4 The prevalence of MetS in PCOS is about 45%, which is twice that of the background population.[9] Even more women than this may have individual components of MetS.[10] Prevalence of hypertension and other MetS-related risk factors increases markedly with body weight. Weight management is an important goal in women with PCOS. Women with PCOS are more likely to suffer complications during pregnancy, including hypertensive disorders.[11]

Conclusions

 While mortality from CV disease has decreased for men over the past two decades, mortality among women has increased. Prognosis, in general, following a CV event is worse for a woman than for a man. Hypertension in young women needs to be effectively managed as it increases risk of vascular events and also increases risk to both mother and baby during pregnancy. The oestrogen component of OCPs leads to a fairly consistent increase in BP, particularly SBP. The ideal agent for the above patient, if lifestyle measures fail, would be one which is compatible with her plans for pregnancy and which is not associated with increased metabolic side effects (given the diagnosis of PCOS). Weight management should be central to treatment of PCOS. Other interventions depend on whether fertility is required, the presence of features of hyperandrogenism (hirsutism and acne), and need to improve CV risk.

References

1   Curtis KM, Mohllajee AP, Martins SL, Peterson HB. Combined oral contraceptive use among women with hypertension: a systematic review. *Contraception* 2006; **73**: 179–88.

2   Lo JC, Feigenbaum SL, Yang J, Pressman AR, Selby JV, Go AS. Epidemiology and adverse cardiovascular risk profile of diagnosed polycystic ovary syndrome. *J Clin Endocrinol Metab* 2006; **91**: 1357–63.

3   Chen M-J, Yang W-S, Yang J-H, Chen C-L, Ho H-N, Yang Y-S. Relationship between androgen levels and blood pressure in young women with polycystic ovary syndrome. *Hypertension* 2007; **49**: 1442–7.

4   Girouard J, Giguere Y, Moutquin J-M, Forest J-C. Previous hypertensive disease of pregnancy is associated with alterations of markers of insulin resistance. *Hypertension* 2007; **49**(5): 1056–62.

5   Kharazmi E, Kaaja R, Fallah M, Luoto R. Pregnancy-related factors and the risk of isolated systolic hypertension. *Blood Press* 2007; **16**: 50–5.

6   Oelkers WHK. Drospirenone in combination with estrogens: for contraception and hormone replacement therapy. *Climacteric* 2005; **8** (Suppl 3): 19–27.

7   Pizzolo F, Pavan C, Corrocher R, Olivieri O. Laboratory diagnosis of primary aldosteronism, and drospirenone-ethinylestradiol therapy. *Am J Hypertens* 2007; **20**: 1334–7.

8   Du Y, Melchert H-U, Schafer-Korting M. Use of oral contraceptives in Germany: prevalence, determinants and use-associated health correlates. Results of National Health Surveys from 1984 to 1999. *Eur J Obstet Gynecol Reprod Biol* 2007; **134**: 57–66.

9   Essah PA, Nestler JE. The metabolic syndrome in polycystic ovary syndrome. *J Endocrinol Invest* 2006; **29**: 270–80.

10 Soares EMM, Azevedo GD, Gadelha RGN, Lemos TMAM, Maranhao TMO. Prevalence of the metabolic syndrome and its components in Brazilian women with polycystic ovary syndrome. *Fertil Steril* 2008; **89**: 649–55.

11 Boomsma CM, Fauser BCJM, Macklon NS. Pregnancy complications in women with polycystic ovary syndrome. *Semin Reprod Med* 2008; **26**: 72–84.

16 Hypertension and the Menopause

Case History

Alice is 52 years old. Her medical history is unremarkable apart from hypertension during both of her pregnancies. She takes no medications. Her blood pressure (BP) has not been checked for some years but is now consistently increased at about 146/92. Her periods have been less frequent over the past 18 months. High levels of luteinizing hormone and follicle-stimulating hormone confirm that she is menopausal. She has severe vasomotor symptoms (flushing and sweating), which are impacting on her quality of life.

What is the effect of menopause on BP?

Is hormone replacement therapy (HRT) contraindicated in a hypertensive woman?

If not, does hypertension influence the choice of agent?

Background

Apart from puberty, which affects both genders, pregnancy and the menopause are the two most significant influences on human physiology in the absence of disease. Cardiovascular (CV) events increase drastically in women over the perimenopausal years (age 45–55), and much of this is due to altered BP regulation. A postmenopausal woman is more than twice as likely to have hypertension as her premenopausal counterpart. While it is hard to disentangle the effects of age and menopause, it seems clear that BP consistently increases over the menopausal years – by 5 mmHg systolic over the 5 years around menopause. Prior to menopause, the BP of women is generally lower than that of men. In a cross-sectional study of 18 326 women aged 46–59 years, Zanchetti *et al.*[1] estimated that menopause was associated with a 3.4 mmHg increase in systolic BP and a 3.1 mmHg increase in diastolic BP. These changes were independent of age, body mass index, smoking status, and use of oral contraceptive pill or hormone replacement therapy (HRT).

At present, HRT is only indicated for the control of troublesome menopausal symptoms. Women with an intact uterus should use a combined preparation (Table 16.1). Oral preparations are most cost-effective and control symptoms with minimum side effects in 90% of women. Use the lowest dose of oestrogen to control symptoms. The C19 progestagens (norethisterone, norgestrel, levonorgestrel) are more likely to cause side effects (e.g. headache, hirsutism and fluid retention) but may be most useful for some women, e.g. where lack of libido is a problem. C21 progestagens (medroxyprogesterone acetate, dydrogesterone) are better tolerated by some. For those women without a uterus

Table 16.1 Available combined hormone replacement therapies

Oestrogen	Progestagen
Conjugated equine	Medroxyprogesterone acetate (O)
Oestradiol valerate	Norethisterone (O)
Oestradiol valerate	Levonorgestrel (O)
Oestradiol-17β	Norethisterone (T)
Oestradiol-17β	Norethisterone (O)
Oestradiol-17β (T)	Norethisterone (O)
Oestradiol-17β	Dydrogesterone (O)
Oestradiol-17β	Drospirenone (O)

Oestrogen preparation is oral unless otherwise stated. O, oral; T, transdermal.

the options are: conjugated equine oestrogen (oral), oestradiol-17β (oral, transdermal patch or gel, nasal, implant), oestriol (oral), estopiprate (oestrone, oral). With combined HRT, cyclical agents should be used for the first 2 years, after which no-bleed regimens may be preferred. There is no justification for prescribing HRT routinely for bone or CV protection. HRT is not contraindicated in women with hypertension, and there is no evidence that current agents significantly increase BP.

Selective oestrogen receptor modulators are agents that share properties with native oestrogen but have distinct properties because of their selective action against some receptor types or in some tissues. Tamoxifen and clomiphene have been the most widely used. Raloxifene is used for bone protection and also protects against breast cancer. However, it provokes menopausal type symptoms and predisposes to venous thromboembolism. The RUTH (Raloxifene Use for The Heart) study in 2003 demonstrated that, like native oestrogen, it did not have significant cardioprotective properties. Other agents in the pipeline include droloxifine and lasofoxifene.

By the age of 60 years, 80% of women will have hypertension. BP is the major modifiable risk factor in postmenopausal women. Effective treatment will decrease the risk of stroke by 38%, and myocardial infarction by 19%.[2] While a cut-off value of 140/90 (in the absence of diabetes or chronic kidney disease) is appropriate, it is important to recognize that there is no safe threshold value – risk increases linearly with BP and target-organ damage can occur at BP <140/90. Of women aged 45 with normal BP, one-third will develop hypertension in the next 10 years. Of women with borderline high BP, half will be hypertensive in 5 years, and two-thirds in 10 years. The risk of CV events in a middle-aged woman with normal BP is 1.62 per 1000 person-years, compared with 2.92/1000 person-years with prehypertension, and 4.32/1000 person-years with hypertension.[3] Systolic BP is a better predictor of CV events than diastolic BP.

Following withdrawal of oestrogen, a variety of mechanisms contribute to increases in BP (Figure 16.1). The renin–angiotensin system (RAS) is activated, with increased renin release and increased secretion of aldosterone. Oestrogen decreases expression of the AT_1 receptor and may also diminish renin secretion. Thus, angiotensin-converting enzyme inhibitors or angiotensin receptor blockers are ideal choices of agents for hypertension around the menopause. Increased activity of the sympathetic nervous system also

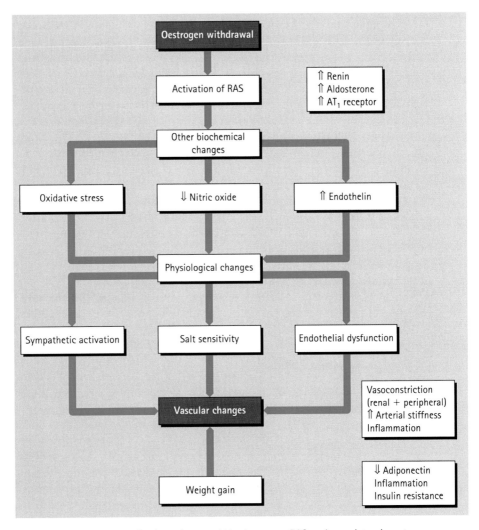

Figure 16.1 Changes contributing to increased blood pressure. RAS, renin–angiotensin system.

contributes to RAS activation and salt retention. However, β-blockers should not be used unless specifically indicated, as there is a high chance of glucose intolerance and dyslipidaemia. Salt sensitivity increases with age but also following oestrogen withdrawal. One consequence is decreased endothelial nitric oxide release. Furthermore, there are increased levels of the endogenous nitric oxide synthase inhibitor asymmetric dimethyl-L-arginine after menopause. Endothelial dysfunction has been reported in studies that have either used flow-mediated dilatation or vasodilatory response to acetylcholine. This phenomenon strongly correlates with increased risk of CV events, and abnormalities are reversed either with oestrogen replacement or with effective treatment of elevated BP. Arterial stiffness is increased as evidenced by increased carotid-femoral or brachial-ankle pulse wave velocity.

There is a tendency for weight gain in the perimenopausal years, although the influence of age is more powerful than that of menopause. Increased adiposity, particularly visceral fat, is associated with decreased adiponectin (which contributes to insulin sensitivity and lowers CV risk), increased expression of inflammatory markers, oxidative stress and endothelial dysfunction. Unlike in men, body mass index is a poor correlate of CV risk – peripheral fat in the typical female distribution contributes to body mass index but does not increase CV risk – indeed, it may be protective, partly through its ability to secrete adiponectin. Increased visceral fat may exaggerate any potentially harmful effect of mixed HRT on the vasculature. Genetic influences almost certainly contribute to increased BP after menopause. Polymorphisms related to RAS, aldosterone synthase, nitric oxide synthase, β_1- and α_{2A}-adrenoreceptors, follicle-stimulating hormone receptor and the aromatase gene (*CYP19A1*) are all determinants of BP responses in women.

The various components of metabolic syndrome become more prevalent in women after the menopause. Women with hypertension are less likely to have the condition effectively controlled. Of the 93 876 subjects in the Women's Health Initiative, 32% were hypertensive. Of those, only 57% were on antihypertensive drugs, but only 36% reached target BP. Only 21% of subjects with diabetes were at target BP.[3] For every increase in BP of 20 mmHg (systolic or diastolic), there is a doubling of the risk of a cardiac event. Although pharmacological doses of oestrogen can be associated with increases in BP, the role of replacement doses is not clear.

In the last two decades, studies appeared to support the notion that HRT might be cardioprotective. Oestrogen was noted to increase high-density lipoprotein cholesterol and decrease low-density lipoprotein cholesterol, to induce some favourable changes in coagulation, and to act as a vasodilator. Some of the potential benefits were offset by progestogens, particularly medroxyprogesterone acetate. Furthermore, there were also non-favourable changes with oestrogen-increased venous thromboembolism and increased inflammatory markers, both of which are more marked with oral compared with transdermal oestrogen. In 1998, one study, HERS (Heart and Estrogen Progestin Replacement Study), recruited women with pre-existing CV disease. Combined HRT was not protective against CV. The definitive trial in women without CV disease was the Women's Health Initiative trial (2004), which suggested that women exposed to combined HRT were not protected from CV events and might actually be at increased risk, particularly ischaemic stroke. Those who started HRT within the early years after menopause and those who used HRT for 5 years or less were not at increased risk. The RR of breast cancer was also increased (1.24; 95% CI 1.01 to 1.34), a risk comparable with that of obesity or high alcohol intake.

Recent Developments

1 Following menopause, oestrone is the predominant circulating oestrogen and is derived from peripheral conversion of androstenedione in adipose tissue. If BP increases following the menopause, as it does in many women, this must be due to the loss of a protective effect, i.e. oestrogen. There is no evidence that treating women with oestrogen at the doses in common HRT preparations increases BP. Steiner *et al.*[4] reported a slight decrease in BP in both normotensive and hypertensive women with 1 mg/day of micronized oestradiol-17β. Oestrogen treatment did not

affect carotid intima-media thickness. In a similar study, Kaya et al.[5] noted a slight reduction in mean arterial pressures with oestradiol (2.0 ± 0.8 mmHg). The night-time systolic and mean arterial pressures were decreased.

2   Drosiprenone, as an aldosterone blocker, can decrease BP by diminishing salt and water retention.[6] The minimum effective dose for BP reduction is 2 mg daily; 3 mg drosiprenone is equivalent to 25 mg spironolactone. The HRT preparation Angeliq contains 0.5 mg drosiprenone with 1 mg oestradiol-17β. While the dose is insufficient on its own to reduce BP, it is a logical choice for women with hypertension requiring HRT. In hypertensive menopausal women taking hydrochlorthiazide 25 mg daily, 3 mg drosiprenone with 1 mg oestradiol-17β decreased systolic BP by 7.2 mmHg and diastolic BP by 4.5 mmHg.[7] Furthermore, drosiprenone had a potassium-sparing effect.

3   The aromatase gene, which converts androgen to oestrogen, is responsible for what oestrogen there is after the menopause. Polymorphisms associated with increased aromatase activity may be associated with higher levels of oestrogen, and thus a greater protective effect, following menopause.[8] Adiposity, especially visceral fat, after the menopause leads to the development of an adverse CV risk profile, and is at least partly genetically determined.[9]

4   Because of the age of subjects, those undergoing surgical oophorectomy typically are not prone to hypertension until 5–10 years later. However, the physiological changes that predispose to hypertension, including increased salt sensitivity, occur at an early stage after oophorectomy.[10] This emphasizes the need for HRT to be considered early – in general, the risks are far outweighed by potential benefits.

Conclusions

Most women will develop hypertension at some stage. Those who develop it earlier are at increased risk as are those in whom it is either unrecognized or undertreated. The menopause is a powerful stimulus for increased BP. Opportunities to screen for hypertension should be taken wherever possible, and BP assessed in the context of their overall CV risk (e.g. using SCORE charts[2]). Lifestyle modifications have the potential to delay onset of hypertension (Figure 16.2). HRT is not contraindicated in menopausal women with hypertension. Indeed, it may protect women from developing hypertension, or at least minimize the impact of the menopause on BP. There is no evidence of any benefit from a particular HRT preparation in terms of BP control or CV risk. Drosiprenone is effective in lowering BP, but not at the doses presently used. Given the central role of the RAS in pathogenesis of menopausal hypertension, blockade with either angiotensin-converting enzyme inhibitors or angiotensin receptor blockers is a logical first step in the treatment of hypertension. Furthermore, these agents do not predispose to the development of diabetes or dyslipidaemia, and may even be protective.

References

1   Zanchetti A, Facchetti R, Cesana GC, Modena MG, Pirrelli A, Sega R, et al. Menopause-related blood pressure increase and its relationship to age and body mass index: the SIMONA epidemiological study. J Hypertens 2005; 23: 2269–76.

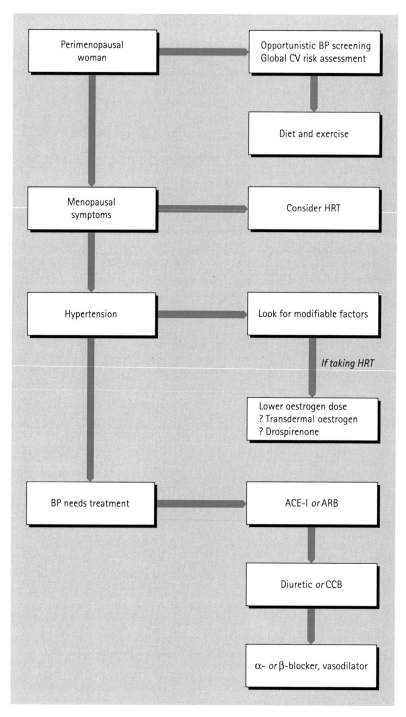

Figure 16.2 Menopause and hypertension. ACE-I, angiotensin-converting enzyme inhibitor; ARB, angiotensin receptor blocker; CCB, calcium channel blocker.

2   Collins P, Rosano G, Casey C, Daly C, Gambacciani M, Hadji P, *et al.* Management of cardiovascular risk in the peri-menopausal woman: a consensus statement of European cardiologists and gynaecologists. *Eur Heart J* 2007; **28**: 2028–40.

3   Coylewright M, Reckelhoff JF, Ouyang P. Menopause and hypertension: an age-old debate. *Hypertension* 2008; **51**: 952–9.

4   Steiner AZ, Hodis HN, Lobo RA, Shoupe D, Xiang M, Mack WJ. Postmenopausal oral estrogen therapy and blood pressure in normotensive and hypertensive subjects: the Estrogen in the Prevention of Atherosclerosis Trial. *Menopause* 2005; **12**: 728–33.

5   Kaya C, Dincer Cengiz S, Cengiz B, Akgun G. The long-term effects of low-dose 17beta-estradiol and dydrogesterone hormone replacement therapy on 24-h ambulatory blood pressure in hypertensive postmenopausal women: a 1-year randomized, prospective study. *Climacteric* 2006; **9**: 437–45.

6   Mallareddy M, Hanes V, White WB. Drospirenone, a new progestogen, for postmenopausal women with hypertension. *Drugs Aging* 2007; **24**: 453–66.

7   Preston RA, Norris PM, Alonso AB, Ni P, Hanes V, Karara AH. Randomized, placebo-controlled trial of the effects of drospirenone-estradiol on blood pressure and potassium balance in hypertensive postmenopausal women receiving hydrochlorothiazide. *Menopause* 2007; **14**: 408–14.

8   Ramirez-Lorca R, Grilo A, Martinez-Larrad MT, Manzano L, Serrano-Hernando FJ, Moron FJ, *et al.* Sex and body mass index specific regulation of blood pressure by CYP19A1 gene variants. *Hypertension* 2007; **50**: 884–90.

9   Casiglia E, Tikhonoff V, Caffi S, Martini B, Guidotti F, Bolzon M, *et al.* Effects of the C825T polymorphism of the GNB3 gene on body adiposity and blood pressure in fertile and menopausal women: a population-based study. *J Hypertens* 2008; **26**: 238–43.

10 Schulman IH, Aranda P, Raij L, Veronesi M, Aranda FJ, Martin R. Surgical menopause increases salt sensitivity of blood pressure. *Hypertension* 2006; **47**: 1168–74.

17 Hypertension in an Older Man

Case History

Robert is a 74-year-old man who is fit and active. He has had hypertension and hyperlipidaemia for at least 10 years. He takes hydrochlorthiazide 25 mg OD, atenolol 50 mg OD and simvastatin 20 mg OD. Blood pressure (BP) is not perfectly controlled – the latest being 164/96. He lives with his wife. Lately, he has developed urinary frequency, getting up twice a night to pass urine and his urinary stream has declined. He smokes five cigarettes per day and drinks very little alcohol. He has been feeling more tired recently and his capacity for physical activity has decreased.

Are there particular factors that contribute to hypertension in elderly men?

What are the particular considerations for antihypertensive treatment?

Which drugs are the most useful?

Background

Recent statistics from the USA estimate that 79 400 000 US adults (1:3) have cardiovascular disease (CVD).[1] Of those with CVD, 37 500 000 are aged 65 years or older. Among American subjects with CVD, hypertension is highly prevalent with an estimated 72 million reaching the current thresholds for diagnosing hypertension. Thirty-three million men have hypertension and in the USA the annual cost of treating hypertension and its complications (men and women) is 66.4 billion dollars. The lifetime risks of developing CV risk factors and CVD are presented in Table 17.1. The majority of men and women will develop hypertension. Unlike other CV risk factors (diabetes, obesity and hyperlipidaemia), if hypertension has not developed by the age of 70 it is just as likely to develop after the age of 70. At all ages, the incidence of CVD is higher in men than in women (Figure 17.1). CVD develops, on average, 10 years later in women.

Data from the Framingham Study,[2] confirm that the lifetime risk for hypertension in both men and women is 90%. While there has been no change in this since 1952 for women, the figure for men has increased by 60%. It appears that the control of hypertension has improved as the prevalence of stage 2 and above hypertension has declined. Presumably, the rising prevalence of obesity and decline in general level of physical activity has contributed to the increase in hypertension in men. Analysis of the NHANES (National Health and Nutrition Examination Survey) database[3] confirms that hypertension control has improved. However, prevalence remains high: 7.3 ± 0.9% in the

Table 17.1 Lifetime risk of developing cardiovascular disease (CVD) and risk factors

| | At Age 40 | | At Age 70 | |
	Men	Women	Men	Women
Any CVD	2 in 3	>1 in 2	>1 in 2	1 in 2
CHD	1 in 2	1 in 3	1 in 3	1 in 4
Stroke	1 in 6	1 in 5	1 in 6	1 in 5
Dementia	–	–	1 in 7	1 in 5
Lung cancer	1 in 12	1 in 17	–	–
Breast cancer	1 in 1000	1 in 8	–	1 in 14
Prostate cancer	1 in 6	–	–	–
Colon cancer	1 in 16	1 in 17	–	–
Diabetes	1 in 3	1 in 3	1 in 9	1 in 7
Hypertension	9 in 10	9 in 10	9 in 10	9 in 10

Adapted from Rosamond et al.[1]

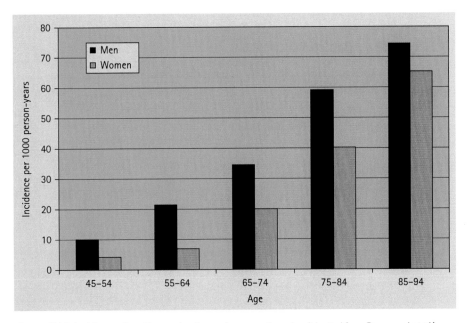

Figure 17.1 Incidence of cardiovascular disease by age and gender. Adapted from Rosamond et al.[1]

18–39 age group, 32.6 ± 2.0% in those aged 40–59, and 66.3 ± 1.8% in those aged 60 or more. Recent data from the Ontario Survey[4] showed similar results with hypertension present in 23.8% of men and 19.0% of women overall. There was a similar pattern of increase with age in the prevalence of hypertension. Women are more likely than men to attend for hypertension screening and follow-up. The increased prevalence of hypertension and lower rates of effective treatment for men extends across different ethnic groups.

Oestrogen is responsible for the relative protection of premenopausal women against vascular disease. Castrated men are relatively protected from hypertension, whereas oophorectomized women treated with androgen are at increased risk. Thus, the ratio of androgen to oestrogen may be important. Furthermore, the pattern of BP elevation is different with men having higher increases in systolic BP and pulse pressure compared with women. Furthermore, for a given level of BP, the atherosclerotic process is more likely to be accelerated in men. Obstructive sleep apnoea/hypopnoea syndrome is associated with a three-fold increase in risk of hypertension, and is twice as common in men. Dietary factors are probably equally important in men and women. Among dietary factors that have been shown to be important in studies involving older men (i.e. the Honolulu Heart Program) is the increased risk of stroke with high coffee consumption and the protective effect of fruit and berry consumption in relation to atherosclerosis progression.

Benign prostatic hyperplasia is common, giving rise to symptoms in up to 30% of men over 60 years. These include hesitancy, urgency, frequency and nocturia, and poor urinary stream with incomplete feeling of bladder emptying. Up to 80% of prostatic hyperplasia is fibromuscular tissue, α_1-adrenergic stimulation of this tissue partly obliterating the urethral lumen at the bladder neck, while α_1-blockade improves urine flow. This makes α-blockade a logical choice in older men with hypertension and prostatic symptoms. Doxazosin (Cardura) and terazosin (Hytrin) have been widely used and can also alleviate prostatic symptoms. They may also cause postural hypotension and erectile dysfunction (ED) and/or ejaculatory dysfunction. Other α_1-blockers have been developed to have a more specific effect on the prostate – tamsulosin (Flomax) was the first selective α_{1a}-adrenergic blocker and has minimal effect on BP.

ED is common in older men, and may lead to impaired quality of life. There is an association between ED, hypertension and endothelial dysfunction. The sinusoids of the corpora cavernosa are lined with endothelial cells, which release smooth muscle relaxant mediators including nitric oxide in response to sexual stimuli acting through somatic and parasympathetic innervation. This smooth muscle relaxation is critical for the net blood inflow, which leads to penile erection. Many of the antihypertensive drugs contribute to ED. This includes thiazides, β-blockers, α-blockers and spironolactone. ED is also commoner with other chronic diseases, including diabetes, chronic obstructive pulmonary disease and cardiac disease.

Dementia is slightly more common in older men (Table 17.1). There is a strong correlation between dementia risk and macrovascular disease.[5] Defects in memory and information processing may be present for up to 10 years before a diagnosis of dementia becomes apparent. The practitioner should be aware that patients with hypertension, and particularly those with multiple CV risk factors, are at risk. It is widely accepted that cognitive decline is underdiagnosed and not sufficiently managed. We are not clear that managing hypertension effectively prevents cognitive decline (except that due to multi-infarct dementia), but it seems prudent to treat risk factors vigorously when a patient is at risk of cognitive decline. β-blockers can contribute to cognitive problems and are probably best avoided in those with memory and other cognitive defects unless there are other reasons to prescribe them.

Recent Developments

1. Higher levels of oestradiol have been associated with an increased risk of stroke in older men. This could be due to increased thrombotic tendency but the relationship is also present with haemorrhagic stroke. Increased adiposity leads to increased conversion of androgen to oestrogen, and may be linked to other risk factors, including hypertension. Low testosterone and high oestrogen have also been linked to increased risk of peripheral vascular disease.[6] A study[7] following older men for nearly 12 years has reported that low testosterone is associated with increased mortality. Those in the lowest quartile had a 40% increased risk compared with those with higher testosterone.

2. The contribution of disordered BP regulation to cognitive impairment has been confirmed in a recent study of elderly men.[8] Those with the lowest dip in nocturnal BP had the lowest cerebral blood flow. Also, regional cerebral blood flow was decreased, and systolic BP increased, in those with extreme nocturnal dips in diastolic BP.

3. Thiazides decrease calcium excretion and have been reported to increase bone density and to decrease risk of fragility fracture. Loop diuretics, on the other hand, increase calcium excretion and have been reported[9] to lead to bone loss at the hip in elderly men. Offloading sodium and water overload with diuretics is important in managing hypertension. The minimum dose and potency needed should be used and loop diuretics should be confined to conditions where there is a specific indication.

4. Classic CV risk factors, including increased BP, account for only part of the CV risk. More accurate prediction may come from the use of multiple biomarkers. For example, adiponectin is decreased in patients at high risk of CVD and numerous studies support its potential use as a risk marker.[10] Other markers that may be of use include those for the failing myocardium, and markers of inflammation, endothelial dysfunction or oxidative stress.[11]

Conclusions

Hypertension is very common in elderly men, who are less likely to seek advice and receive effective treatment to lower BP than elderly women are. While the pathogenesis of hypertension and its treatment are very similar in both genders, there are some differences. Presumably because of vascular properties (including size and geometry), systolic BP and pulse pressures are more likely to be elevated in males. The change in sex steroid status with ageing is emerging as a CV risk factor for men and may be a determinant of BP responses to ageing. The presence of prostatic symptoms and ED, both of which are common in elderly men, help to determine the most appropriate treatment. As with older women, thiazides and calcium channel blockers are first-line treatments (Figure 17.2). In older men with hypertension, relative hypogonadism and cognitive decline are determinants of health status and quality of life and should be considered when making an overall assessment.

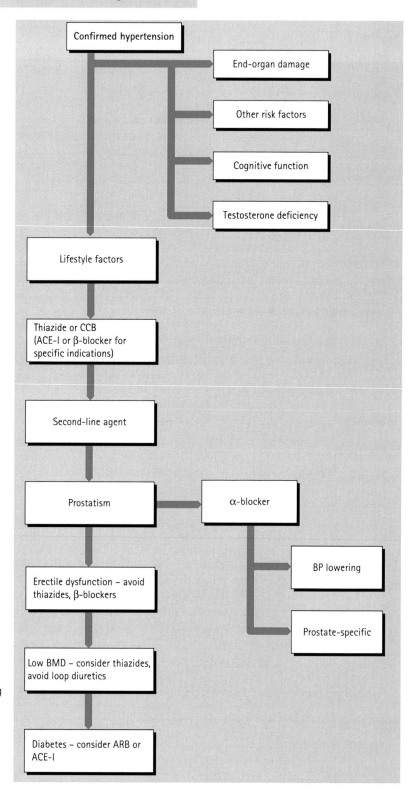

Figure 17.2 An elderly man with hypertension. ACE-I, angiotensin-converting enzyme inhibitor; ARB, angiotensin receptor blocker; BMD, bone mineral density; CCB, calcium channel blocker.

References

1   Rosamond W, Flegal K, Friday G, Furie K, Go A, Greenlund K, *et al.* Heart disease and stroke statistics – 2007 update: a report from the American Heart Disease Association Statistics Committee and Stroke Statistics Subcommittee. *Circulation* 2007; **115**: e69–e171.

2   Vasan RS, Beiser A, Seshadri S, Larson MG, Kannel WB, D'Agostino RB, Levy D. Residual lifetime risk for developing hypertension in middle-aged women and men. *JAMA* 2002; **287**: 1003–10.

3   Ong KL, Cheung BMY, Man YB, Lau CP, Lam KSL. Prevalence, awareness, treatment, and control of hypertension among United States adults 1999–2004. *Hypertension* 2007; **49**: 69–75.

4   Leenen FHH, Dumais J, McInnis NH, Turton P, Stratychuk L, Nemeth K, *et al.* Results of the Ontario Survey on the prevalence and control of hypertension. *Can Med Assoc J* 2008; **178**: 1441–9.

5   Muller M, Grobbee DE, Aleman A, Bots M, van der Schouw YT. Cardiovascular disease and cognitive performance in middle-aged and elderly men. *Atherosclerosis* 2007; **190**: 143–9.

6   Tivesten A, Mellstrom D, Jutberger H, Fagerberg B, Lernfelt B, Orwoll E, *et al.* Low serum testosterone and high serum estradiol associate with lower extremity peripheral arterial disease in elderly men. The MrOS Study in Sweden. *J Am Coll Cardiol* 2007; **50**: 1070–6.

7   Laughlin GA, Barrett-Connor E, Bergstrom J. Low serum testosterone and mortality in older men. *J Clin Endocrinol Metab* 2008; **93**: 68–75.

8   Siennicki-Lantz A, Reinprecht F, Axelsson J, Elmstahl S. Cerebral perfusion in the elderly with nocturnal blood pressure fall. *Eur J Neurol* 2007; **14**: 715–20.

9   Lim LS, Fink HA, Kuskowski MA, Taylor BC, Schousboe JT, Ensrud KE, *et al.* Loop diuretic use and increased rates of hip bone loss in older men: the Osteoporotic Fractures in Men Study. *Arch Intern Med* 2008; **168**: 735–40.

10 Frystyk J, Berne C, Berglund L, Jensevik K, Flyvbjerg A, Zethelius B. Serum adiponectin is a predictor of coronary heart disease: a population-based 10-year follow-up study in elderly men. *J Clin Endocrinol Metab* 2007; **92**: 571–6.

11 Zethelius B, Berglund L, Sundstrom J, Ingelsson E, Basu S, Larsson A, *et al.* Use of multiple biomarkers to improve the prediction of death from cardiovascular causes. *N Engl J Med* 2008; **358**: 2107–16.

18 Hypertension in the Elderly

Case History

Connie is a 72-year-old widow who enjoys an active life. She has been somewhat limited in recent years by osteoarthritis and late-onset asthma. She stopped smoking 5 years ago and her symptoms are controlled with non-steroidal anti-inflammatory drugs and bronchodilators. She has a strong family history of increased blood pressure (BP). Recently her BP has been persistently increased, the latest value being 174/98. She would like to know if it is really worth treating this.

What are the risks and benefits of treating her BP?

Which agent(s) are most appropriate?

Does her age put her at any particular risk from medication?

Background

Systolic BP (SBP) rises continuously with age. Diastolic BP (DBP) rises typically until about the age of 60, after which it tends to decrease. This means that, with ageing, there is a tendency to develop isolated systolic hypertension and that there is a widening of the pulse pressure (difference between SBP and DBP). Data from a number of studies, including Framingham and MRFIT (Multiple Risk Factor Intervention Trial), show that the risk of cardiovascular (CV) disease and particularly stroke increase linearly with BP.[1] Hypertension is the single most important modifiable risk factor for vascular disease in the elderly. The relationship between ageing and increased BP is modified by the presence of chronic disease states such as respiratory disease and cancer, which may attenuate the age-related increase. Type 2 diabetes is very commonly accompanied by hypertension. The combination of the two greatly increases susceptibility to vascular complications.

The disproportionate rise in SBP with ageing is due to decreased compliance (increased stiffness) in arteries and arterioles. This leads to increased transmission of the pressure wave that accompanies ventricular systole, and is due to atherosclerosis and vascular calcification. Prior to 60 years of age, increased peripheral resistance caused by increased vascular tone increases both SBP and DBP. Changes in salt sensitivity, enhanced sympathetic nervous system activity, and decreased baroreceptor responsiveness contribute, along with structural vascular changes, to the increased BP with ageing. Up to 90% of elderly people are hypertensive. With an ageing population, an increasing number will fall into the BP categories that are defined as hypertension.

Postural hypotension may be present in 10–20% of those aged 70 years and over. It is defined as a decrease in SBP of ≥20 mmHg or DBP of ≥10 mmHg within 3 minutes of standing up from the recumbent position. Decreases in BP, including with standing, are more common in the postprandial period, especially first thing in the morning. BP is more labile in the elderly leading to increased variability in office measures of BP. On ambulatory BP monitoring, the normal night-time decrease in BP may be attenuated in the elderly. Office hypertension is also very common,[1] occurring in up to 25% of elderly patients with apparently increased BP. Office measurements of BP do not necessarily reflect sustained hypertension. There is a danger that patients could be unnecessarily exposed to the risk of hypotensive drugs. The elderly are more prone to side effects of antihypertensive drugs due to the use of concurrent medications, renal impairment, susceptibility to postural change in BP, and comorbidities. While trial data suggest that older subjects are at least as likely to benefit from treatment as younger subjects – perhaps more because of the high risk of events – the risks and benefits of treatment should be carefully considered and discussed in each case. Also, the potential benefit of lifestyle changes should not be neglected.

The benefits of treating hypertension in the elderly include decreased risk of heart failure by 50%, stroke by 35%, myocardial infarction by 25%, and a slower progression of cognitive decline. As in younger people, increased BP should be verified on at least two occasions. Assessment should include consideration of underlying causes (particularly renovascular disease), screening for modifiable causes, assessment of target-organ damage, and global CV risk assessment. A careful review of all medications should be undertaken in each case. Drugs that tend to increase BP include non-steroidal anti-inflammatory drugs and cyclo-oxygenase-2 inhibitors, sympathomimetics (e.g. decongestants), steroids, erythropoietin and cyclosporine. High alcohol intake and use of illicit drugs (particularly cocaine) also increase BP. Electrocardiogram (ECG) will help identify cardiac ischaemia and left ventricular hypertrophy. Plasma levels of B-type natriuretic peptide (BNP) or NT-proBNP are helpful in identifying heart failure – those who are positive should have an echocardiogram. Renal function and measurement of protein excretion should be undertaken in all cases. The fundi should be inspected for retinopathy. Causes of secondary hypertension in the elderly are summarized in Box 18.1.

Box 18.1 Causes of secondary hypertension in the elderly

- Obstructive sleep apnoea
- Renovascular disease or chronic kidney disease
- Endocrine:
  - Mineralocorticoid excess
  - Thyroid disease
  - Hyperparathyroidism
  - Steroid use or Cushing's syndrome
- High alcohol intake
- Medications (non-steroidal anti-inflammatory drugs, decongestants, etc.)

The target BP is widely accepted as 140/90, but this is often difficult to achieve in the elderly without exposing the patient to complex drug regimens with risks of poor compliance and side effects. A BP of 130/80 is considered the goal in high-risk patients, including those with diabetes or chronic kidney disease. Treatment should particularly aim to decrease SBP, as this is more likely to be increased than DBP and increases correlate more closely with risk of vascular events. Exercise, weight reduction, balanced diet and salt restriction are all just as likely to be beneficial as in younger age groups. Medications are often overprescribed for the elderly – they are often already taking medications, they are fearful of complications of hypertension, and lifestyle modification may be harder to achieve.

In uncomplicated hypertension, thiazides are usually the first-line treatment. Disadvantages include worsening of diabetes, gout and hypokalaemia. Dihydropyridine calcium channel blockers are probably as effective. Angiotensin-converting enzyme inhibitors (ACE-Is) or angiotensin receptor blockers (ARBs) should be considered first-line if there is another reason to prescribe them, such as heart failure, post-myocardial infarction, chronic kidney disease or diabetes. β-blockers are not usually considered first-line treatment in the elderly unless otherwise indicated (angina or following myocardial infarction). Unless there is evidence of developing complications, hypotensive medication should be stepped up more gradually in the elderly to avoid side effects. Most patients will require two or more drugs to control their BP. Home BP monitoring is helpful to improve engagement and assess treatment response.

A 1998 Cochrane review[2] identified 15 trials with 21 908 patients. At that time, thiazides and β-blockers were the most widely used first-line agents. Treatment for 5 years decreases CV morbidity and mortality from 177 to 126 events per 1000 patients. The trials considered included some of the landmark studies showing the benefit of treating hypertension in the elderly: SHEP (Systolic Hypertension in the Elderly Program) 1991; Syst-Eur (Systolic Hypertension in Europe) 1991; STOP (Swedish Trial in Old Patients – with Hypertension) 1991. Further support for the use of thiazides as first-line agents came from ALLHAT (Antihypertensive and Lipid-Lowering Treatment to Prevent Heart Attack Trial) (2002), which showed chlorthalidone to be superior to amlodipine, lisinopril and doxazosin in older people.[2] Chlorthalidone has a higher incidence of metabolic side effects than other thiazides because of its long duration of action. In other trials,[2] amlodipine, felodipine and extended release nifedipine have all been shown to lower BP and to protect against CV events. ACE-Is or ARBs are also safe in the elderly and are most conveniently used in combination preparations with thiazides. Renin–angiotensin system blockade may have benefits beyond CV and renal protection with recent studies suggesting that it may protect against cognitive and physical decline with ageing.

Recent Developments

1 ACE-Is and ARBs are very well tolerated in the elderly, and patients may be more inclined to persist with these agents than with diuretics or β-blockers.[3] Recent data from NHANES III suggest that older patients are more likely to persist with treatments, and that those who do not visit their doctor regularly are unlikely to persist.[4]

2 Data from the Dublin outcome study of 1144 elderly subjects confirm that ambulatory BP is an important predictor of CV mortality.[5] Ambulatory BP monitoring provides information on night-time and early morning BPs, both of which are highly predictive

of risk. Hypertension interacts with other metabolic syndrome (MetS) components to increase risk, but optimal cut-offs need to be clarified for the elderly. A recent study[6] where 3257 older subjects were followed-up for 12 years suggests that pulse pressure was more predictive of CV events than SBP or DBP when considered with other MetS variables. A cut-off of 75 mmHg for men and 80 mmHg for women was suggested.

3 MetS is highly prevalent and strongly predictive of CV events. Carotid intima-media thickness is widely used as a surrogate marker for developing atherosclerosis. Of MetS variables, hypertension is the most strongly associated with increased intima-media thickness in the elderly.[7] Hypertension needs to be assessed in the context of other risk factors. MetS has proved to be a useful concept and correlates with both the presence and severity of coronary atherosclerosis in the elderly.

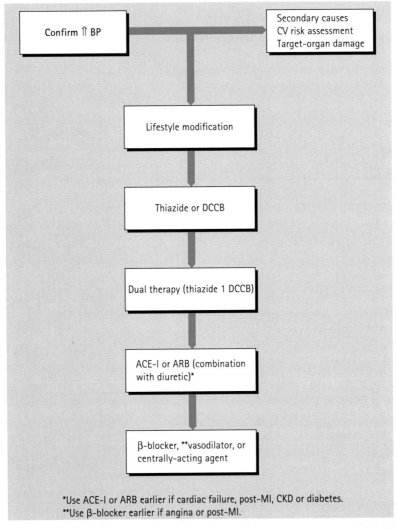

*Use ACE-I or ARB earlier if cardiac failure, post-MI, CKD or diabetes.
**Use β-blocker earlier if angina or post-MI.

Figure 18.1 Hypertension in the elderly. CKD, chronic kidney disease; DCCB, dihydropyridine calcium channel blocker.

4   Macrovascular events are a major cause of morbidity and mortality in older people. Microvascular changes also contribute to cognitive decline and dementia. Data from the Cardiovascular Health Study show a correlation between retinal microvascular abnormalities and risk of cognitive impairment.[8] Another surrogate marker for developing dementia is white matter and other lesions on magnetic resonance imaging. The presence of these correlates with increased arterial stiffness,[9] and decreasing BP may prevent their development.

Conclusions

Hypertension is very common in the elderly and treatment is effective in preventing CV and renal disease. However, only 1:5 elderly persons with high BP reach the target of 140/90, even with treatment. Hypertension is a critical determinant of CV risk in the elderly with a linear increase in risk with increasing BP. SBP is particularly likely to be higher, mainly because of decreased arterial compliance. Older patients are at increased risk of side effects from antihypertensive medications. These include postural hypotension, worsening renal function, electrolyte abnormalities, gout and hyperglycaemia. A treatment flow is suggested in Figure 18.1. On the basis of published evidence, there is most evidence to support thiazide diuretics and dihydropyridine calcium channel blockers as first-line agents. Evidence is accumulating that ACE-Is and ARBs are not only well tolerated in the elderly but may have benefits beyond BP control and renal protection.

References

1   Pinto E. Blood pressure and ageing. *Postgrad Med J* 2007; **83**: 109–14.

2   Mulrow C, Lau J, Cornell J, Brand M. Pharmacotherapy for hypertension in the elderly. *Cochrane Database System Rev* 1998; CD000028.

3   Pannarale G. Optimal drug treatment of systolic hypertension in the elderly. *Drugs Aging* 2008; **25**: 1–8.

4   Borghi C, Veronesi M, Dormi A, Prandin MG, Cosentino E, Strocchi E. Persistence of treatment and blood pressure control in elderly hypertensive patients treated with different classes of antihypertensive drugs. *Am J Geriatr Cardiol* 2007; **16**: 280–6.

5   Burr ML, Dolan E, O'Brien EW, O'Brien ET, McCormack P. The value of ambulatory blood pressure in older adults: the Dublin outcome study. *Age Ageing* 2008; **37**: 201–6.

6   Mazza A, Zamboni S, Tikhonoff V, Scarpa R, Cuppini S, Zennaro R, *et al.* Pulse hypertension: a new component of the metabolic syndrome in elderly women? *J Hum Hypertens* 2007; **21**: 934–41.

7   Empana J-P, Zureik M, Gariepy J, Courbon D, Dartigues JF, Ritchie K, *et al.* The metabolic syndrome and the carotid artery structure in noninstitutionalized elderly subjects: the three-city study. *Stroke* 2007; **38**: 893–9.

8   Baker ML, Marino Larsen EK, Kuller LH, Klein R, Klein BEK, Siscovick DS, *et al.* Retinal microvascular signs, cognitive function, and dementia in older persons: the Cardiovascular Health Study. *Stroke* 2007; **38**: 2041–7.

9   Ohmine T, Miwa Y, Yao H, Yuzuriha T, Takashima Y, Uchino A, *et al.* Association between arterial stiffness and cerebral white matter lesions in community-dwelling elderly subjects. *Hypertens Res* 2008; **31**: 75–81.

19 The Very Elderly

Case History

JS is a sprightly 82-year-old woman, who manages well at home and looks after her elderly husband. She suffered a stroke 2 years ago, and has mild residual left-sided weakness. She is mobile with a walking stick, and manages all normal activities of daily living. Her only medications are a thiazide diuretic, inhalers for chronic obstructive pulmonary disease and aspirin 100 mg OD. She has persistent systolic hypertension (typical BP 160/74). She is a non-smoker, and is not overweight. The estimated glomerular filtration rate is 48, and electrolytes are normal.

Is it beneficial to treat this level of BP at her age?

Are there any risks from drug treatments to lower her BP?

Which agents are most useful in this age group?

Background

The number of very elderly people is increasing, and more people are reaching their 80s and above with relatively good health. Currently, in the USA, there are about 15 million people, aged ≥80 years, accounting for 4.5% of the population. Although BP tends to fall with age, hypertension is highly prevalent in the elderly and is associated with considerable morbidity and mortality. Complications of hypertension account for a considerable proportion of healthcare spending on the elderly. Hypertension trials have focused on younger people, and we have had to extrapolate the results of these to older people. Early clinical trials in the elderly have suggested that treatment of hypertension could reduce strokes and heart failure by 30–40% and myocardial infarction by 20% but the treatment was itself associated with increased mortality.

The strength of the association between hypertension and adverse events is diminished in the extremely elderly. There is good evidence for a correlation between BP and survival in the very elderly.[1] Low BP, particularly low diastolic (DBP), is associated with increased risk of death. The threshold for treatment should almost certainly be higher than in younger groups and we should not be aiming for too low a treatment target. It seems reasonable that treatment should be considered when systolic BP (SBP) is above 160, and we should aim to keep SBP above 140. Antihypertensive treatment is not without risk at any age, but many risks are increased in very old subjects (Table 19.1).

Table 19.1 Risks of antihypertensive treatment in the very elderly	
Effect	Drugs implicated
Postural hypotension	Any drug(s), diuretic, α-blocker, vasodilator
Falls	As above
Bradycardia	β-blocker
Renal impairment	ACE-I, ARB, diuretic
Hypokalaemia	Diuretic
Hyperkalaemia	ACE-I, ARB, spironolactone
Hyponatraemia	Diuretic
Hyperglycaemia	Diuretic, β-blocker
Dyslipidaemia	Diuretic, β-blocker
Sleep or mood disturbance	β-blocker

ACE-I, angiotensin-converting enzyme inhibitor; ARB, angiotensin receptor blockers

Early studies generally used diuretic-based regimens. Diuretics thus became the cornerstones of hypotensive regimens in the elderly. However, they do have a range of potential side effects. Arrhythmias and sudden death due to hypokalaemia may have contributed to the increased mortality in this age group with antihypertensives. Patients taking diuretics should have regular checks of renal function and electrolytes, and these should also be checked during intercurrent illness. Some classes of drugs may have a protective effect on end organs independent of BP lowering. Calcium channel blockers (CCBs) may protect against stroke, and aldosterone-blockers protect the myocardium, although there are no specific data relating to the very elderly. Two important recent trials with renin–angiotensin system-blocking drugs are:

- ANBP-2 (Second Australian National Blood Pressure Study)[2] which recruited 6083 hypertensive subjects aged 65–84 years. Patients were randomized to enalapril or hydrochlorthiazide and followed for a median of 4.1 years. Compared with diuretic, the hazard ratio for any cardiovascular (CV) event or death was 0.89 (95% CI: 0.79 to 1.00, $P = 0.005$). The protective effect of angiotensin-converting enzyme inhibitors was significant for men but not women.

- SCOPE (Study on COgnition and Prognosis in the Elderly)[3] which recruited 4964 subjects aged 70–89 years with SBP 160–179 or DBP 90–99 mmHg. Those randomized to candesartan had a decrease in BP of 21.7/10.8 compared with 18.5/9.2 in controls. There was a marked decrease in risk of stroke with candesartan, but no significant decrease in overall CV event rate. Cognitive function (mini mental state examination) did not significantly decline in either group over the 3.7 years of follow-up.

The very recent HYVET trial (Hypertension in the Very Elderly Trial)[4] provides definitive information on treating hypertension in the very elderly. An international study involving 3845 patients aged over 80 years with SBP >160 mmHg, HYVET randomized patients to indapamide sustained release 1.5 mg or placebo. If needed, perindopril (2 or 4 mg OD) was added to achieve the target BP of 150/80. Indapamide exerts most of its antihypertensive effect by direct vasodilatation. It protects against end-organ damage including left ventricular hypertrophy, and is less likely to produce metabolic side effects than are standard thiazides. After follow-up of 2 years, BP in the treatment group was 15.0/6.1 mmHg lower than that in the placebo group. Active treatment was associated with reductions of:

- Death from any cause by 21% (95% CI: 4 to 35; $P = 0.02$)
- CV deaths by 23% (95% CI: 1 to 40; $P = 0.06$)
- Fatal or non-fatal stroke by 30% (95% CI: -1–51; $P = 0.06$)
- Stroke death by 39% (95% CI: 1 to 62; $P = 0.05$)
- Heart failure by 64% (95% CI: 42 to 78; $P < 0.001$).

The pilot HYVET study suggested that treatment of hypertension in the very elderly age group was associated with an increased risk of death. This was not borne out in the full study. Patients in this study were acknowledged to be healthier than the average octogenarian. HYVET demonstrates that treating hypertension with indapamide and the higher SBP target than would be used for younger groups is safe. The BP reductions in the HYVET cohort over 5 years are shown in Figure 19.1. It is apparent that the major benefit of treatment is on SBP, and that this is apparent within 2 years. In this age group, BP naturally decreases with time, as shown.

While lifestyle factors should always be considered, the potential for management of these factors to be of tangible benefit in the extreme elderly is somewhat limited. As

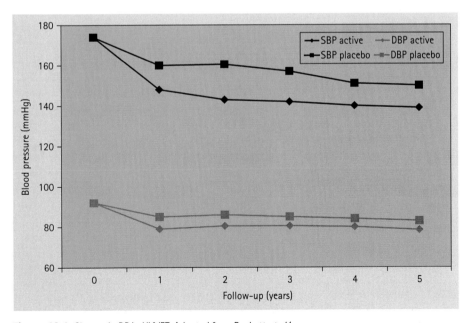

Figure 19.1 Change in BP in HYVET. Adapted from Beckett et al.[4]

diuretic therapy is most often used as a first-line drug treatment, it is prudent to limit salt intake so that the diuretics can have maximum benefit. Care needs to be exercised when suggesting weight loss in the elderly, as dieting might lead to loss of muscle as well as fat with a consequent compromise of physical function. Elderly hypertensives should be encouraged to maintain as active a lifestyle as possible, but the capacity for benefit from exercise is often quite limited. With data from HYVET, we should perhaps consider inda-pamide more often. Also, the newer vasodilating β-blockers may offer benefits in the elderly without exposing them to risk of extreme α- or β-blockade. CCBs are also safe and effective. Changes in mechanical properties of blood vessels are extremely important in the pathogenesis of hypertension in the elderly, while neurohumoral mechanisms are relatively more important in younger patients. Angiotensin-converting enzyme inhibitors and angiotensin receptor blockers have important end-organ protective effects.

Recent Developments

1 The link between higher BP and decreased risk of mortality has been confirmed in a recent study[5] involving 4071 hypertensive patients aged at least 80 years. This study and earlier observations suggest that caution is warranted in lowering BP in very elderly subjects. Caution should be particularly exercised when DBP is lowered. Another smaller study[6] has recently failed to find a relationship between SBP and mortality in subjects aged over 80 years.

2 Data from the Leiden 85-plus study[7] suggests that hypertension is not associated with decline in renal function in the very elderly. On the contrary, those with lower DBP at baseline showed an accelerated decline in renal function, as did those in whom SBP decreased during follow-up. Other recent data[8] suggest that CCBs can protect against cognitive decline independent of ability to lower BP. These data are in agreement with Syst-Eur, and together these studies argue strongly for CCBs as first-line agents in managing hypertension in elderly subjects at high risk of cognitive decline.

3 Genetic markers may be important even in very elderly subjects. The apolipoprotein-E ε4 allele is associated with an increased risk of Alzheimer's disease. Hypertensive patients with this allele appear to be relatively protected from cognitive decline if they are treated with BP-lowering drugs.[9]

4 Many stroke trials either do not specify the type of stroke or focus on thrombotic strokes that are about four times more common than haemorrhagic strokes. In the very elderly, haemorrhagic strokes tend to occur at lower levels of SBP and DBP than in the young.[10] Also, obesity and diabetes are less prominent risk factors for haemorrhagic stroke.

Conclusions

It appears that the greatest benefit of hypertension treatment in those at the upper age extreme of life is in preventing disability from stroke or heart failure. However, com-pared with younger subjects, the benefit of treating hypertension is less apparent and the

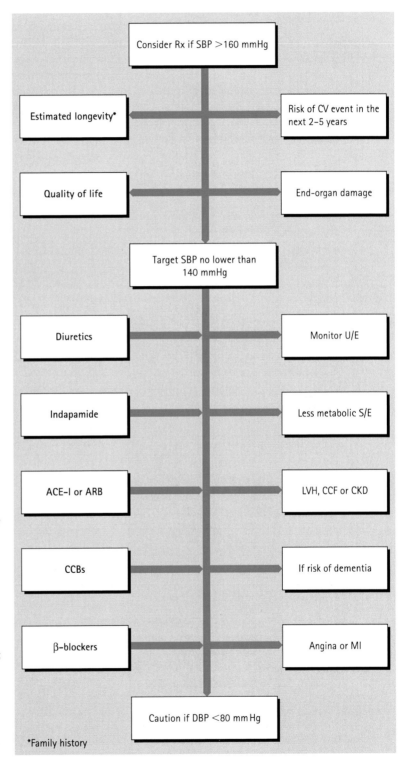

Figure 19.2
Hypertension in the very elderly. ACE-I, angiotensin-converting enzyme inhibitor; ARB, angiotensin receptor blocker; CCB, calcium channel blocker; CCF, congestive cardiac failure; CKD, chronic kidney disease; DBP, diastolic blood pressure; LVH, left ventricular hypertrophy; Rx, treatment; S/E, serum electrolytes; SBP, systolic blood pressure; U/E, urea and electrolytes.

relationship between high BP and adverse CV events is attenuated. A scheme for managing hypertension is proposed in Figure 19.2. Caution should be exercised in treating the above patient's BP – SBP is high but the DBP is on the low side. Lower DBP has been associated with increased mortality and renal decline in this age group. There are also increased risks with individual BP-lowering drugs in the very elderly. Although diuretics have been the most widely used front-line drugs, recent evidence suggests that we should be considering indapamide, CCBs and other drugs with vasodilatory action. Treatment decisions should consider estimates of the patient's longevity and the short-term likelihood of an event if they are not treated.

References

1 Goodwin JS. Embracing complexity: a consideration of hypertension in the very old. *J Gerontol Ser A* 2003; **58**: 653–8.

2 Wing LMH, Reid CM, Ryan P, Beilin LJ, Brown MA, Jennings GLR, *et al.* A comparison of outcomes with angiotensin-converting enzyme inhibitors and diuretics for hypertension in the elderly. *N Engl J Med* 2003; **348**: 583–92.

3 Lithell H, Hansson L, Skoog I, Elmfeldt D, Hofman A, Olofsson B, *et al.* The Study on Cognition and Prognosis in the Elderly (SCOPE): principal results of a randomized double-blind intervention trial. *J Hypertens* 2003; **21**: 875–86.

4 Beckett NS, Peters R, Fletcher AE, Staessen JA, Liu L, Dumitrascu D, *et al.* Treatment of hypertension in patients 80 years of age or older. *N Engl J Med* 2008; **358**: 1887–98.

5 Oates DJ, Berlowitz DR, Glickman ME, Silliman RA, Borzecki AM. Blood pressure and survival in the oldest old. *J Am Geriatr Soc* 2007; **55**: 383–8.

6 Kagiyama S, Fukuhara M, Ansai T, Matsumura K, Soh I, Takata Y, *et al.* Association between blood pressure and mortality in 80-year-old subjects from a population-based prospective study in Japan. *Hypertens Res* 2008; **31**: 265–70.

7 van Bemmel T, Woittiez K, Blauw GJ, van der Sman-de Beer F, Dekker FW, Westendorp RGJ, *et al.* Prospective study of the effect of blood pressure on renal function in old age: the Leiden 85-Plus Study. *J Am Soc Nephrol* 2006; **17**: 2561–6.

8 Trompet S, Westendorp RGJ, Kamper AM, de Craen AJM. Use of calcium antagonists and cognitive decline in old age. The Leiden 85-plus study. *Neurobiol Aging* 2008; **29**: 306–8.

9 Hestad KA, Engedal K. Antihypertensive medication is associated with less cognitive impairment in the very old with apolipoprotein-E epsilon4 allele. *Drugs Aging* 2006; **23**: 723–31.

10 Chiquete E, Ruiz-Sandoval MC, Alvarez-Palazuelos LE, Padilla-Martinez JJ, Gonzalez-Cornejo S, Ruiz-Sandoval JL. Hypertensive intracerebral hemorrhage in the very elderly. *Cerebrovasc Dis* 2007; **24**: 196–201.

Hypertension in Special Groups

20 Hypertension in Pregnancy

Case History

Mary is 32 years old and 29 weeks into her first pregnancy. To date, the pregnancy has been uncomplicated and recent ultrasound scans confirmed normal foetal size for estimated gestation, and that there were no foetal abnormalities. She attends for routine review and her blood pressure (BP) is 150/95. Her BP was also high the previous week. Her pre-pregnancy health was excellent, and there is no history of hypertension. Her mother has hypertension. Urinalysis is negative for protein.

How should this be investigated further?

What is the threshold for starting antihypertensive treatment?

What is the target BP for this patient?

Which agents are safe and effective in pregnancy?

Background

Hypertensive complications are present in 6–8% of pregnancies, representing the commonest medical disorder in pregnancy. BP should be measured with the patient rested and sitting with the arm horizontal and supported. Diastolic BP (DBP) is defined as disappearance of the Korotkoff V sound. High values should be repeated on a separate occasion. Hypertension is defined as:

- Mild: systolic BP (SBP) 140–159 mmHg, DBP 90–109 mmHg
- Severe: SBP ≥160 mmHg, DBP ≥110 mmHg

Gestational hypertension occurs after 20 weeks and usually resolves before 12 weeks postpartum. By definition, there are no vascular complications of established hypertension nor are there signs or symptoms of pre-eclampsia. There is an increased risk of pre-eclampsia – the earlier hypertension develops, the greater the risk. About 6% of pregnant women are affected.

Chronic hypertension occurs when there is pre-pregnancy hypertension, or sustained increase in BP prior to 20 weeks of gestation. It complicates 3–5% of pregnancies.

Mild pre-eclampsia when the following criteria apply:

- SBP >140 mmHg and/or DBP >90 mmHg *or* SBP 20 mmHg greater than pre-pregnancy or early pregnancy value and/or DBP increased by >10 mmHg above pre-pregnancy or early pregnancy
- >20 weeks of gestation
- Proteinuria – albumin/creatinine ratio >25 mg/mmol on spot testing or >300 mg/24 h on timed collection
- Absence of neurological complications

Severe pre-eclampsia – when the above criteria are fulfilled but:

- SBP >170 mmHg and/or DBP is >110 mmHg

but consider with lesser degrees of hypertension when there is:

- severe proteinuria (>5000 mg per 24 h);
- oliguria (<400 ml/24 h);
- thrombocytopenia (<100 000/ ml);
- elevated liver enzymes (>3 × normal);
- neurological symptoms (headache, blurred vision, impaired consciousness);
- pulmonary oedema; and
- intrauterine growth restriction (IUGR).

Eclampsia – the patient fulfils the criteria for pre-eclampsia and convulsions (in the absence of pre-existing epilepsy or predisposition to epilepsy).

HELLP (Haemolytic anaemia, Elevated Liver enzymes and Low Platelets) is a form of severe pre-eclampsia where there is a high risk of maternal mortality.

Gestational hypertension implies a temporary disorder related to pregnancy. This diagnosis is often only clear in retrospect when BP returns to normal following delivery. It is an important diagnosis as 20–40% of patients develop pre-eclampsia. The latter is more likely when hypertension is severe, there has been previous pregnancy hypertension, a history of miscarriage, or where hypertension develops early. When hypertension develops late in pregnancy, the proven benefits of treatment are mainly to the mother rather than the foetus. When diagnosed very late in pregnancy it is not clear that aggressive treatment of hypertension rather than expectant treatment with careful timing of delivery is warranted.[1]

Incidence and severity of chronic hypertension varies between racial groups, and is particularly high in African Americans. For women with mild to moderate hypertension and no end-organ damage, the risk during pregnancy is low and they often do not need change to their pre-pregnancy treatment. There is, in any case, a physiological lowering of BP during pregnancy. Risks to the mother include pre-eclampsia, abruptio placentae, renal impairment, stroke and pulmonary oedema. Of these pre-eclampsia is by far the commonest (50–75% of women with severe hypertension). There is no evidence that any specific therapeutic agent or achievement of any specific BP target prevents pre-eclampsia. Risks to the foetus are miscarriage (with early pregnancy hypertension), prematurity and intrauterine growth retardation (IUGR). The presence of hypertension greatly increases the cost of pregnancy with increased clinic visits and tests, medications, greater likelihood of hospital admission and operative delivery.

Thresholds for treating hypertension and treatment targets vary between guidelines.[2,3] It is reasonable to initiate treatment when SBP is >150 mmHg and when DBP is >95 mmHg. A target of 130/85 seems reasonable and can frequently be achieved. These thresholds may need to be varied according to the perceived risk of the patient. SBP is often relatively more increased in pregnancy than is DBP. Monitoring is required to detect foetal distress related to decreased placental perfusion, and its presence will affect timing and mode of delivery. Drug treatment is generally based on long experience with drugs known to be safe, rather than on extensive trials. Methyldopa and labetalol are still considered the first-line agents, followed by nifedipine and hydralazine. Angiotensin-converting enzyme inhibitors and angiotensin receptor blockers are contraindicated in pregnancy (Box 20.1).

All women with hypertension in pregnancy should have measurement of proteinuria, defined as protein excretion ≥300 mg per day in a timed 24-h collection, or ≥30 mg/mmol creatinine in a spot collection. Plasma creatinine and electrolytes should also be measured. ECG and fundoscopy will exclude end-organ damage in patients with chronic hypertension. A routine chest X-ray is not justified.

Box 20.1

Angiotensin-converting enzyme inhibitors and angiotensin receptor blockers are contraindicated in pregnancy because of risk of cardiac and renal defects, oligohydramnios and IUGR.

Methyldopa is converted to α-methylnoradrenaline, which acts as a central α_2-adrenergic agonist. There is no evidence of teratogenicity or cognitive defects in children exposed to this agent *in utero*. It may cause fatigue, depression, sleep disturbances and dry mouth. A minority (5%) have increased liver enzymes. Long-term use can cause more serious hepatic side effects, antinuclear factor positivity and Coombs' positive haemolytic anaemia. Usual daily dose is 500–3000 mg in two to four doses.

Labetalol and other β-blockers This class of drugs has been widely used in pregnancy, and is not thought to be teratogenic. There is risk of IUGR, perhaps because of decreased placental blood flow. β-blockers are almost certainly more effective than methyldopa at lowering BP. Atenolol is probably best avoided because of risk of decreased placental function leading to decreased placental weight and IUGR, as well as the risk of foetal bradycardia and neonatal hypoglycaemia. Labetalol combines peripheral β-blocking activity with α_1-blocking activity. It is effective and safe, though not completely devoid of potential to cause IUGR and neonatal hypoglycaemia. Side effects include fatigue, mood and sleep disturbance, and bronchoconstriction. A usual daily dose is 200–1200 mg in two to three doses.

Calcium channel blockers Nifedipine is the most widely used of these drugs in pregnancy. Nicardipine, felodipine and verapamil have also been used. Neuromuscular blockade leading to profound weakness and myocardial depression have been reported when used with magnesium as a prophylactic treatment for eclamptic fits. Common side effects are flushing, headache, tachycardia and peripheral oedema. Long-acting preparations are preferred with a total daily dose of 30–120 mg.

Hydralazine acts as a direct vasodilator and has been used widely, both in the management of chronic hypertension in pregnancy and in the acute management of severe hypertension. Side effects include headache, nausea, flushing and palpitations. Long-term use can lead to peripheral neuropathy or drug-induced lupus. A usual daily dose is 50–300 mg in two to four divided doses.

Diuretics, e.g. hydrochlorthiazide 12.5 or 25 mg daily is thought to be safe. It may decrease the fluid retention experienced with vasodilator drugs.

When BP is >160/110, particularly with encephalopathy, end-organ damage (cardiac or renal failure) or eclampsia, BP should be reduced urgently by 25%, and thereafter more gradually to less than 160/100. Management should be undertaken in hospital with careful maternal and foetal monitoring. The commonly used agents are:

1 Labetalol, 10–20 mg IV followed by 20–80 mg infusions every 30 min to a maximum of 200 mg.

2 Hydralazine, 5 mg IV followed by 5–10 mg every 30 min.

3 Nifedipine, 10–30 mg orally or sublingually (short-acting capsules).

Patients should continue to be monitored and, where necessary, receive treatment following delivery. For patients with gestational hypertension or pre-eclampsia, hypertension is usually improved within days but may take up to a few weeks. Similarly, chronic hypertension often improves within weeks of delivery. Women should be encouraged to

---

Box 20.2 Antihypertensive drugs safe during breast-feeding

1 Angiotensin-converting enzyme inhibitors: captopril, enalapril
2 β-blockers: labetalol, propranolol, nadolol, oxprenolol and timolol
3 Vasodilators: hydralazine and minoxidil
4 Calcium channel blockers: diltiazem, verapamil and nifedipine
5 Centrally-acting: methyldopa
6 Other: spironolactone

breast-feed where possible. Many drugs are safe and not concentrated in breast milk (Box 20.2). Atenolol and metoprolol should be avoided.

Recent Developments

1   There has been recent concern about the outcome of pregnancies in women who receive fertility treatments. Two recent analyses[1,2] confirm the association with hypertensive complications but also demonstrate that much of the excess relates to women with multiple pregnancies. In the study by Schieve et al.,[4] the relative risk (RR) of hypertensive disorders in singleton pregnancies was 1.5 (95% CI: 1.04 to 2.2) in women who had received fertility treatment compared with those who had not. Hypertension was associated with an increased risk of preterm delivery and low birth weight. Hernandez-Diaz et al.[5] reported an incidence of hypertensive disorders of 8.9% in normal pregnancies compared with 15.8% in those who had received fertility treatment, a RR of 1.9 (95% CI: 1.4 to 2.6). This risk was lower when the analysis was confined to singleton pregnancies.

2   Women with low, as opposed to normal (20–25 kg/m^2) body mass index have decreased risk of hypertensive complications, while those who are overweight or obese have increased risk. An analysis by Samuels-Kalow et al.[6] included 13 722 women recruited in 1975–76. Compared with those in the recommended body mass index range, those who were overweight had a RR of hypertensive disorders of 2.82 (95% CI: 2.40 to 3.31), while those who were obese had a RR of 5.51 (95% CI 4.15 to 7.31). Furthermore, there was an association between hypertensive disorders and premature death within the following 15 years. Bodnar et al.[7] studied a cohort of 38 188 women. Again, there was a strong relationship between body mass index and risk of hypertensive disorders. Risk was particularly high in black women who were overweight or obese.

3   Asthma is a common disorder in young women of child-bearing age. Optimal control is important during pregnancy. Martel et al.[8] have shown, in a nested case–control study involving 4593 pregnancies in 3505 women, that use of short-acting β_2-agonists is actually associated with decreased risk of hypertensive disorders in pregnancy. This study confirms the safety of these agents in pregnancy but does not explain their apparent protective effect.

4   There is increasing evidence that hypertensive disorders of pregnancy are associated with adverse cardiovascular risk factor profile longer term.[9] In the years that follow pregnancy, markers of insulin resistance are increased in women who have been hypertensive,[10] and those with hypertension in pregnancy have greater subsequent weight gain and risk of diabetes. Callaway et al.[11] reported a risk of diabetes at 21 years after pregnancy of 7.4% in women who did not have hypertension in pregnancy compared with 15.3% in those who did, equating to an odds ratio (OR) of 2.03 (95% CI 1.42 to 2.91).

Conclusions

Women planning pregnancy should be encouraged to maintain as near normal body weight as possible and should be screened for hypertension. Management of hypertension in pregnancy is summarized in Figure 20.1. There is no internationally recognized threshold for starting treatment– this depends on a number of factors, including the stage of gestation and the woman's overall health. A guide of 150/95 is reasonable. Likewise, there is no universally recognized target BP, although it seems reasonable to aim for about 130/85. Methyldopa and labetalol remain the drugs of first choice. While most cases of chronic hypertension relate to underlying essential hypertension, and most

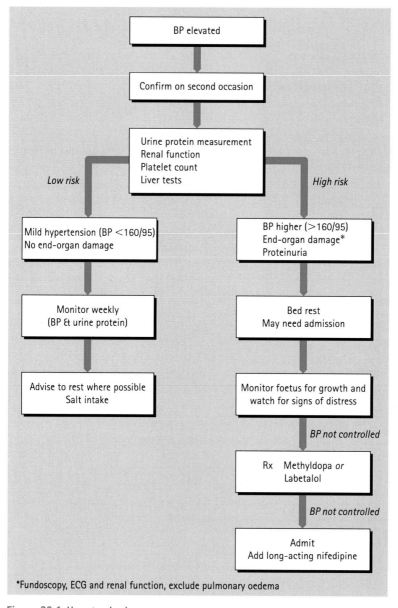

*Fundoscopy, ECG and renal function, exclude pulmonary oedema

Figure 20.1 Hypertension in pregnancy.

cases of apparent gestational hypertension resolve within a few weeks of delivery, the possibility of underlying causes for hypertension (e.g. Cushing's syndrome, renovascular disease) should be borne in mind. These should be considered particularly in those with refractory hypertension or electrolyte disturbances. Hypertension in pregnancy is emerging as an important marker for future health. Patients should be advised of this and followed-up accordingly.

References

1   Magee LA, Ornstein MP, von Dadelszen P. Management of hypertension in pregnancy. *BMJ* 1999; **318**: 1332–6.

2   Podymow T, August P. Update on the use of antihypertensive drugs in pregnancy. *Hypertension* 2008; **51**: 960–9.

3   Magee LA, Helewa M, Moutquin J-M, von Dadelszen P. Diagnosis, evaluation, and management of the hypertensive disorders of pregnancy. *J Obstet Gynaecol Can* 2008; **30** (Suppl 1): S1–48.

4   Schieve LA, Cohen B, Nannini A, Ferre C, Reynolds MA, Zhang Z, *et al.* A population-based study of maternal and perinatal outcomes associated with assisted reproductive technology in Massachusetts. *Matern Child Health J* 2007; **11**: 517–25.

5   Hernandez-Diaz S, Werler MM, Mitchell AA. Gestational hypertension in pregnancies supported by infertility treatments: role of infertility, treatments, and multiple gestations. *Fertil Steril* 2007; **88**: 438–45.

6   Samuels-Kalow ME, Funai EF, Buhimschi C, Norwitz E, Perrin M, Calderon-Margalit R, *et al.* Prepregnancy body mass index, hypertensive disorders of pregnancy, and long-term maternal mortality. *Am J Obstet Gynecol* 2007; **197**: 490.e1–6.

7   Bodnar LM, Catov JM, Klebanoff MA, Ness RB, Roberts JM. Prepregnancy body mass index and the occurrence of severe hypertensive disorders of pregnancy. *Epidemiology* 2007; **18**: 234–9.

8   Martel M-J, Rey E, Beauchesne M-F, Perreault S, Forget A, Maghni K, *et al.* Use of short-acting beta2-agonists during pregnancy and the risk of pregnancy-induced hypertension. *J Allergy Clin Immunol* 2007; **119**: 576–82.

9   Garovic VD, Hayman SR. Hypertension in pregnancy: an emerging risk factor for cardiovascular disease. *Nat Clin Pract Nephrol* 2007; **3**: 613–22.

10 Girouard J, Giguere Y, Moutquin J-M, Forest J-C. Previous hypertensive disease of pregnancy is associated with alterations of markers of insulin resistance. *Hypertension* 2007; **49**: 1056–62.

11 Callaway LK, Lawlor DA, O'Callaghan M, Williams GM, Najman JM, McIntyre HD. Diabetes mellitus in the 21 years after a pregnancy that was complicated by hypertension: findings from a prospective cohort study. *Am J Obstet Gynecol* 2007; **197**: 492.e1–7.

21 Pre-eclampsia

Case History

A 30-year-old woman presents for routine review. She is at 32 weeks of her first pregnancy. When she came last week, her blood pressure (BP) was 135/85 and urine was 1+ for protein. On this review, she has BP of 145/95 and urine is 2+ positive for protein on stick testing. She feels entirely well and her pregnancy has been, to date, uncomplicated. She would like to know what the implications of these findings are.

Do we have sufficient information to diagnose pre-eclampsia?

How should she be managed?

What does this mean for her pregnancy and for health of her baby?

Does it have any implications for future pregnancies and her future health?

Background

Pre-eclampsia is new onset of hypertension and proteinuria after 20 weeks' gestation, and occurs in 5–7% of pregnancies (Figure 21.1).[1,2] The aetiology is not completely understood. Oedema is no longer a diagnostic criterion. In women with chronic hypertension, pre-eclampsia is diagnosed if there is a sudden increase in BP or proteinuria develops (or previous proteinuria worsens). Eclampsia is defined as new-onset seizures in a woman who fulfils the criteria for pre-eclampsia and has no other reason for seizures. It occurs in <1% of women with pre-eclampsia. Seizures may occur before (40%), during (40–50%) or after delivery (15%). In the clinic, proteinuria is routinely assessed by stick testing (Box 21.1). When urine is positive for protein on stick testing, this should always be confirmed on a separate occasion at least 48 hours later, and when urinary tract infection has been excluded. Protein excretion should then be quantified precisely. Diagnostic criteria are:

- Pre-eclampsia
  - Systolic BP ≥140 mmHg and/or diastolic BP ≥90 mmHg
  - Patient had previous normal BP and is >20 weeks' gestation
  - Proteinuria >300 mg in 24 h

- Severe pre-eclampsia
  - Systolic BP ≥160 mmHg and/or diastolic BP ≥110 mmHg
  - Proteinuria >3000 mg in 24 h

● Other features – oliguria (<400 ml in 24 h), headache, visual disturbance, pulmonary oedema, low platelets (<100 000 per ml), liver enzymes more than twice normal, intrauterine growth restriction (IUGR).

Elevated BP should always be confirmed on a second occasion at least 6 hours later after the patient is rested. Low-dose (75–100 mg daily) aspirin is not routinely recommended for women at low risk of pre-eclampsia, but may modestly decrease risk in those who are predisposed. Low calcium intake is associated with high BP in pregnancy and supplementation (1000 mg per day) should be considered where dietary intake is low. The patient should abstain from alcohol and smoking, and maintain physical activity. Severe salt or calorie restriction should be avoided.

Box 21.1 Urinary protein excretion

● Normal: <150 mg per 24 h
● Microalbuminuria: 30–300 mg per 24 h
● 1+ positive: >300 mg/litre
● 2+ positive: >1000 mg/litre
● 3+ positive: >3000 mg/litre

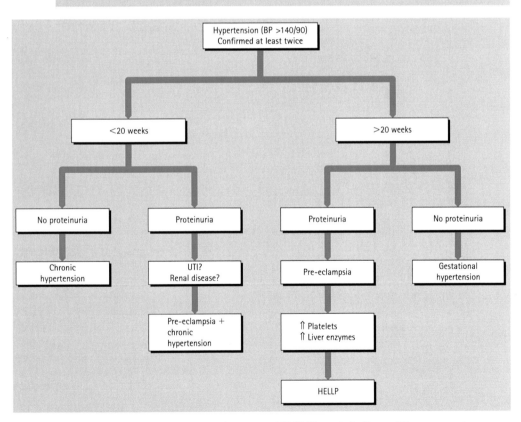

Figure 21.1 Hypertensive disorders of pregnancy. HELLP, (Haemolysis, Elevated Liver enzymes, Low Platelets); UTI, urinary tract infection.

The initiating event is thought to be decreased placental perfusion with resultant ischaemia and hypoxia,[3] leading to the release of vasoactive substances including soluble fms-like tyrosine kinase 1 (sFlt1), autoantibodies to angiotensin II receptor and cytokines (tumour necrosis factor-α). Endothelial dysfunction decreases nitric oxide release and increases endothelin-1, leading to increased total peripheral resistance and decreased natriuresis. Endothelial dysfunction also causes increased generation of reactive oxygen species (oxidative stress).

There is no diagnostic test. All women should be assessed for potential risk factors (Box 21.2). The only identified paternal risk factor is past history of fathering a pregnancy with pre-eclampsia. When hypertension and proteinuria is confirmed, further investigation should include full blood count (FBC) and coagulation screen (including platelet count), electrolytes and creatinine, and liver enzymes. Plasma urate is often increased, but this is not a specific marker. Biomarkers have been sought including markers of endothelial damage and dysfunction, inflammatory markers, markers of placental function and trophoblast invasion, and markers of maladaptation to paternal antigens. Uterine artery Doppler studies show increased resistance index and the presence of a diastolic notch.

Box 21.2 Risk factors for pre-eclampsia

Maternal factors	Pregnancy-associated
Age >35 or <20 years	Chromosomal abnormalities
Black race	Congenital anomalies
Nulliparous	Molar pregnancy
Previous or family history of pre-eclampsia	Multi-foetal pregnancy
Diabetes	Oocyte donation/donor insemination
Chronic hypertension	
Renal disease	
Connective tissue disease	
Antiphospholipid syndrome	

Uncomplicated pre-eclampsia does not require admission. Methyldopa and labetalol are the most widely used first-line drugs with nifedipine (long-acting) and hydralazine as second line. For urgent treatment of severe hypertension, IV labetalol or hydralazine are most frequently used, along with oral/sublingual short-acting nifedipine. Magnesium sulphate has now superseded phenytoin or diazepam for prophylactic treament of seizures. Typically, a 4–6 g loading dose is followed by an infusion of 1–2 g/h. Signs of magnesium toxicity include decreased conscious level, respiratory depression, absent deep tendon reflexes. The foetus should be carefully monitored for IUGR (weekly biophysical profile) or foetal distress (cardiotocography). Women with pre-eclampsia before 34 weeks of gestation should receive oral steroids to accelerate foetal lung maturation.

The condition resolves soon after delivery. Foetal indications for early delivery include severe IUGR or oligohydramnios. Maternal indications include suspected placental abruption, deteriorating renal or hepatic function, low platelets, eclamptic fits, symptoms (headache, visual disturbance, abdominal pain). Vaginal delivery is preferred where possible. Where Caesarean section is required, regional anaesthesia carries lower risk, except where there is a low platelet count or other coagulopathy. Platelet transfusion may be required before delivery. Also, high-dose dexamethasone (10 mg IV every 12 h) may used in HELLP (Haemolytic anaemia, Elevated Liver enzymes and Low Platelets) syndrome. Both mother and child should be carefully monitored following delivery. Hypertension may develop and seizures may occur in the days or weeks after delivery.

Recent Developments

1   Impaired endothelial function and vascular remodelling are major factors in the local and systemic effects of pre-eclampsia. Circulating anti-angiogenic factors increased in pre-eclampsia include sFlt1 (the soluble VEGF receptor-1) and soluble endoglin, a component of the transforming growth factor-β receptor complex.[4] The soluble VEGF receptor-2 has been reported to be decreased.[5] Vascular endothelial growth factor (VEGF) has recently been shown to have potential to improve features of pre-eclampsia in animal models.

2   A biomarker for developing pre-eclampsia would assist greatly in managing women at high risk. To date, no consistent protein marker has emerged. Recent studies[6,7] using antibodies to CD146 have demonstrated increased circulating levels.

3   Up to 1:5 women with pre-eclampsia may develop autoantibodies that activate the angiotensin II type 1 receptor.[8] These may arise because of disordered immune function in the foeto-placental unit during pregnancy and may contribute to the development of hypertension.

4   Pre-eclampsia is associated with increased future risk of cardiovascular disease. A meta-analysis[9] reported RR of hypertension of 3.70 (95% CI: 2.70 to 5.03), of ischaemic heart disease 2.16 (95% CI: 1.86 to 2.52) and stroke 1.81 (95% CI: 1.45 to 2.27). The latter finding is contrary to that of other studies including a very recent one[10] in which breast cancer was also reported to be decreased in women with previous pre-eclampsia.

5   Presence of chronic hypertension remains the most powerful predictor of pre-eclampsia. Chappell *et al.*[11] reported pre-eclampsia to occur in 22% of women with chronic hypertension. Half of these occurred before 34 weeks' gestation, and the risk was amplified in women who had previous pre-eclampsia or renal impairment.

6   Vitamin D deficiency in early pregnancy has recently been considered a risk factor.[12] Furthermore, vitamin D supplementation in infancy may protect against future development of pre-eclampsia.[13] This could be through its immunomodulatory effect, which is also thought to be responsible for the protective effect of vitamin D in relation to type 1 diabetes.

Conclusions

The level of BP (if confirmed) in this woman is sufficient to diagnose pre-eclampsia. Also, her proteinuria should be quantified by a timed collection of urine. An algorithm for managing pre-eclampsia is shown in Figure 21.2. The condition has significant

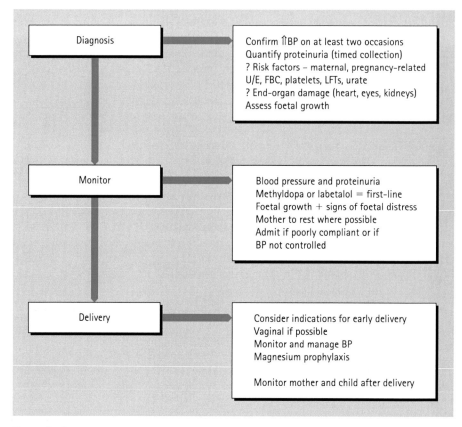

Figure 21.2 Monitoring a patient with pre-eclampsia. FBC, Full blood count; LFTs, liver function tests; U/E, urea and electrolytes.

implications for maternal and perinatal health. Pre-eclampsia affects more than 8 million women worldwide every year. It is associated with future development of insulin resistance and hypertension, and thus with increased cardiovascular risk. Patients with pre-eclampsia should be aware of this and have periodic monitoring of glucose, lipids and BP. They should avoid undue weight gain (compared with pre-pregnancy weight) following delivery and maintain physical fitness). Although pre-eclampsia is most likely to occur in a first pregnancy, those who have it once are more likely to develop it in a subsequent pregnancy.

References

1 Podymow T, August P. Update on the use of antihypertensive drugs in pregnancy. *Hypertension* 2008; **51**: 960–9.

2 Magee LA, Helewa M, Moutquin J-M, von Dadelszen P. Diagnosis, evaluation, and management of the hypertensive disorders of pregnancy. *J Obstet Gynaecol Can* 2008; **30** (Suppl 1): S1–48.

3 Gilbert JS, Ryan MJ, LaMarca BB, Sedeek M, Murphy SR, Granger JP. Pathophysiology of hypertension during pre-eclampsia: linking placental ischemia with endothelial dysfunction. *Am J Physiol* 2008; **294**: H541–50.

4 Maynard S, Epstein FH, Karumanchi SA. Pre-eclampsia and angiogenic imbalance. *Annu Rev Med* 2008: **59**: 61–78.

5 Chaiworapongsa T, Romero R, Gotsch F, Espinoza J, Nien JK, Goncalves L, *et al.* Low maternal concentrations of soluble vascular endothelial growth factor receptor-2 in pre-eclampsia and small for gestational age. *J Matern Fetal Neonat Med* 2008; **21**: 41–52.

6 Canbakan B, Keven K, Tutkak H, Danisman N, Ergun I, Nergizoglu G. Circulating endothelial cells in pre-eclampsia. *J Hum Hypertens* 2007; **21**: 558–63.

7 Grundmann M, Woywodt A, Kirsch T, Hollwitz B, Oehler K, Erdbruegger U, *et al.* Circulating endothelial cells: a marker of vascular damage in patients with pre-eclampsia. *Am J Obstet Gynecol* 2008; **198**: 317.e1–5.

8 Hubel CA, Wallukat G, Wolf M, Herse F, Rajakumar A, Roberts JM, *et al.* Agonistic angiotensin II type 1 receptor autoantibodies in postpartum women with a history of pre-eclampsia. *Hypertension* 2007; **49**: 612–17.

9 Bellamy L, Casas J-P, Hingorani AD, Williams DJ. Pre-eclampsia and risk of cardiovascular disease and cancer in later life: systematic review and meta-analysis. *BMJ* 2007; **335**: 974–80.

10 Terry MB, Perrin M, Salafia CM, Zhang FF, Neugut AI, Teitelbaum SL, *et al.* Pre-eclampsia, pregnancy-related hypertension, and breast cancer risk. *Am J Epidemiol* 2007; **165**: 1007–14.

11 Chappell LC, Enye S, Seed P, Briley AL, Poston L, Shennan AH. Adverse perinatal outcomes and risk factors for pre-eclampsia in women with chronic hypertension. *Hypertension* 2008; **51**: 1002–9.

12 Bodnar LM, Catov JM, Simhan HN, Holick MF, Powers RW, Roberts JM. Maternal vitamin D deficiency increases the risk of pre-eclampsia. *J Clin Endocrinol Metab* 2007; **92**: 3517–22.

13 Hypponen E, Hartikainen AL, Sovio U, Jarvelin MR, Pouta A. Does vitamin D supplementation in infancy reduce the risk of pre-eclampsia? *Eur J Clin Nutr* 2007; **61**: 1136–9.

PROBLEM

22 Patients of African Descent

Case History

Charles is a fit 53-year-old man of African descent. He is worried about his blood pressure (BP) – systolic BP currently consistently >160 mmHg and diastolic BP >100 mmHg. His 74-year-old mother is disabled following a stroke and his father died in his 60s from coronary artery disease. Charles has a very strong family history of hypertension and many members of his family have had difficulties in obtaining good BP control. He has tried antihypertensive treatment on two previous occasions but stopped because his pressure was not controlled. He has normal renal function and his ECG is within normal limits.

Why are black patients more susceptible to hypertension?

Are lifestyle interventions as effective in this racial group?

Do black subjects need a different approach to treatment?

Background

The prevalence of hypertension among black Americans is among the highest of any racial group, and appears to be increasing. Black subjects develop hypertension at an earlier stage in life and typically have higher levels of BP. Compared with Americans of European descent, African Americans have:[1]

- 50% higher mortality from coronary artery disease;

- Two times the incidence of stroke, and

- Four times the incidence of chronic kidney disease due to hypertension.

As in other populations, control of hypertension is only obtained in a minority, many are undiagnosed and the risk from hypertension has been amplified in recent years by the rising prevalence of obesity and diabetes. The prevalence of hypertension in the US black population is shown in Figure 22.1. Hawaiian/Pacific Islander and American Indian populations also have a high prevalence of hypertension and cardiovascular (CV) disease. Paradoxically, in spite of the high prevalence of hypertension, the prevalence of coronary artery disease is actually lower in black men compared with white American men. However, the prevalence is higher in black women compared with white women: in 2004, coronary artery disease was present in 9.4% and 6.0% of white men and women respectively, while comparable figures for the black population were 7.1% and 7.8%. The overall

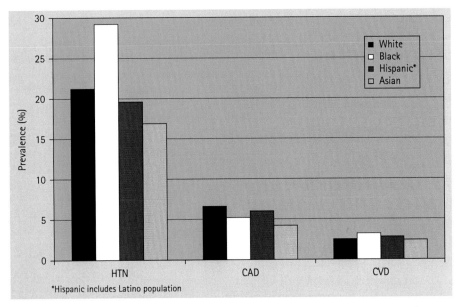

Figure 22.1 Prevalence of CVD in the USA. CAD, coronary artery disease; CVD, cardiovascular disease; HTN, hypertension.

Table 22.1 Cardiovascular disease prevalence and death rates in the USA

	Cardiovascular disease prevalence (%)	Annual death rate*
White female	35.0	115.4
White male	37.2	194.4
Black female	49.0	148.6
Black male	44.6	222.2

*Per 100 000 population.

prevalence of CV disease (including hypertension) and death rates from CV causes are shown in Table 22.1.

As in the USA, those of African descent in the UK also have a three- to four-fold risk of hypertension.[2] Also, the higher prevalence of hypertension translates into a higher incidence of stroke and chronic kidney disease. Prehypertension is also commoner in younger black people but not in older subjects because of the very high prevalence of hypertension. There is evidence that black subjects are more likely to have their hypertension detected than other racial groups, and this is attributed to an increased awareness of risk. However, the increased severity of hypertension in black subjects means that, in spite of early detection, they are no more likely to have well-controlled BP than other racial groups. This underlines the need for specific knowledge about the aetiology and treatment for this group, and need for specific treatment guidelines.

Hypertension is, to an extent, heritable but no single gene or combination of genes has yet been linked to the high prevalence of hypertension in this population. Renin levels tend to be low in black hypertensive subjects. This may suggest salt and water overload or that the renin–angiotensin system (RAS) is not involved. However, more recent studies have suggested that enhanced local RAS activity may contribute to the high prevalence of chronic kidney disease. Hypertension in the black population is characteristically salt-sensitive. No physiological basis for this has been adequately documented, although there is a strong association between salt sensitivity and obesity – over 70% of African American men and women are overweight. Abnormalities have been sought in the renal epithelial sodium channel, but there are no consistent data suggesting that this is involved in pathogenesis of hypertension. Some of the aetiological factors that have been documented in the general hypertensive population show a slightly exaggerated contribution. These include endothelial and nitric oxide mediated vasodilatation, enhanced sympathetic nervous system activity and increased endothelin generation. Low socio-economic status is a major contributor. This is strongly associated with obesity, low intake of fruit, vegetables and dairy produce, and compliance problems. Evidence suggests that lifestyle interventions are as effective in black as in white subjects.

An analysis[3] of 28 trials that reported results by racial subgroup has pulled together a very useful body of information. In ALLHAT (Antihypertensive and Lipid-Lowering Treatment to Prevent Heart Attack Trial), there was no difference between black and other racial groups for overall outcome (fatal and non-fatal coronary heart disease) but black participants derived a benefit from chlorthalidone for CV disease prevention ($P = 0.04$) and stroke ($P = 0.01$). The diuretic was modestly more effective than lisinopril in decreasing BP but this may not entirely account for the difference in risk reduction between the two drugs. In the LIFE (Losartan Intervention For Endpoint reduction) study, the preventative benefits of losartan were not apparent in the subgroup of black participants. Trial data suggest that the major antihypertensive classes have similar effects in decreasing systolic BP (except β-blockers) and all classes are similar in their effect on diastolic BP. β-blockers exert their beneficial effects partly through RAS and, in general, RAS-inhibiting drugs are not first-line choices for black patients although their organ-protecting effect is similar to that for other racial groups.

Recent Developments

1   In the ARIC (Atherosclerosis Risk in Communities) study,[4] 14 162 middle-aged adults free of CV disease at baseline were followed for 13 years. African Americans had higher rates of CV events than white people did. This was reflected in a higher prevalence of risk factors – 80% of African Americans had at least one risk factor compared with 60% of white people. Hypertension is particularly prominent as a risk factor in black populations. Data from the South London stroke register[5] has recently confirmed that the incidence of haemorrhagic stroke is higher in the black Caribbean and African populations.

2   AASK (African American Study of Kidney Disease and Hypertension)[6] compared metoprolol, amlodipine and ramipril in 1094 subjects with hypertensive kidney disease followed for a mean of 4.1 years. Patients were assigned to either a usual BP goal or a lower BP target. None of the groups differed in terms of CV events during follow-up. The study was relatively small for the complex design, and illustrates the need for good outcome studies in this population at high risk of hypertensive complications.

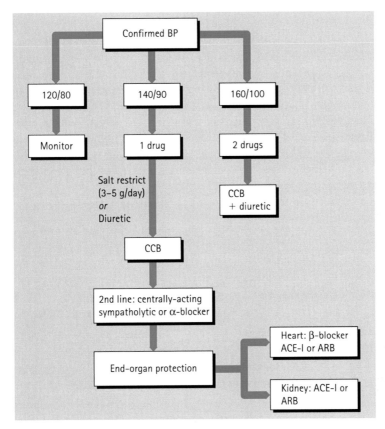

Figure 22.2 Hypertension in black subjects. ACE-I, angiotensin-converting enzyme inhibitor; ARB, angiotensin receptor blocker; CCB, calcium channel blocker.

3 The metabolic syndrome, prevalent in 1:4 adults, is equally present in black and white subjects. Hypertension makes a proportionately higher contribution to the metabolic syndrome in black subjects compared with white. The presence of metabolic syndrome components is strongly related to the presence of obesity. In MESA (the Multi-Ethnic Study of Atherosclerosis),[7] 60–85% of black subjects were overweight or obese. The high prevalence of metabolic syndrome factors among the overweight correlated with the presence of coronary artery calcification, increased carotid intima-media thickness, and Left Ventricular Mass Index.

4 Low-grade inflammation is present in overweight/obese subjects and correlates with risk of vascular disease. C-reactive protein levels are higher in black subjects, as shown in a recent report from SWAN (Study of Women's Health Across the Nation).[8] A substudy of AASK has documented that increased NT-proBNP (a marker for heart failure) predicts CV events in African Americans with hypertensive kidney disease.[9] Finally, a population-based, cross-sectional study of over 1400 middle-aged African Americans has shown a correlation between generalized or focal narrowing of retinal arteries and left ventricular hypertrophy.[10] These markers could be useful in clinical practice to identify high-risk patients.

Conclusions

The pathogenesis of hypertension in this racial group is incompletely understood. Many of the mechanisms implicated are similar to those generally documented, with the exception of increased salt sensitivity and lesser activation of RAS. The importance of socioeconomic factors in the high prevalence of hypertension and the apparent poor response to treatment should not be forgotten. Lifestyle interventions are at least as effective in black subjects – in particular, salt restriction and weight reduction are likely to have an impact. Drugs that have a principal effect on RAS are not first-line in this ethnic group, although are indicated where end-organ protection is required (Figure 22.2). Diuretics and calcium channel blockers are regarded as first-line agents. From trials, most agents will decrease systolic BP by 3–15 mmHg, and diastolic BP by 2–10 mmHg. Combination treatments are generally required.

References

1   Gadegbeku CA, Lea JP, Jamerson KA. Update on the disparities in the pathophysiology and management of hypertension: focus on African Americans. *Med Clin North Am* 2005; **89**: 921–33.

2   Yip GYH, Barnett AH, Bradbury A, Cappuccio FP, Gill PS, Hughes E, *et al.* Ethnicity and cardiovascular disease prevention in the United Kingdom: a practical approach to management. *J Hum Hypertens* 2007; **21**: 183–211.

3   Park IU, Taylor AL. Race and ethnicity in trials of antihypertensive therapy to prevent cardiovascular outcomes: a systematic review. *Ann Fam Med* 2007; **5**: 444–52.

4   Hozawa A, Folsom AR, Sharrett AR, Chambless LE. Absolute and attributable risks of cardiovascular disease incidence in relation to optimal and borderline risk factors: comparison of African American with white subjects – Atherosclerosis Risk in Communities Study. *Arch Intern Med* 2007; **167**: 573–9.

5   Smeeton NC, Heuschmann PU, Rudd AG, McEvoy AW, Kitchen ND, Sarker SJ, *et al.* Incidence of hemorrhagic stroke in black Caribbean, black African, and white populations: the South London stroke register, 1995–2004. *Stroke* 2007; **38**: 3133–8.

6   Norris K, Bourgoigne J, Gassman J, Hebert L, Middleton J, Phillips RA, *et al.* Cardiovascular outcomes in the African American Study of Kidney Disease and Hypertension (AASK) Trial. *Am J Kidney Dis* 2006; **48**: 739–51.

7   Burke GL, Bertoni AG, Shea S, Tracy R, Watson KE, Blumenthal RS, *et al.* The impact of obesity on cardiovascular disease risk factors and subclinical vascular disease: the Multi-Ethnic Study of Atherosclerosis. *Arch Intern Med* 2008; **168**: 928–35.

8   Kelley-Hedgepeth A, Lloyd-Jones DM, Colvin A, Matthews KA, Johnston J, Sowers MR, *et al.* Ethnic differences in C-reactive protein concentrations. *Clin Chem* 2008; **54**: 1027–37.

9   Astor BC, Yi S, Hiremath L, Corbin T, Pogue V, Wilkening B, *et al.* N-terminal prohormone brain natriuretic peptide as a predictor of cardiovascular disease and mortality in blacks with hypertensive kidney disease: the African American Study of Kidney Disease and Hypertension (AASK). *Circulation* 2008; **117**: 1685–92.

10 Tikellis G, Arnett DK, Skelton TN, Taylor HW, Klein R, Couper DJ, *et al.* Retinal arteriolar narrowing and left ventricular hypertrophy in African Americans. The Atherosclerosis Risk in Communities (ARIC) study. *Am J Hypertens* 2008; **21**: 352–9.

23 Patients of Asian Indian Descent

Case History

Jagdeep is 42 years old and accepts that the time has come to start drug treatment for hypertension. He is an accountant who has a busy working and family life. He is not currently taking any medications. ECG and renal function are normal. He tries to keep fit but has become moderately overweight in the past 5 years. He has a strong family history of hypertension. His father and two uncles developed coronary artery disease in their 50s.

Are there particular considerations in managing hypertension in Indian patients?

What drugs should be used as first-line treatments?

Are there specific treatment goals?

Background

Hypertension is a major public health problem in India and in Indian migrant populations. As in other populations, hypertension is considered to be present when systolic blood pressure (BP) is >140 mmHg or diastolic BP is >90 mmHg. Cardiovascular (CV) disease accounted for about 2.3 million deaths in India in 1990, and this is projected to double by 2020. In India, hypertension accounts for the equivalent of 57% of all strokes and 24% of all coronary artery disease. It is present in 25% of adult urban and 10% of rural populations. In all, 60.4 million Indian men and 52.6 million Indian women have hypertension. This has risen steadily over the past five decades, and by 2025 there will be 107.3 million Indian men and 106.2 million Indian women with hypertension.

The increased risk of rural dwelling Asians in recent years is also being seen in migrant populations. In the UK, 7.9% of the population are from minority ethnic groups, accounting for a total of 4.6 million people.[1] Asian or British Asian subjects account for just over 50% of the total ethnic minority population. Despite ethnic minority populations having a younger age structure than the general British population, they have a 50% increased risk of premature CV death. Furthermore, the death rate from CV disease is not falling as rapidly as it is in the general population, meaning that the disparity is increasing. Between the 1970s and the 1990s, the risk of CV death in the 20–69-year-old general British population fell by 29% and 17% for men and women, respectively, while the corresponding figures for the British Asian population were only 20% and 7%. The prevalence of hypertension is slightly higher in the Asian population, but the prevalence of the metabolic syndrome, impaired glucose tolerance and obesity are markedly increased. The age-standardized rate of diabetes is increased by three- to six-fold compared with Caucasians, meaning that diabetes is diagnosed in up to 17% of Indian Asian adults. Recent studies of Indian migrants in Singapore, North America, and the UK[2] suggest that the increased CV risk of migrant populations relates largely to increased fat consumption and increased obesity. In Asians, increased fat mass translates readily into insulin resistance, obesity and prediabetic/prehypertensive states.

Box 23.1 A simple risk calculator

Risk factors	Target-organ damage	Associated clinical
Age >55	Left ventricular hypertrophy	Stroke/transient ischaemic attack
Male gender	Albuminuria	Coronary heart disease
Postmenopausal	Carotid stenosis	Chronic kidney disease
Diabetes	Retinopathy	Peripheral vascular disease
Family history of coronary artery disease		Advanced retinopathy
Increased waist–hip ratio		
Dyslipidaemia		
High C-reactive protein		
Estimated glomerular filtration rate <60		

Other history	Blood pressure (mmHg)		
	Stage 1	Stage 2	Stage 3
	SBP 140–159	SBP 160–179	SBP ≥180
	DBP 90–99	DBP 100–109	DBP ≥110
No other risk factors	Low	Medium	High
1–2 risk factors	Medium	Medium	Very high
3 or more risk factors, target-organ damage or diabetes	High	High	Very high
Macrovascular disease present	Very high	Very high	Very high

Risk strata (10-year risk of myocardial infarction or stroke):

- low: <15%
- medium: 15–20%
- high: 20–30%
- very high: ≥30%

Globally, stroke is the most common cause of adult disability and the third most common cause of death. Incidence of stroke closely parallels the prevalence of hypertension. A total of 3.5 million of the 5.5 million strokes that occur annually in the world occur in developing countries. The high incidence of stroke in Indian Asians is a matter of major concern. Generally, the age-adjusted incidence of stroke is 100–300/100 000 of the population per annum. This is increased by up to 50% in Indian populations. The cost of acute care, rehabilitation and ongoing social care is enormous. The majority of strokes are thromboembolic. In Caucasians, 8–15% of strokes are haemorrhagic. The proportion of strokes that are lacunar (small vessel) or haemorrhagic is about two-fold higher in Indians. This reflects the high prevalence respectively of glucose intolerance and hypertension.

The principles of non-pharmacological management of hypertension are similar to those in other groups. Even modest weight loss can improve BP control. Adherence to a DASH (Dietary Approaches to Stop Hypertension)-type diet and restriction of alcohol intake are important. Smoking is the most potent single modifiable risk factor. Salt should be restricted to 6 g (<2.4 g sodium) per day in a temperate climate but this may be relaxed in warmer climates. Indian cooking typically involves high salt usage. Patients should be advised to curtail this and to restrict foods high in salt such as pickles, chutneys, processed foods, or those with a large amount of baking powder. Barriers to, and inhibitions about, exercise are gradually lifting. Heavy isometric exercises such as weight-lifting should be avoided in those with poorly controlled BP. Yoga, meditation and biofeedback may all help to lower BP.

For pharmacotherapy, five classes are considered suitable as first-line agents – diuretics, β-blockers, calcium channel blockers, angiotensin-converting enzyme (ACE) inhibitors and angiotensin receptor blockers. Large-scale drug trials focusing on Asians are lacking. Considerations about choice of drug do not differ substantially from those for Caucasians. Low-dose diuretic is generally the first line. There is a tendency to hyperglycaemia and dyslipidaemia, but the strong evidence base suggesting that diuretics protect against CV events offsets this. β-blockers are no longer favoured as first-line agents and their combination with diuretics should be avoided in this population because of risk of inducing or worsening diabetes. Younger patients are more likely to have high renin–angiotensin system activity and thus benefit from ACE inhibitors or angiotensin receptor blockers. Calcium channel blockers are indicated in the elderly, including those with isolated systolic hypertension. α-blockers have particular appeal as second- or third-line agents in Indians as they may improve insulin resistance. Where needed, specific drugs for organ protection should be used in high-risk patients including those with diabetes, cardiac disease or chronic kidney disease. Long-acting agents and fixed dose combinations should be considered to improve compliance. To avoid side effects synergistic low-dose combinations are preferred to using high doses of single drugs.

Recent Developments

1   The relative contribution of genetic and environmental factors to hypertension in Indians has not been extensively studied. A study[3] involving 508 families with 1250 non-twin sibpairs and 463 spouse pairs has addressed this. Concordance rates for diabetes, hypertension and metabolic syndrome among sibs were 11%, 14% and 23%, respectively. Corresponding figures among spouse pairs were 4.8%, 6.3% and 28.1%. Type 2 diabetes and hypertension have strong genetic influences, whereas metabolic syndrome appears to be predominantly environmental. Among possible genetic influences, polymorphisms in the ACE and MTHFR genes have been studied in Indians. The T allele of the MTHFR gene is associated with decreased enzyme

activity and therefore increased homocysteine levels. An association with stroke was documented. The ACE DD allele is associated with higher plasma ACE and increased risk of hypertension.

2   The prevalence of hypertension in Indian children and adolescents is increasing as being overweight or obese becomes more common.[4] BP begins to increase steeply at a body mass index above 20 in boys and 21.5 in girls. Given the CV risk of the Indian population, screening at-risk children for hypertension should be undertaken and lifestyle factors need to be addressed from an early stage.

3   Dietary salt intake is a major issue. In the Chennai Urban Rural Epidemiology Study (CURES),[5] detailed dietary histories were taken from 2220 subjects. The mean salt intake was 8.5 g/day – well above the recommended level. High income and older age were both associated with higher salt intake. Both systolic BP and diastolic BP increased with quintiles of increasing salt intake. Focus on this alone could significantly impact on the prevalence of hypertension.

4   In Asian populations, there is a strong relationship between the presence of hypertension or diabetes and the risk of CV death,[6] irrespective of whether the individual is in their country of ethnic origin or overseas. Indeed dietary change in the latter circumstance may lead to increased risk. Although awareness of the risk of hypertension has increased among Indian Asians, many patients still have undetected or undertreated hypertension.[7]

5   Polycystic ovary syndrome presents in a variable way with menstrual disturbances, subfertility and hirsutism. There is increased risk of hypertensive and hyperglycaemic complications of pregnancy, and increased CV risk through these factors in later life. In the Indian subcontinent, as in other parts of the world, polycystic ovary syndrome is being increasingly diagnosed, partly through increased awareness, but also because of increasing prevalence of obesity.[8]

Conclusions

There is considerable concern about the high prevalence of hypertension and diabetes in patients of Indian origin, whether they are living in India or as migrants. The high prevalence places this ethnic group at particular risk of chronic kidney disease, stroke and other CV complications. While the broad principles of managing hypertension are similar to those in other ethnic groups, several factors should be borne in mind: (1) dietary intake of salt is high, and if this cannot be decreased then appropriate diuretic therapy should be initiated; (2) diuretics and β-blocker treatment should be monitored because of the high risk of diabetes. The two should not be used together unless there is a specific indication for both; and (3) there is a particular risk from hypertension and other metabolic syndrome components in this population. A target BP of 140/90 is reasonable but a lower target is appropriate for high-risk (e.g. diabetic or chronic kidney disease). An algorithm for BP management in Indian subjects is presented in Figure 23.1.

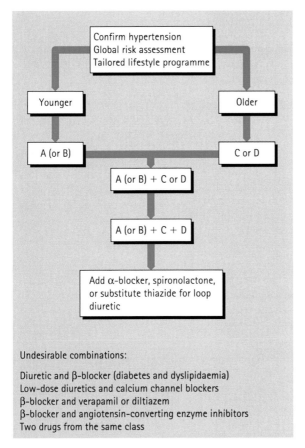

Figure 23.1 Treatment of hypertension in Indians. A = angiotensin-converting enzyme inhibitor or angiotensin receptor blocker; B = β-blocker; C = calcium channel blocker; D = diuretic.

References

1   Lip GYH, Barnett AH, Bradbury A, Cappuccio FP, Gill PS, Hughes E, *et al.* Ethnicity and cardiovascular disease prevention in the United Kingdom: a practical approach to management. *J Hum Hypertens* 2007; **21**: 183–211.

2   Patel JV, Vyas A, Cruikshank JK, Prabhakaran D, Hughes E, Reddy KS, *et al.* Impact of migration on coronary heart disease risk factors: comparison of Gujaratis in Britain and their contemporaries in villages of origin in India. *Atherosclerosis* 2006; **185**: 297–306.

3   Shnaker J, Kanjilal S, Rao VS, Perumal G, Khadrinarasimhiah NB, Mukerjee M, *et al.* Adult nontwin concordance rates for type 2 diabetes, hypertension and metabolic syndrome among Asian Indians: The Indian Atherosclerosis Research Study. *Vasc Health Risk Manage* 2007; **3**: 1063–8.

4   Rao S, Kanade A, Kelkar R. Blood pressure among overweight adolescents from urban school children in Pune, India. *Eur J Clin Nutr* 2007; **61**: 633–41.

5   Radhika G, Sathya RM, Sudha V, Ganesan A, Mohan V. Dietary salt intake and hypertension in an Urban South Indian Population – CURES-53. *J Assoc Physicians India* 2007; **55**: 405–10.

6   Nakagami T, Qiao Q, Tuomilehto J, Balkau B, Tajima N, Hu G, *et al.* Screen-detected diabetes, hypertension and hypercholesterolemia as predictors of cardiovascular mortality in five populations of Asian origin: the DECODA study. *Eur J Cardiovasc Prev Rehab* 2006; **13**: 555–61.

7   Mohan V, Deepa M, Farooq S, Datta M, Deepa R. Prevalence, awareness and control of hypertension in Chennai – The Chennai Urban Rural Epidemiology Study (CURES-52). *J Assoc Physicians India* 2007; **55**: 326–32.

8   Allahbadia GN, Merchant R. Polycystic ovary syndrome in the Indian Subcontinent. *Semin Reprod Med* 2008; **26**: 22–34.

Complications and Emergencies

PROBLEM

24 Hypertensive Emergency

Case History

Mrs AH is 48 years old and has been treated for hypertension for 6 years. She complies irregularly with her medication (hydrochlorthiazide, candesartan and amlodipine). Clinic blood pressures (BPs) are usually high. She presents with a 2-day history of headache and blurring of vision. BP is 220/140 and she has flame haemorrhages and papilloedema on fundoscopy. She has no chest pain or breathlessness and her lungs are clear on auscultation. She is obese (body mass index 31 kg/m²) but her general health is good.

What is the definition of hypertensive emergency?

What are the common precipitating factors?

How should the condition be managed acutely?

What follow-up treatment and investigation is required?

Background

It is probably reasonable to regard the terms of 'malignant hypertension', 'hypertensive crisis', 'hypertensive emergency' and 'accelerated (phase) hypertension' as being synonymous. Although now a relatively uncommon medical emergency thanks to the general improvement in hypertension management in recent years, it still occurs. Hypertensive emergency affects less than 1% of hypertensive patients, but this is up to 500 000 patients in the USA alone. The term implies severe hypertension (diastolic BP >120 mmHg) with end-organ damage (cerebral, renal or cardiac) and necessitates urgent admission and acute lowering of BP.[1,2] Where severe hypertension is not accompanied by end-organ damage, the term 'hypertensive urgency' has been used and implies a less acute state in which BP can be lowered over 24–48 h.

Hypertensive emergency most commonly occurs with pre-existing hypertension. Aetiological factors are summarized in Box 24.1. The condition is an acute failure of autoregulation with an increase in systemic vascular resistance. Decreased tissue perfusion, which is worsened by platelet deposition, places end organs at risk of ischaemia. Although uncommon, it is serious, and makes effective outpatient management of hypertension mandatory, particularly if BP is very high.

Box 24.1 **Causes of hypertensive emergency**

- Withdrawal from antihypertensive drugs (especially clonidine)
- Alcohol withdrawal
- Sympathomimetics (cocaine, amphetamines, lysergic acid diethylamide LSD)
- Renovascular or renal parenchymal disease, acute glomerulonephritis
- Scleroderma, vasculitic
- Phaeochromocytoma
- Renin or aldosterone secreting tumours
- Pre-eclampsia, eclampsia
- Autonomic hyperactivity (Guillain–Barré and other spinal syndromes)
- Head injury

Fundoscopy is almost always abnormal, and may reveal haemorrhages (flame-shaped, blot), changes in arteriolar calibre with arteriovenous nipping, exudates (hard and soft), or papilloedema. Left ventricular failure is the most common cardiovascular manifestation (increased jugular venous pressure, bilateral crackles, added heart sounds). The patient should be asked about chest pain, and signs of ischaemia sought on the electrocardiogram (ECG). Aortic dissection and gastrointestinal ischaemia should also be considered. Neurological manifestations include disorientation, decreased consciousness, focal neurological signs, and seizures. The term 'hypertensive encephalopathy' is used where there is generalized neurological deficit. Cerebral infarction and pulmonary oedema each occur in about 25% of hypertensive emergencies. Encephalopathy, heart failure and unstable angina/myocardial infarction are about half as common. Intracerebral bleed including subarachnoid haemorrhage occurs in about 1:20.

Electrolytes and renal function should be checked. Secondary hyperaldosteronism occurs in up to 50% and may lead to hypokalaemia. Full blood count (FBC) may reveal microangiopathic haemolytic anaemia. Metabolic acidosis may occur where there is renal impairment. ECG may show left ventricular hypertrophy where there has been previous sustained hypertension. All patients should be monitored in a high-dependency area with telemetry. A chest X-ray should be requested to assess cardiac size, exclude dissection and to diagnose pulmonary oedema. Urinalysis will show proteinuria – an important clue to the diagnosis of hypertensive emergency. Haematuria or urine casts are strongly suggestive of glomerular disease. Specialized investigations are not generally required in the acute phase. Computed tomography should be carried out if aortic dissection is suspected. Renal artery Doppler, magnetic resonance angiogram, or contrast angiogram should be considered in patients with suspected renovascular disease.

Untreated, a mortality rate of up to 90% is estimated. The condition requires urgent treatment. Management is highly dependent on the clinical setting. Aim to decrease BP by 20% over 1–2 h, slower if there is cardiac or cerebral ischaemia. The following agents are used acutely.

- Sodium nitroprusside: IV at a dose of 0.3–10 μg/kg per min. Use for no longer than 2 days as it may cause cyanide toxicity. Rash and flushing may occur, and increased intracerebral pressure has been described. Nitroprusside is a direct vasodilator. Continuous arterial BP monitoring is advised. Prolonged or excessive use can lead to thiocyanate toxicity (nausea, vomiting, clouding of consciousness and lactic acidosis).

- Fenoldopam mesylate (Corlopam): IV at an initial rate of 0.03–0.1 μg/kg per min. This agent, is a dopamine D_{1A} receptor antagonist, which through renal receptors stimulates natriuresis and through its vascular receptor decreases afterload. Reflex tachycardia is common.

- Glyceryl trinitrate (GTN): IV at an initial rate of 5 μg/min, increased by 5μg/min every 10 min until there is an effect. GTN is particularly indicated when there is ischaemic chest pain or cardiac failure.

- Esmolol (Brevibloc): a short-acting cardioselective β_1-blocker is given as an IV loading dose of 500 μg/kg per min over 1–2 min, followed by a maintenance dose of 50 μg/kg/min for up to 24 hours.

These agents are potent and should be used in the intensive care setting. Enalaprilat (Vasotec IV) is available in some countries, and is the active form of enalapril. Given as a slow injection of 1.25 mg every 6 hours, it is useful where there is pulmonary oedema. Other agents that may be useful are:

- Labetalol: given as an IV bolus of 20–80 mg over 10 min. More potent and cardio-specific β-blockers are indicated in acute coronary syndrome. Oral labetalol is useful in hypertensive urgency where 100–200 mg can be administered initially and repeated at 6 hours. Labetalol also has a rapid onset (10–15 minutes).

- Nicardipine (2–10 mg/h) or nimodipine (1–2 mg/h): short-acting β-blockers are useful in cerebral ischaemic emergencies and in hypertensive encephalopathy, and also to decrease vasospasm after subarachnoid haemorrhage.

- Methyldopa (250–1000 mg) and hydralazine 10–20 mg): direct vasodilators that can be administered by IV bolus every 6 hours. Used in pregnancy as they are known to be safe.

Management is summarized in Figure 24.1. When the need to decrease the BP within a few hours is not critical, the term 'hypertensive urgency' has been used. This does not

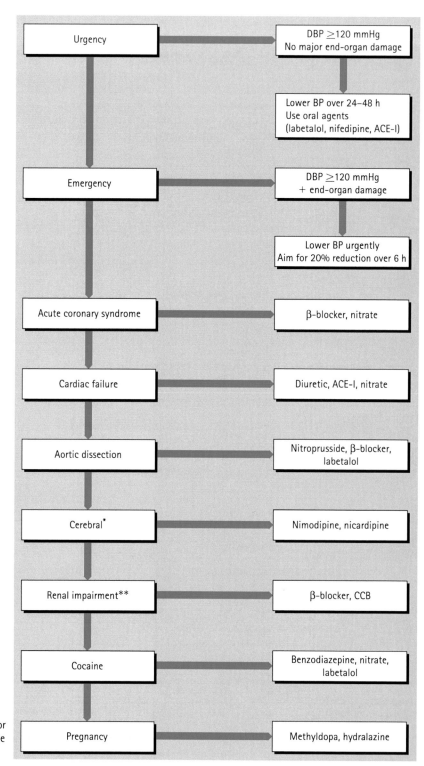

Figure 24.1 Management of hypertensive urgency and emergency. ACE-I, angiotensin-converting enzyme inhibitor; *Ischaemia, haemorrhage or encephalopathy. **Avoid ACE-Is or angiotensin receptor blockers in the acute phase

necessarily require use of IV agents. Oral agents that are useful include labetalol, short-acting nifedipine, and angiotensin-converting enzyme inhibitors. The aim is to achieve reasonable BP control (<160/100 mmHg) within 24–48 h.

Recent Developments

1 Cocaine use has increased rapidly over the past two decades such that it is now the most commonly used illicit drug. Cocaine, as the hydrochloride salt, is either sniffed or dissolved in water. Crack cocaine is not acid neutralized and can be smoked or inhaled when heated. In the USA, there are an estimated 2 million cocaine users and 0.5 million crack cocaine users, with over 30 million having used the drugs at one time. Cocaine causes intense sympathetic overdrive with vasoconstriction, and is an increasing cause of hypertensive emergency. Thrombotic microangiopathy with intravascular haemolysis and thrombocytopenia occurs in hypertensive emergency. It has been recognized with cocaine-induced hypertensive crisis,[3] as has acute aortic dissection.[4]

2 There are ethnic differences in the incidence of hypertensive emergency, being more common in black subjects.[5] This is partly biological as hypertension is commoner in black subjects and often harder to control. There may also be underlying socio-economic factors that lead to poorer medication compliance.

3 Renin and aldosterone are often markedly elevated in hypertensive emergency, and this correlates with markers of microvascular haemolysis and renal impairment. Increased aldosterone with suppressed renin is strongly suggestive that primary mineralocorticoid excess may be the cause.[6] A genetic predisposition to hypertensive crisis may also operate through the renin–angiotensin system. The TT genotype of the M235T polymorphism in the angiotensinogen gene has been linked with risk of hypertensive crisis.[7]

4 Computer-based methods to analyse the retinal vasculature on digital images show considerable promise for predicting severe hypertension. Subtle changes in vascular geometry are predictive of hypertensive crisis.[8] While some of these can be appreciated during ophthalmoscopic examination, precise quantification of vessel length, diameter, wall thickness, tortuosity and branching may yield a more quantitative index.

5 Oral phosphodiesterase 5 inhibitors (PDE5) are widely used for the treatment of erectile dysfunction, and work by inhibiting the breakdown of cyclic guanosine monophosphate. Hypotension occurs occasionally with use of these agents because of vasodilatation. This can be used to good effect in hypertensive emergency – sildenafil has a synergistic effect with sodium nitroprusside.[9] The combined approach may help minimize the dose of nitroprusside, and thus lessen the risk of thiocyanate accumulation.

Conclusions

Hypertensive crisis is an emergency where severe hypertension is accompanied by cere-bral, cardiac or renal impairment. It occurs in up to 1% of patients with hypertension, and demands urgent treatment to lower BP within minutes to hours. It usually occurs in patients with pre-existing hypertension and is associated with poor compliance and withdrawal of medications (clonidine, β-blockers). Where possible, the patient should be urgently admitted to a high dependency area. IV medication is needed if there is clouding of consciousness or evolving end-organ damage. Choice of agent depends on circumstances (Figure 24.1). Diuretics are best avoided unless there is evidence of volume expansion. The patient should be closely followed-up. Renal and cardiac function should be monitored closely, and the treatment kept as simple as possible to ensure maximum compliance. While it is not a common medical emergency now, it does carry a high risk of mortality or end-organ damage.

References

1   Aggarwal M, Khan IA. Hypertensive crisis: hypertensive emergencies and urgencies. *Cardiol Clin* 2006; **24**: 135–46.

2   Flanigan JS, Vitberg D. Hypertensive emergency and severe hypertension: what to treat, who to teat, and how to treat. *Med Clin North Am* 2006; **90**: 439–51.

3   Gu X, Herrera GA. Thrombotic microangiopathy in cocaine abuse-associated malignant hypertension: report of 2 cases with review of the literature. *Arch Pathol Lab Med* 2007; **131**: 1817–20.

4   Singh S, Trivedi A, Adhikari T, Molnar J, Arora R, Khosla S. Cocaine-related acute aortic dissection: patient demographics and clinical outcomes. *Can J Cardiol* 2007; **23**: 1131–4.

5   van den Born B-JH, Koopmans RP, Groeneveld JO, van Montfrans GA. Ethnic disparities in the incidence, presentation and complications of malignant hypertension. *J Hypertens* 2006; **24**: 2299–304.

6   Labinson PT, White WB, Tendler BE, Mansoor GA. Primary hyperaldosteronism associated with hypertensive emergencies. *Am J Hypertens* 2006; **19**: 623–7.

7   van den Born B-JH, van Montfrans GA, Uitterlinden AG, Zwinderman AH, Koopmans RP. The M235T polymorphism in the angiotensinogen gene is associated with the risk of malignant hypertension in white patients. *J Hypertens* 2007; **25**: 2227–33.

8   van den Born B-JH, Koopmans RP, van Montfrans GA. The renin–angiotensin system in malignant hypertension revisited: plasma renin activity, microangiopathic hemolysis, and renal failure in malignant hypertension. *Am J Hypertens* 2007; **20**: 900–6.

9   Bahadur MM, Aggarwal VD, Mali M, Thamba A. Novel therapeutic option in hypertensive crisis: sildenafil augments nitroprusside-induced hypotension. *Nephrol Dial Transplant* 2005; **20**: 1254–6.

25 Coronary Artery Disease

Case History

Albert is 59 years old and has recovered well from his first myocardial infarction (MI) 8 months ago. He has occasional mild chest pain with exertion, readily relieved by inhaled nitrate. The MI was uncomplicated, and he was discharged taking aspirin 100 mg OD, metoprolol 25 mg BD and simvastatin 20 mg OD. His blood pressure (BP) is persistently elevated at >150/95. He is a non-smoker and, although he used to be a heavy drinker, he now takes very little alcohol. Renal function is normal and there is no evidence of heart failure. He is stressed as he looks after his wife who is quite disabled by multiple sclerosis.

What is the best way to control his BP?

Are there any drugs we should be cautious about in this situation?

Do long-acting nitrates contribute to BP control?

Background

Globally, coronary artery disease (CAD) is responsible for over 3.3 million deaths annually.[1] Death rate is 254 per 100 000 per year, with higher rates in poorer and underdeveloped parts of the world. It is estimated that 54% of strokes and 47% of coronary events are attributable to high BP, half of this being due to hypertension and half due to increased BP in the range currently regarded as normal. An estimated 79.4 million people (1:3 adults) in the USA alone have cardiovascular (CV) disease. Among these, 72 million are hypertensive. An estimated 15.8 million Americans have CAD with 7.9 million having had previous MI and 8.9 million suffering from angina. CAD accounts for 1:5 deaths in developed countries and in the USA each year there are 840 000 patients admitted with acute coronary syndrome. The average age at first MI is 65.8 years for men and 70.4 years for women. At age 40, the lifetime risk for a coronary event is 49% for a man and 30% for a woman. The prevalence of both hypertension and CAD varies between racial groups (Table 25.1).

Managing hypertension is only one aspect of secondary prevention after acute MI. A number of guidelines are available, e.g. http://www.nice.org.uk/CG048, the main features of which are as follows:

1 Lifestyle factors:
   a Physical activity, 20–30 min/day at submaximal intensity.
   b Quit smoking.

Table 25.1 Prevalence of hypertension and coronary artery disease		
	Hypertension (%)	Coronary artery disease (%)
Caucasians	21.2	6.6
Black	29.2	5.2
Hispanic	19.6	6.0
Asian	16.9	4.2
Hawaiians, Pacific Islanders	20.7	13.8
American Indians	25.4	7.6

Data shown are from US statistics 2006.

c Mediterranean type diet.
d At least 7 g of omega-3 fatty acids/week (2–4 portions of oily fish). If not possible, consider 1 g/day of omega-3 acid ethyl esters.
e Limit alcohol intake: 21 units/week for men, 14 units/week for women.
f Maintain body weight as near the desired range as possible.

2 Cardiac rehabilitation (may be offered as a home programme, should involve partners and carers and take into account the overall needs of the patient):
a Physical activity guidance.
b Health education.
c Stress management.
d Advice on employment and return to work.

3 Drug treatment:
a Antiplatelet drugs: low-dose aspirin (with clopidogrel for 12 months after non-STEMI (non-ST Elevation Myocardial Infarction), for 4 weeks after STEMI). For those who are intolerant, consider warfarin, aiming for INR in the range 2–3.
b Angiotensin-converting enzyme inhibitors.
c β-blocker.
d Statin.

Many of the lifestyle modifications recommended after MI are helpful in maintaining BP control. Clearly, both the angiotensin-converting enzyme inhibitors (ACE-Is) and the β-blocker will favourably influence BP. β-blockers are initiated early after MI, but are no longer routinely used intravenously. β-blockers are less effective in decreasing BP in elderly subjects, and no longer considered to be first-line agents for hypertension control. Numerous trials including GISSI-3 (Gruppo Italiano per lo Studio della Sopravvivenza nell'Infarto Miocardico-3), ISIS-4 (Fourth International Study of Infarct Survival), SAVE (Survival and Ventricular Enlargement), AIRE (Acute Infarction Ramipril Efficacy) and CONSENSUS-II (Cooperative North Scandinavian Enalapril Survival Study II) have confirmed the value of ACE-Is in decreasing mortality after MI.[2] This benefit is not entirely due to the BP-lowering effect of ACE-Is. Even early after an acute MI, first dose hypotension is not a major problem. However, care should be taken in those who might have depleted intravascular volume because of diuretics and in elderly people who might have renal artery stenosis. Calcium channel blockers decrease coronary and peripheral vascular resistance. Early studies suggested that short-acting nifedipine was associated with increased reflex sympathetic activity that might predispose to arrhythmias. The longer-acting dihydropyridines amlodipine and felodipine are safe options for managing hypertension following MI. Similarly, verapamil and diltiazem can be considered if myocardial function is well preserved.

Very high BP (>200/120 mmHg) is a contraindication to thrombolysis. BP should be reduced to <160/110 mmHg before thrombolysis. For those in whom BP cannot be safely reduced, primary angioplasty is an option. Thrombolysis is also contraindicated where there are haemorrhagic complications of hypertension – retinopathy or haemorrhagic stroke. For urgent BP reduction in a patient with recent MI, IV nitrate or labetalol should be considered. BP should not be decreased too abruptly.

The largest trial involving subjects with non-acute CAD is the International Verapamil-Trandolapril Study,[3] involving 22 576 subjects with hypertension and CAD at 862 sites in 14 countries. Patients were randomized to a strategy based on verapamil with trandolapril added as needed or one based on atenolol with hydrochlorthiazide. Primary outcome was all-cause death or non-fatal MI or stroke. Mean follow-up was 2.7 years. There was no difference between the two groups either in primary outcome or in BP control. In each group, about 71% of patients achieved systolic BP <140 mmHg and diastolic BP <90 mmHg.

Endothelial dysfunction with loss of nitric oxide-mediated vasodilatation and consequent arterial stiffness is an important contributor to systolic hypertension in the elderly. The potential benefit of nitrate (nitric oxide donor) as an antihypertensive agent has been neglected. The major concern has been that nitrate tolerance will develop. However, with currently used preparations of long-acting nitrate this does not occur. Isorbide mononitrate at doses of 60–120 mg OD improves systolic BP and pulse wave reflection, with a benefit sustained for up 2 years.[4] Long-acting nitrates are often underprescribed and should certainly be considered when angina is accompanied by refractory hypertension.

Recent Developments

1   The VALIANT (VALsartan in Acute myocardial INfarcTion) study[5] has focused on young survivors of MI. While most MIs occur in older subjects, about 10% occur in patients under 45 years, with increased risk for males, smokers and those who are obese. The adjusted relative risk (RR) for a recurrent event with hypertension was 1.82 (95% CI: 1.3 to 2.6) for young subjects compared with 1.21 (95% confidence interval [CI]: 1.1 to 1.3) for older subjects.

2   A follow-up study (8.7 years) of hypertensive patients from the Skaraborg project[6] suggested that markers of end-organ damage (microalbuminuria and left ventricular hypertrophy) are more predictive of MI mortality in men, while markers of impaired glucose tolerance are more important in women. Further data from the VALIANT study[7] emphasized the importance of hypertension. Patients with uncontrolled BP were more likely to suffer stroke and other CV following MI.

3   CV risk factors, including hypertension, are highly prevalent among the first-degree relatives of patients with premature CV disease.[8] Variations in the genes that regulate BP are important determinants. Recent studies suggest that variations in the genes for angiotensinogen and the β_1-adrenoreceptor are implicated in susceptibility to CAD.

4 Patients at risk of CAD have abnormal vascular remodelling. Biomarkers reflecting this abnormality may be useful in predicting onset of CAD in high-risk patients. Recently, angiopoietin-2 (a mediator of angiogenesis) levels have been shown to be predictive of MI in hypertensive subjects.[9]

5 Patients with multiple CV risk factors are at increased risk of CV events and subsequent complications. For example, those with diabetes and hypertension are twice as likely to develop heart failure and other complications following MI compared with those with hypertension alone.[10]

Conclusions

 All patients should receive a β-blocker following MI. These are particularly beneficial with large infarcts, chronic circulatory failure or ventricular arrhythmia. β-blockers are

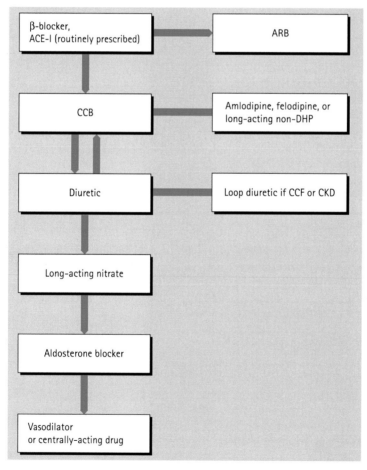

Figure 25.1 Hypertension following myocardial infarction. ACE-I, angiotensin-converting enzyme inhibitor; ARB, angiotensin receptor blocker; CCB, calcium channel blocker; CCF, congestive cardiac failure; CKD, chronic kidney disease; DHP, dihydropyridine

also useful for patients who have angina but have not suffered MI. Routine prescription of an ACE-I is also recommended following MI. An angiotensin receptor blocker is a suitable alternative where an ACE-I is not tolerated. However, many patients do not reach target BP and uncontrolled hypertension is an important risk factor for further CV events. Lifestyle factors should not be neglected. There is no antihypertensive class contraindicated in patients with CAD (Figure 25.1) – caution should be exercised with drugs that worsen the metabolic profile (hyperglycaemia and dyslipidaemia).

References

1   Lawes CMM, Vander Hoorn S, Rodgers A, International Society of Hypertension. Global burden of blood-pressure-related disease, 2001. *Lancet* 2008; **371**: 1513–18.

2   Lip GY, Lydakis C, Beevers DG. Management of patients with myocardial infarction and hypertension. *Eur Heart J* 2000; **21**: 1125–34.

3   Pepine CJ, Handberg EM, Cooper-DeHoff RM, Marks RG, Kowey P, Messerli FH, *et al.* A calcium antagonist vs a non-calcium antagonist hypertension treatment strategy for patients with coronary artery disease. The International Verapamil-Trandolapril Study (INVEST): a randomized controlled trial. *JAMA* 2003; **290**: 2805–16.

4   Stokes GS, Bune AJ, Huon N, Barin ES. Long-term effectiveness of extended-release nitrate for the treatment of systolic hypertension. *Hypertension* 2005; **45**: 380–4.

5   Anderson RE, Pfeffer MA, Thune JJ, McMurray JJV, Califf RM, Velazquez E, *et al.* High-risk myocardial infarction in the young: the VALsartan In Acute myocardial iNfarcTion (VALIANT) trial. *Am Heart J* 2008; **155**: 706–11.

6   Bog-Hansen E, Larsson CA, Gullberg B, Melander A, Bostrom K, Rastam L, *et al.* Predictors of acute myocardial infarction mortality in hypertensive patients treated in primary care: a population-based follow-up study in the Skaraborg Project. *Scand J Prim Health Care* 2007; **25**: 237–43.

7   Thune JJ, Signorovitch J, Kober L, Velazquez EJ, McMurray JJV, Califf RM, *et al.* Effect of antecedent hypertension and follow-up blood pressure on outcomes after high-risk myocardial infarction. *Hypertension* 2008; **51**: 48–54.

8   Hurrell C, Wietlisbach V, Jotterand V, Volet M, Lenain V, Nicod P, *et al.* High prevalence of major cardiovascular risk factors in first-degree relatives of individuals with familial premature coronary artery disease – the GENECARD project. *Atherosclerosis* 2007; **194**: 253–64.

9   Patel JV, Lim HS, Varughese GI, Hughes EA, Lip GYH. Angiopoietin-2 levels as a biomarker of cardiovascular risk in patients with hypertension. *Ann Med* 2008; **40**: 215–22.

10 Colivicchi F, Mettimano M, Genovesi-Ebert A, Schinzari F, Iantorno M, Melina G, *et al.* Differences between diabetic and non-diabetic hypertensive patients with first acute non-ST elevation myocardial infarction and predictors of in-hospital complications. *J Cardiovasc Med* 2008; **9**: 267–72.

26 Hypertension and Cardiac Failure

Case History

RW is a 72-year-old woman who experiences severe dyspnoea on moderate exertion. She has suffered two myocardial infarctions, but is not troubled with angina. She takes aspirin 100 mg OD, atenolol 25 mg BD and frusemide 40 mg omni mane. On examination, you find that she has bilateral basal crackles in her lungs and that her blood pressure (BP) is 170/92. She has cardiomegaly and mild pulmonary oedema on chest X-ray. Electrocardiogram (ECG) shows that she has voltage criteria for left ventricular (LV) hypertrophy with lateral ST depression. Her plasma B-type or brain natriuretic peptide (BNP) is elevated at 240 pg/ml. Echocardiogram reveals that she has a normal ejection fraction (EF) at 54%.

How would you assess and manage this patient?

Is hypertension an important component of her overall clinical picture?

What agents should be used to treat her BP, and what target should we aim for?

Background

Heart failure (HF) arises when the heart is unable to meet the metabolic demands of tissues, usually because of decreased cardiac function but sometimes because of increased demands. The annual cost of managing HF in the USA is $60 billion with the 1 million or so hospital admissions each year costing a total of about $23 billion. The cost of managing HF accounts for about 2% of the total healthcare budget. Men and women are equally affected but women tend to develop HF at an older age. It is commoner in subjects of African or Hispanic descent compared with Caucasians, and prevalence is also increased in many indigenous minority populations. Population prevalence of HF is about 4 per 1000 adults, rising to 3% of those aged ≥65 and over, and to 7% of those aged ≥75. In all, 5 million people in the USA are affected. The common causes are coronary artery disease, diabetes, hypertension, cardiomyopathy, valvular heart disease, pericardial disease and infection (including rheumatic fever). As causes of HF, coronary artery disease and diabetes have increased in recent years while hypertension and valvular heart disease have decreased. Although hypertension is the primary cause in much less than 10% of cases of HF, it is present in at least 40%. In spite of advances in management of HF, mortality remains high with about 60% dying within 5 years of diagnosis. This is worse than the overall prognosis from malignant disease (about 50% mortality in 5 years).

The cardinal symptoms of left ventricular failure are exertional dyspnoea, orthopnoea, paroxysmal nocturnal dyspnoea, cough, fatigue and weakness, along with decreased mental function and quality of life. Patients with advanced left ventricular failure (Box 26.1) experience dyspnoea at rest. Right ventricular failure is characterized by peripheral oedema, hepatomegaly, gastrointestinal congestion and elevated venous pressure.

Box 26.1 Staging of heart failure

1 New York Heart Association (NYHA) Classification
- Class I: No limitations. Ordinary physical activity does not cause undue fatigue, dyspnoea or palpitations.
- Class II: Slight limitation of physical activity. Comfortable at rest but ordinary activity results in fatigue, dyspnoea, palpitations or angina.
- Class III: Marked limitation of physical activity. Comfortable at rest but symptoms are provoked by less than ordinary levels of activity.
- Class IV: Symptomatic at rest. Symptoms increase with physical activity.

2 Goldman Activity Classification
- Class I: Able to perform any physical activity up to 7 metabolic equivalents (METS).
- Class II: Can perform any activity up to 5 METS, but cannot perform activities ≥ 7 METS.
- Class III: Can perform any activity up to 2 METS, but unable to complete any activity ≥ 5 METS.
- Class IV: Cannot perform activities ≥ 2 METS.

Routine investigations in patients with suspected congestive heart failure should include electrolytes, creatinine, estimated glomerular filtration rate, full blood count (FBC), lipids, thyroid tests, urinalysis, chest X-ray and ECG. The latter does not diagnose congestive heart failure but will exclude ischaemic change and left ventricular hypertrophy. BNP is a 32 amino acid molecule with a 17 amino acid ring structure. Unlike atrial natriuretic peptide (ANP), it is predominantly secreted and stored in the ventricles. Increased BNP levels are indicative of ventricular disorders. Levels normally increase with age and are higher in women than in men. Plasma BNP >100 pg/ml is more than 98% sensitive and 95% specific for HF. N-terminal pro BNP (NT-proBNP) is more stable and has a longer half-life. Doppler 2D echocardiogram should be performed to assess systolic and diastolic LV function, and to exclude valve disease or intracardiac shunts, where this is available. Normal echocardiography does not exclude HF and, in the face of symptoms, may suggest diastolic dysfunction. Systolic and diastolic HF are distinguished according to the EF. The two do not differ in symptomatology but there are differences in cardiac remodelling, perhaps reflecting the different disease processes involved (Box 26.2). In systolic HF, there is eccentric remodelling with ventricular dilatation and decreased EF. Diastolic HF is associated with concentric remodelling, normal end diastolic volume but abnormalities of ventricular relaxation and stiffness.

> **Box 26.2 Systolic and diastolic heart failure***
>
> | *Predominantly systolic* | *Predominantly diastolic* |
> |---|---|
> | Coronary artery disease | Hypertension |
> | Diabetes | Aortic stenosis |
> | Alcohol | Hypertrophic cardiomyopathy |
> | Valvular heart disease | Restrictive cardiomyopathy |
> | Drugs (cocaine, doxorubicin) | Some coronary artery disease |
> | Some cardiomyopathies | |
> | Atrial and ventricular septal defect, congenital heart disease | |
>
> *Distinguished on the basis of ejection fraction (<50% = systolic heart failure).

Where possible, regular aerobic or resistance exercise should be undertaken. All patients who smoke should be strongly advised to quit. Angiotensin-converting enzyme inhibitors (ACE-Is) or angiotensin receptor blockers (ARBs) should be commenced in all patients with systolic dysfunction. Diuretics should be administered to abolish or decrease pulmonary and peripheral oedema. Those with diastolic dysfunction should generally be treated with relatively low doses of diuretic (<80 mg frusemide per day). Patients with LV systolic dysfunction should be prescribed a suitable β-blocker once ACE-I/ARB and diuretic therapy have been optimized. Only two β-blockers are generally licensed for use in HF – bisoprolol and carvedilol. These should be started at low dose (1.25 mg bisoprolol OD, 3.25 mg carvedilol BD) and increased gradually at no less than 2-weekly intervals to a maximum dose (10 mg bisoprolol OD, 25 mg carvedilol BD). Nebivolol is being increasingly used. Heart rate, BP and symptoms should be carefully monitored as the dose is titrated upwards. Digoxin or spironolactone are often added to the above if patients have continuing symptoms or signs. Amlodipine should be considered for persistent hypertension but verapamil and diltiazem should be avoided because of their negative inotropic effects, and short-acting dihydropyridines should also be avoided. When indicated, coronary revascularization, resynchronization therapy, implantable defibrillator or cardiac transplantation should be considered. The increase in HF in the elderly in recent years is almost entirely due to increased diastolic HF, which is invariably accompanied by systolic hypertension. If pulmonary or peripheral oedema is absent, the management of diastolic HF and systolic hypertension are identical. ACE-Is, ARBs and calcium channel blockers have proved particularly effective in lowering central aortic pressure.[1] Management of hypertension in patients with HF is summarized in Figure 26.1.

Recent Developments

1   Both albuminuria and LV strain pattern on ECG are important predicators of HF in hypertensive patients. Okin *et al.*[2] followed 7786 subjects free of HF at baseline for an average of 5 years. The incidence of HF was 4.9% in those with increased albumin/creatinine ratio at baseline, 8.0% in those with LV strain alone, and 10.4% in patients who had both surrogate markers.

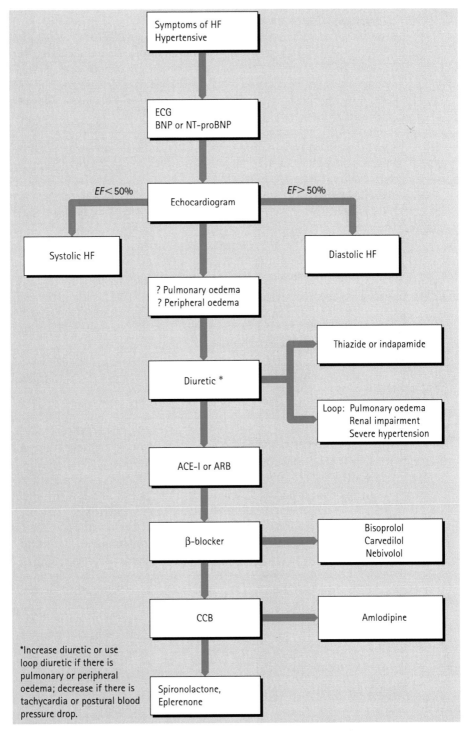

Figure 26.1 Management of hypertension and HF. ACE-I, angiotensin-converting enzyme inhibitor; ARB, angiotensin receptor blocker; BNP, brain natriuretic peptide; CCB, calcium channel blocker; EF, ejection fraction; HF, heart failure

2 Hypertension is more common in women with HF than in men with HF. There is a suggestion that ARBs might be more effective than ACE-Is for women with HF.[3] Lenzen *et al.*[4] studied large cohorts of men and women from the Euro Heart Survey on Heart Failure. Despite HF being equally common in both genders, women were less likely to have investigation of LV function and less likely to receive evidence-based drug treatment. We must be aware that gender differences exist, and fully investigate all patients with suspected HF.

3 While obesity is associated with increased morbidity and mortality, a paradox has been noted in a study of 22 576 hypertensive patients treated with either verapamil- or atenolol-based strategies.[5] The primary end-point was death, non-fatal myocardial infarction or stroke. The relative risk (RR) for overweight subjects was 0.77 (95% CI: 0.70 to 0.86, $P<0.001$), for class I obese subjects 0.68 (95% CI: 0.59 to 0.78, $P<0.001$), and for class II/III obese subjects 0.76 (95% CI: = 0.65 to 0.88, $P<0.001$). The reason for this apparent protective effect of increased body weight is not clear.

4 Renin–angiotensin system-blocking drugs have been immensely important in recent years. However, it is uncertain to what degree their protection is mediated through BP lowering. In a recent meta-analysis[6] involving 146 838 patients in 26 large-scale trials, there was no evidence for a BP-independent effect of either ACE-Is or ARBs in protecting against stroke or HF. A recent small trial focused on patients with diastolic dysfunction,[7] and again concluded that the beneficial effect of valsartan was mediated solely through BP lowering.

Conclusions

The above patient has predominantly systolic hypertension with probable diastolic HF. Measurement of BNP is extremely helpful in identifying such patients, management of which is summarized in Figure 26.1. The prevalence of diastolic HF is increasing in the elderly and it is almost invariably accompanied by hypertension although other factors may be important – e.g. up to 40% of patients have diabetes or impaired glucose tolerance. In the absence of marked pulmonary or peripheral oedema, the management is really just the management of hypertension. Diuretics (the lowest dose necessary) are often used as first-line treatment and renin–angiotensin system-blocking drugs have become the cornerstone. Existing guidelines would suggest that the target for this group is 140/90. There are two cautionary aspects: (1) brachial artery pressure may not entirely reflect central arterial pressure, and (2) lowering systolic BP to target may unduly lower diastolic BP in the elderly. This may further decrease myocardial perfusion. In the absence of specific guidelines, clinical judgement needs to be exercised in determining to what extent BP should be lowered.

References

1 Susic D, Frohlich ED. Optimal treatment of hypertension with diastolic heart failure. *Heart Fail Clin* 2008; **4**: 117–24.

2 Okin PM, Wachtell K, Devereux RB, Nieminen MS, Oikarinen L, Viitasalo M, *et al.* Combination of the electrocardiographic strain pattern and albuminuria for the prediction of

new-onset heart failure in hypertensive patients: the LIFE study. *Am J Hypertens* 2008; **21**: 273–9.

3   Hudson M, Rahme E, Behlouli H, Sheppard R, Pilote L. Sex differences in the effectiveness of angiotensin receptor blockers and angiotensin converting enzyme inhibitors in patients with congestive heart failure – a population study. *Eur J Heart Fail* 2007; **9**: 602–9.

4   Lenzen MJ, Rosengren A, Scholte op Reimer WJM, Follath F, Boersma E, Simoons ML, *et al.* Management of patients with heart failure in clinical practice: differences between men and women. *Heart* 2008; **94**: e10.

5   Uretsky S, Messerli FH, Bangalore S, Champion A, Cooper-Dehoff RM, Zhou Q, *et al.* Obesity paradox in patients with hypertension and coronary artery disease. *Am J Med* 2007; **120**: 863–70.

6   Blood Pressure Lowering Treatment Trialists' Collaboration, Turnbull F, Neal B, Pfeffer M, Kostis J, Algert C, *et al.* Blood pressure-dependent and independent effects of agents that inhibit the renin-angiotensin system. *J Hypertens* 2007; **25**: 951–8.

7   Solomon SD, Janardhanan R, Verma A, Bourgoun M, Daley WL, Purkayastha D, *et al.* Effect of angiotensin receptor blockade and antihypertensive drugs on diastolic function in patients with hypertension and diastolic dysfunction: a randomised trial. *Lancet* 2007; **369**: 2079–87.

27 Hypertension and Stroke

Case History

GM is a 70-year-old man whose hypertension is not perfectly controlled. He takes atenolol 50 mg OD, hydrochlorthiazide 25 mg OD, ramipril 5 mg OD, aspirin and omeprazole. Lately, he has been stressed as his wife is undergoing treatment for breast cancer. His clinic blood pressure (BP) is 164/94 mmHg. Electrocardiogram (ECG) shows sinus rhythm with no left ventricular hypertrophy. His parents both lived into their 80s. He is a non-smoker and is very active, walking regularly and playing bowls twice a week. He feels well, and in the light of his current stress, he is reluctant to increase or change his present treatment.

What is the relationship between high BP and stroke risk?

To what extent does effective treatment of hypertension protect against stroke?

Which are the most useful agents?

Background

In the USA, there are more than 700 000 strokes annually, accounting for over 160 000 deaths.[1] Evidence suggests that mortality from stroke has declined over the past four decades, but stroke incidence has increased. It remains the third most common cause of death, and a major cause of morbidity and disability. There are 4.8 million stroke survivors in the USA. Direct and indirect cost of caring for stroke victims probably approaches $60 billion. Hypertension is the leading modifiable risk factor, accounting for an estimated two-thirds of total stroke burden, particularly in younger subjects.

Non-modifiable risk factors include age, race (higher in black and Hispanic subjects), gender (commoner in men), low birth weight and family history. The major modifiable risk factors are summarized in Table 27.1. These factors have been combined in a number of predictive tools to estimate the risk of first stroke, including the Framingham stroke profile. None of these has found widespread usage in clinical practice. Less well documented risk factors include metabolic syndrome, high alcohol intake, hypercoagulability (factor V Leiden, anti-phospholipid antibodies, etc.), oral contraceptive use, low-grade inflammation, infectious agents (*Chlamydia pneumoniae*, *Helicobacter pylori* and cytomegalovirus), and obstructive sleep apnoea/hypopnoea syndrome.

Patients with BP >140/90 are at increased risk of stroke. The relative risk (RR) is higher in younger age groups, although the absolute risk increases with age. The relationship between increased BP and stroke is continuous and log-linear with no threshold

Table 27.1 Modifiable risk factors for stroke

	Relative risk
Coronary heart disease	
men	1.7
women	1.6
Hypertension	
age 50	4.0
age 60	3.0
age 70	2.0
age 80	1.4
age 90	1.0
Atrial fibrillation	3.5
Smoking	1.8
Diabetes	4.0
Dyslipidaemia	2.0

Adapted from Goldstein, et al.[1]

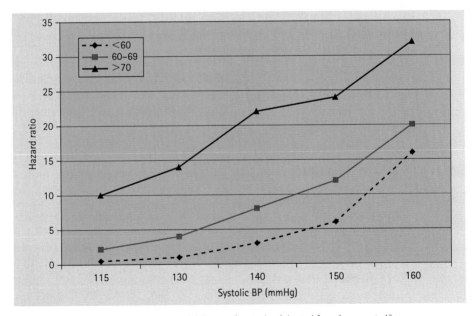

Figure 27.1 Age and blood pressure as risk factors for stroke. Adapted from Lawes, et al.[2]

value. There is an important interaction with age, BP and stroke risk (Figure 27.1). The RR of stroke with hypertension is most increased. However, the absolute risk increases markedly with age and there is a synergy between age and high BP as risk factors. BP control is as important in older subjects.

Effective treatment of hypertension is often not achieved, but when it is it decreases the risk of stroke by 35–45%. Although the major evidence for stroke prevention is with diuretics and β-blockers, other classes of drug may be as effective. The most important issue, by far, is BP reduction. Lifestyle modifications are often not pushed hard enough in decreasing hypertension. Each 10 mmHg reduction in systolic BP (SBP) is associated with one-third reduction in risk of stroke. Each 5 mmHg reduction in diastolic BP similarly decreases stroke risk.

Lawes *et al.*[2] reviewed trial data on hypertension and stroke risk. Data from over 40 trials with almost 200 000 participants were included. The 17 trials, which used either diuretic or β-blockers as primary treatment, included a total of 24 500 patients. The RR of stroke for the treatment wing was 0.65 (95% CI: 0.59 to 0.73). Major landmark trials were included in this analysis including HDFP (Hypertension Detection and Follow-up Program), Medical Research Council and SHEP (Systolic Hypertension in the Elderly Program). Six trials with angiotensin-converting enzyme inhibitors were analysed (including HOPE [Heart Outcomes Prevention Evaluation] and PROGRESS (Perindopril Protection Against Recurrent Stroke Study), involving nearly 9500 patients in treatment and placebo wings. The RR for stroke reduction with active treatment was 0.72 (95% CI: 0.68 to 0.83). Two trials with calcium channel blockers included about 2800 patients. RR for stroke with treatment was 0.61 (95% CI: 0.44 to 0.85). Subgroup analysis showed that, in spite of a relatively modest BP reduction (6–13 mmHg systolic, 1–6 mmHg diastolic), the risk of stroke was decreased irrespective of age and baseline SBP, and in patients with a history of vascular disease. Three trials – ABCD (Appropriate Blood Pressure Control in Diabetes), HOT (Hypertension Optimal Treatment) and UKPDS (UK Prospective Diabetes Study group) – compared more intensive with less intensive treatment to lower BP. More intensive treatment was associated with RR of 0.8 (95% CI: 0.65 to 0.99) compared with less intensive approaches. Fifteen trials involving over 96 000 subjects were identified, which compared the effect of different classes of antihypertensive drug, there was no difference in SBP or diastolic BP reduction between diuretics, β-blockers, calcium channel blockers or angiotensin-converting enzyme inhibitors. The benefits of treatment appear to be similar for haemorrhagic and thromboembolic strokes.

Recent Developments

1   The lifetime risk of stroke is 1:5 for a middle-aged woman and 1:6 for a middle-aged man. A recent study[3] has shown that in an inner city multi-ethnic population, admissions for ischaemic stroke have decreased since 1997 despite an increase in the prevalence of risk factors. This decrease extended across different racial groups. Survival at 30 days was poorer in patients of South Asian origin. A trend toward decreased hospitalization rates for stroke was also reported in a national US study.[4] Rates for men (per 100 000) in 1988, 1997 and 2004 were 287, 352 and 265 respectively. The corresponding rates for women were 252, 293 and 223. About 70% of strokes occurred in patients aged 65 and over, and 16% were classified as haemorrhagic. There was no evidence of a decline in admissions for haemorrhagic stroke.

2   Globally, hypertension is estimated to be responsible for 7.6 million premature deaths annually (13.5% of total) and 92 million disability-adjusted life-years

(DALYs, 6.0% of total).[5] Overall, the equivalent of 54% of strokes and 47% of ischaemic heart disease is attributable to elevated BP. The increased burden of stroke in lower socioeconomic groups is particularly apparent for those who develop stroke at a younger age.[6] Stroke risk is also increased in those with psychological distress or poor overall health status.

3   An extended SHEP cohort[7] confirmed that chlorthalidone-based treatment decreased cardiovascular mortality over 14 years of follow-up. Of patients who developed a stroke during the 14 years, two-thirds died. Patients with a transient ischaemic attack/accident had no increase in risk of death. This confirms that vigorous treatment of patients at risk of stroke is worthwhile.

4   For those who suffer a stroke, uncontrolled hypertension at presentation is a poor prognostic factor.[8] However, low BP (mean arterial pressures <90) is also a risk factor for early demise. We must beware of overenthusiastic treatment of hypertension in the elderly where it can be difficult to effectively treat SBP without unduly lowering diastolic BP. In the acute situation, patients with cardiovascular emergencies and those with diabetes often present with severe hypertension. This must be managed carefully as too rapid or excessive lowering of BP may compromise cerebral, myocardial and renal perfusion.

5   Subcortical white matter hyperintensities and lacunar infarcts are signs of small vessel disease apparent on magnetic resonance imaging scanning. These lesions are common in patients with hypertension,[9] and may contribute to gradual functional and cognitive decline.[10] Lacunar infarcts are particularly common in patients with diabetes. They often do not cause a huge amount of disability compared with large vessel strokes, accounting for the observation that the prognosis after acute stroke is no worse in patients with diabetes than in their non-diabetic counterparts.

6   It is not surprising that both hypertensive and diabetic retinopathy are strongly associated with cerebrovascular lesions, including lacunar infarcts.[11] What is surprising is how infrequently retinal examination is performed in patients with hypertension, particularly as this has now become routine in patients with diabetes. Automated measurements of retinal vascular configuration from digital retinal images may provide indices of stroke risk.

7   Another area of interest is arterial stiffness, which is measured using carotid–femoral pulse wave velocity (direct) or central pulse pressure (indirect). Increased arterial stiffness is associated with a high risk of stroke,[12] and may lead to BP being overestimated with brachial artery measurement leading to inappropriate treatment of systemic arterial pressure.

Conclusions

Hypertension is more strongly related to stroke risk than it is to other macrovascular diseases. There is increasing awareness of masked hypertension, nocturnal hypertension and morning BP surge as risk factors. Stroke is also a microvascular disease (lacunar infarction) and, as such, associated with other microvascular conditions (retinopathy and chronic kidney disease). Management of hypertension is important in both primary and secondary prevention, around the time of the acute event, and in other medical

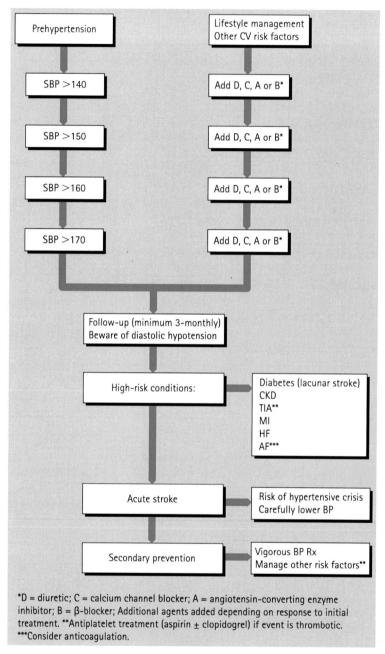

Figure 27.2 Hypertension and stroke. AF, atrial fibrillation; CKD, chronic kidney disease; CV, cardiovascular; HF, heart failure; MI, myocardial infarction; TIA, transient ischaemic attack

emergencies such as myocardial infarction, which increase stroke risk. The protective effect of antihypertensive agents is largely independent of drug class with diuretics, calcium channel blockers, β-blockers and angiotensin-converting enzyme inhibitors all having strong evidence supporting their use. As a rule of thumb, we can anticipate a

10 mmHg reduction in SBP with each agent equating to 30–40% risk reduction. It follows that a patient with a SBP of 170 mmHg may require three agents to render them normotensive (Figure 27.2) but that such treatment may more than halve their risk of subsequent stroke.

References

1 Goldstein LB, Adams R, Alberts MJ, Appel LJ, Brass LM, Bushnell CD, *et al.* Primary prevention of ischaemic stroke: a guideline from the American Heart Association/American Stroke Association Stroke Council. *Circulation* 2006; **113**: e873–923.

2 Lawes CMM, Bennett DA, Feigin VL, Rodgers A. Blood pressure and stroke – an overview of published reviews. *Stroke* 2004; **35**: 1024–33.

3 Gunarathne A, Patel JV, Potluri R, Gill PS, Hughes EA, Lip GYH. Secular trends in the cardiovascular risk profile and mortality of stroke admissions in an inner city, multiethnic population in the United Kingdom (1997–2005). *J Hum Hypertens* 2008; **22**: 18–23.

4 Fang J, Alderman MH, Keenan NL, Croft JB. Declining US stroke hospitalization since 1997: National Hospital Discharge Survey, 1988–2004. *Neuroepidemiology* 2007; **29**: 243–9.

5 Lawes CMM, Vander Hoorn S, Rodgers A, International Society of Hypertension. Global burden of blood-pressure-related disease, 2001. *Lancet* 2008; **371**: 1513–18.

6 Avendano M, Glymour MM. Stroke disparities in older Americans: is wealth a more powerful indicator of risk than income and education? *Stroke* 2008; **39**: 1533–40.

7 Patel AB, Kostis JB, Wilson AC, Shea ML, Pressel SL, Davis BR. Long-term fatal outcomes in subjects with stroke or transient ischemic attack: fourteen-year follow-up of the systolic hypertension in the elderly program. *Stroke* 2008; **39**: 1084–9.

8 Keezer MR, Yu AYX, Zhu B, Wolfson C, Cote R. Blood pressure and antihypertensive therapy as predictors of early outcome in acute ischemic stroke. *Cerebrovasc Dis* 2008; **25**: 202–8.

9 Gouw AA, van der Flier WM, Fazekas F, van Straaten ECW, Pantoni L, Poggesi A, *et al.* Progression of white matter hyperintensities and incidence of new lacunes over a 3-year period: the Leukoaraiosis and Disability study. *Stroke* 2008; **39**: 1414–20.

10 Reitz C, Tang M-X, Manly J, Mayeux R, Luchsinger JA. Hypertension and the risk of mild cognitive impairment. *Arch Neurol* 2007; **64**: 1734–40.

11 Baker ML, Hand PJ, Wang JJ, Wong TY. Retinal signs and stroke: revisiting the link between the eye and brain. *Stroke* 2008; **39**: 1371–9.

12 De Silva D, Woon FP, Chen C, Chang HM, Kingwell B, Cameron J, *et al.* Profile and associations of central pulse wave velocity and central pulse pressure among ischemic stroke patients. *Eur J Neurol* 2008; **15**: 196–8.

Co-morbidities and Associated Disorders

PROBLEM

28 Type 1 Diabetes

Case History

Sally is 28 years old, and has been on insulin since the age of 6. She has two children aged 4 and 2. She had no problems during her pregnancies but does not want more children. She uses a basal bolus insulin regimen. Blood glucose control could be better (HbA$_1$c 8.5%) but she finds this difficult with her busy life (children and part-time job). Recently, her blood pressure (BP) has been high – systolic is about 140 mmHg and diastolic about 90. She has microalbuminuria (albumin/creatinine ratio = 76), which has progressed slowly in recent years. She is reluctant to commence antihypertensive medication.

What BP target should we be aiming for in patients with type 1 diabetes?

Should all patients be given renin–angiotensin system (RAS)–blocking drugs irrespective of BP?

What are the relative contributions of RAS blockade and BP lowering?

Background

Hypertension is present in at least one-third of patients with type 1 diabetes and correlates strongly with the presence of nephropathy. Patients with type 1 diabetes are at increased risk of renal failure and cardiovascular (CV) events (Box 28.1) – these risk factors tend to develop in parallel. Diabetes (type 1 and 2) accounts for about 40% of end-stage renal disease (ESRD), and the proportion is rising due to the increased contribution from type 2 diabetes. In the USA, the annual cost of managing ESRD in patients with diabetes is about $20 billion, with more than $2 billion of that spent on patients with type 1 diabetes. The DCCT (Diabetes Control and Complications Trial), completed in 1993, confirmed the importance of glycaemic control in preventing complications. Since then, numerous studies have reaffirmed the importance of BP control in type 1 diabetes.

Box 28.1

In preventing diabetes complications remember **ABC:**

A = Haemoglobin A₁c

B = Blood pressure

C = Cholesterol

The fact that only 1:20 with diabetic nephropathy develops ESRD is encouraging, but also reflects the high risk of this patient group as many die prematurely from CV disease before they can develop ESRD. Hypertension is a critical, but not the only, factor in the progression of nephropathy and in its association with vascular complications. Early changes leading to nephropathy include increased activity of the renal RAS and sympathetic nervous system, changes in renal salt handling, and loss of nitric oxide-mediated vasodilatation. Increased plasma volume due to salt and water retention results from tubular changes, which may worsen with the development of insulin resistance and also be associated with a diminished response to natriuretic peptides. Insulin resistance, the precursor of type 2 diabetes, also develops in type 1 patients where there is excessive weight gain with insulin therapy. Hyperglycaemia almost certainly initiates the changes of nephropathy causing glomerular hyperfiltration and tubular epithelial hypertrophy. These lead to microalbumin and plasma volume expansion, and with these changes and the consequent hypertension there is glomerular basement membrane thickening and increased mesangial matrix accumulation leading ultimately to glomerulosclerosis and macroalbuminuria. Contributing biochemical changes include activation of protein kinase C and the polyol pathway, accumulation of advanced glycation end-products, and increased expression of transforming growth factor-β. The filtration barrier is partly maintained by specialized epithelial cells called podocytes. These produce their effect mainly through the production of nephrin, a protein whose expression is decreased in developing nephropathy. Activated T cells and macrophages are also involved in the pathogenesis. Common genetic and environmental factors may be involved in pancreatic β-cell and renal damage.[1]

Generally, type 1 diabetes and its association with nephropathy has been less well studied than has the association in type 2 diabetes. Early studies (1990–2000) clearly showed that angiotensin-converting enzyme inhibitors – captopril, enalapril and ramipril – helped prevent the progression from MA to macroalbuminuria. They suggested that lower BP targets might be appropriate, although in many studies the actual decrease in BP with angiotensin-converting enzyme inhibitors was relatively modest showing that this class had a protective effect that was not reflected in its BP-lowering ability. Lifestyle measures – weight control, exercise, salt reduction, limiting alcohol intake – should be considered in all patients and may be sufficient alone in those with a systolic BP of 130–139 or diastolic BP of 80–89. However, high-risk patients in this range should probably have pharmacological management. Angiotensin-converting enzyme inhibitors or angiotensin receptor blockers for those who are intolerant are recommended for all patients with MA. Beyond providing renal protection with a RAS-blocking drug, lowering BP is a more important consideration than the actual choice of drug. Cost and compliance issues should be considered. Although β-blockers and thiazides have a slight hyperglycaemic effect, this is not problematic with type 1 diabetes – at worst, their use may lead to a slightly increased insulin requirement. Masking of hypoglycaemic symptoms with β-blockers is also not usually a major problem but they are best avoided in those with severe or problematic hypoglycaemia.

Patients with diabetes have excess mortality from renal disease during the first 20 years after diagnosis, and thereafter have an increased risk of death from CV disease. Stadler *et al.*[2] performed a record linkage study involving 648 patients with type 1 diabetes identified in 1983–84. Their outcome at 20 years was documented. Albuminuria was more common in those with highest HbA$_1$c. After 20 years, 13% of the patients had died and 5.6% required renal replacement therapy. Poor glycaemic control correlated strongly with both these adverse outcomes. This study did not specifically consider BP as a determinant of outcome, but adds to previous data showing that vigorous management of glucose and BP is required. In recent years, there has been a trend for an improved outlook in type 1 diabetes in European studies and this is also the conclusion of the Pittsburgh Epidemiology of Diabetes Complications Study.[3] Those diagnosed more recently were less likely to develop neuropathy, ESRD, or to die prematurely. However, in this cohort, overt nephropathy, coronary artery disease and proliferative retinopathy did not show decreased prevalence in recent years. Thus, evidence suggests that the management of risk factors in patients with type 1 diabetes has become more effective but there is still a considerable way to go.

Recent Developments

1 In a large observational study, Shankar *et al.*[4] studied the development of two outcomes – proteinuria and estimated glomerular filtration rate <60 – over a 16-year period. Patients were divided into quartiles according to systolic BP and diastolic BP. As expected, there was a strong relationship between baseline BP and renal outcomes. Patients with BP of ≤120/70 were protected. These data suggest that we should consider starting antihypertensives and aim for lower targets than those presently accepted.

2 Decline in renal function may occur relatively early in type 1 diabetes.[5] If detected early, MA is reversible. The measurement of microalbumin over the past two decades has transformed the early identification of nephropathy. However,

the practical difficulties of timed urine collections have partly limited its use. Cystatin C is a low molecular weight protein (13.3 kDa), the serum level of which increases with developing nephropathy. There is increasing evidence that cystatin C measurement might be useful.[5,6]

3　A very large series[7] has emphasized how common CV risk factors are in children, adolescents and young adults with type 1 diabetes. At least one risk factor was present in >50%. Presence of risk factors was strongly age dependent with two or more risk factors being present in 22% of young adults. Increased carotid intima-media thickness is a surrogate marker for developing atherosclerosis, and is increased in young people with diabetes.[8]

4　Simultaneous pancreatic and renal transplantation is increasingly available for patients with type 1 diabetes and ESRD. With a pancreas transplant, the patient can benefit from normal glycaemic control and be free of insulin treatment, albeit at the cost of taking immunosuppressive treatment. Compared with those who undergo renal transplant alone, those with dual kidney and pancreas transplant not only benefit from normalized glycaemic control, but also have lower BP and are less dyslipidaemic.[9]

5　Nephrin is involved in maintaining the integrity of the glomerular filtration barrier and is also expressed in the pancreatic β-cell. As type 1 diabetes is an autoimmune disease, it may not be surprising that circulating anti-nephrin antibodies have been reported to occur in up to 1:4 patients with type 1 diabetes.[10] Such antibodies may be a marker for nephropathy risk and could participate in pathological processes that lead to declining renal function.

Conclusions

Nephropathy is the most costly of diabetic complications, but one in which there is considerable scope for prevention (Figure 28.1). Either retarding its development or its progress will also improve the overall outlook for the diabetic patient because of the association between nephropathy and other vascular complications. The accepted BP target is 130/80. However, there is evidence that even lower levels of BP will protect against nephropathy. As with blood glucose control, the potential risk and benefits of tight BP control should be assessed for, and discussed with, the patient. Hyperglycaemia is responsible for the early changes of nephropathy, and every attempt should be made to obtain the best possible glycaemic control. The prevalence of type 1 diabetes is increasing, and the incidence in adults now equals that in children. The same considerations apply to adult-onset as to childhood-onset type 1 diabetes, but adults are more likely to develop hypertension in the early years after diagnosis. Prescription of angiotensin-converting enzyme inhibitors has become standard for patients at risk of nephropathy. They have an effect on renal protection independent of BP lowering, However, other agents may be required to achieve target BP. It is not possible at present to quantify the relative contributions of BP lowering and RAS inhibition.

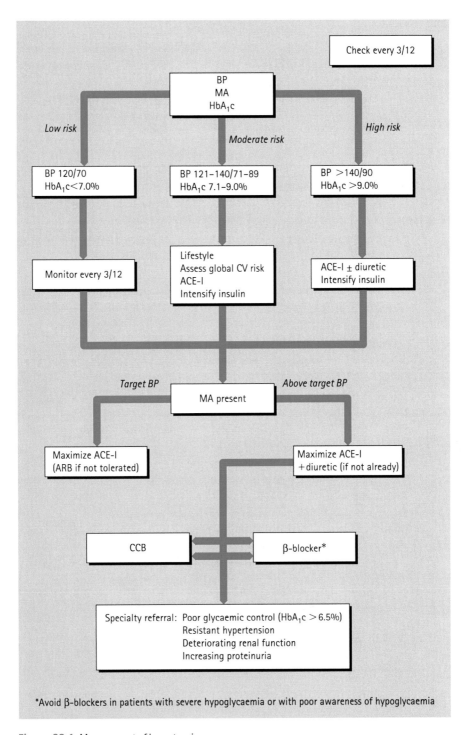

Figure 28.1 Management of hypertension.

References

1   Ichinose K, Kawasaki E, Eguchi K. Recent advancement of understanding pathogenesis of type 1 diabetes and potential relevance to diabetic nephropathy. *Am J Nephrol* 2007; **27**: 554–64.

2   Stadler M, Auinger M, Anderwald C, Kastenbauer T, Kramar R, Feinbock C, *et al.* Long-term mortality and incidence of renal dialysis and transplantation in type 1 diabetes mellitus. *J Clin Endocrinol Metab* 2006; **91**: 3814–20.

3   Pambianco G, Costacou T, Ellis D, Becker DJ, Klein R, Orchard TJ. The 30-year natural history of type 1 diabetes complications: the Pittsburgh Epidemiology of Diabetes Complications Study experience. *Diabetes* 2006; **55**: 1463–9.

4   Shankar A, Klein R, Klein BEK, Nieto FJ, Moss SE. Relationship between low-normal blood pressure and kidney disease in type 1 diabetes. *Hypertension* 2007; **49**: 48–54.

5   Perkins BA, Ficociello LH, Ostrander BE, Silva KH, Weinberg J, Warram JH, *et al.* Microalbuminuria and the risk for early progressive renal function decline in type 1 diabetes. *J Am Soc Nephrol* 2007; **18**: 1353–61.

6   Maahs DM, Ogden LG, Kretowski A, Snell–Bergeon JK, Kinney GL, Berl T, *et al.* Serum cystatin C predicts progression of subclinical coronary atherosclerosis in individuals with type 1 diabetes. *Diabetes* 2007; **56**: 2774–9.

7   Schwab KO, Doerfer J, Hecker W, Grulich-Henn J, Wiemann D, Kordonouri O, *et al.* Spectrum and prevalence of atherogenic risk factors in 27,358 children, adolescents, and young adults with type 1 diabetes: cross-sectional data from the German diabetes documentation and quality management system (DPV). *Diabetes Care* 2006; **29**: 218–25.

8   Dalla Pozza R, Bechtold S, Bonfig W, Putzker S, Kozlik-Feldmann R, Netz H, *et al.* Age of onset of type 1 diabetes in children and carotid intima medial thickness. *J Clin Endocrinol Metab* 2007; **92**: 2053–7.

9   Luan FL, Miles CD, Cibrik DM, Ojo AO. Impact of simultaneous pancreas and kidney transplantation on cardiovascular risk factors in patients with type 1 diabetes mellitus. *Transplantation* 2007; **84**: 541–4.

10 Aaltonen P, Rinta-Valkama J, Patari A, Tossavainen P, Palmen T, Kulmala P, *et al.* Circulating antibodies to nephrin in patients with type 1 diabetes. *Nephrol Dial Transplant* 2007; **22**: 146–53.

29 Metabolic Syndrome

Case History

Raymond is a 48-year-old sales representative. In his busy working life, he spends many hours each week driving. He eats irregularly, often in restaurants and hotels, or fast food while travelling. Outside work, he has little time for exercise. He smokes 20 cigarettes a day, and drinks at least 50 units of alcohol per week. His typical blood pressure (BP) is about 138/88. He is obese with a body mass index of 31.6 kg/m². Fasting cholesterol is 6.1 mmol/l, and fasting glucose is 6.5 mmol/l. He is not taking any regular medications.

Does he need drug treatment for his BP?

Why is hypertension associated with other features of metabolic syndrome (MetS)?

What is the optimal approach to treating hypertension in MetS?

Background

MetS is a cluster of risk factors that now affects 1:4 adults in developed countries. Subjects with MetS are three times more likely to suffer a cardiovascular (CV) event, twice as likely to die from CV disease, and five times more likely to develop type 2 diabetes. Diabetes and hypertension are strongly associated. Only one in three hypertensive patients without diabetes have MetS, and 85% of patients with MetS are hypertensive. MetS is highly associated with overweight and obesity and insulin resistance. Many patients with insulin resistance have increased circulating insulin. This leads to sodium retention, activation of the sympathetic nervous system and loss of the normal vasodilatory effect of insulin. MetS is defined on the basis of classical CV risk factors, but the diagnosis also embraces many non-classical risk factors that are not measured in routine clinical practice. These include endothelial dysfunction, transcapillary leak of albumin and lipoproteins, low-grade inflammation, and coagulation abnormalities (increased tissue factor VII and fibrinogen, plasminogen activator inhibitor-1, and platelet activation).

MetS is not caused by a singular abnormality, and its relationship with macrovascular complications is complex. Although there is general agreement about the major components of MetS, there has been a variety of definitions. Currently, the two most widely used are those from the IDF (International Diabetes Federation) and the ATPIII (Cholesterol Education Program Adult Treatment Panel III). The presence of central obesity, assessed by waist circumference (WC), is at the core of the IDF definition (Box 29.1). Different cutoffs for WC are used in children and adolescents and in different racial groups. Box 29.2

shows the ATPIII definition. As MetS becomes more common with age, isolated systolic hypertension is the commonest form of hypertension associated with it. Isolated diastolic hypertension occurs in younger subjects, while systolic–diastolic hypertension is commoner in middle life. Young women are less likely to develop MetS, and less likely to develop hypertension if they have MetS. Risk from MetS depends not only on age, number and severity of risk factors, but also on duration of exposure. South Asian, Chinese and Japanese races are at increased risk of MetS with only a modest weight gain. Patients of African descent are at particular risk of hypertension with weight gain.

Box 29.1 International Diabetes Federation definition of metabolic syndrome

Central obesity* *plus* any two of the following:

- Increased triglycerides: ≥1.7 mmol/l (150 mg/dl), *or* specific treatment for this
- Decreased high-density lipoprotein cholesterol: <1.03 mmol/l (40 mg/dl) in males, <1.29 mmol/l (50 mg/dl) in females, *or* specific treatment for this
- Increased BP: systolic BP ≥130 mmHg or diastolic BP ≥85 mmHg, *or* treatment for hypertension
- Increased fasting glucose: fasting plasma glucose ≥5.6 mmol/l (100 mg/dl), *or* treatment for type 2 diabetes

*Central obesity is defined by waist circumference:

- Europids: male, ≥94 cm; female, ≥80 cm
- South Asians, Chinese, Japanese: male, ≥90 cm; female, ≥80 cm
- Other races: use Europid values until specific data become available

---

Pathogenesis of hypertension in MetS is complex:[1] high levels of insulin have an anti-natriuretic effect. Salt sensitivity is also related to insulin resistance, with insulin action inhibited in salt-sensitive individuals or with a high salt diet. Insulin also stimulates endothelin secretion and enhances its action. Insulin resistance, increased leptin and increased free fatty acids all contribute to activation of the sympathetic nervous system. Activation of the renin–angiotensin system occurs, and high circulating aldosterone has been identified as an aetiological factor and therapeutic target in MetS-related hypertension. The renin–angiotensin system pathway is also present in fat tissue and increased

---

Box 29.2 ATPIII (Cholesterol Education Program Adult Treatment Panel III) definition of metabolic syndrome

Any three of the following five:

1 Abdominal obesity, as defined by waist circumference: men, >102 cm (>40 inches); women, >88 cm (>35 inches)

2 Triglycerides: ≥150 mg/dl

3 High-density lipoprotein cholesterol: men, <40 mg/dl; women, <50 mg/dl.

4 Blood pressure: ≥130/≥85 mmHg

5 Fasting glucose: ≥110 mg/dl

activation of this in obesity contributes to increased BP. Oxidative stress and low-grade inflammation both contribute to vascular damage.

The need for aggressive treatment of MetS variables is increased if there is target-organ damage – a previous CV event or established CV disease, increased Left Ventricular Mass Index or left ventricular hypertrophy, albuminuria or decreased glomerular filtration rate, or increased carotid intima-media thickness. The choice of agent for hypertension should be one that not only decreases BP but that also does not adversely affect, or indeed

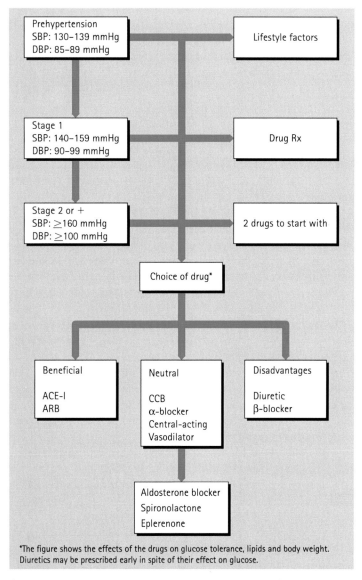

*The figure shows the effects of the drugs on glucose tolerance, lipids and body weight. Diuretics may be prescribed early in spite of their effect on glucose.

Figure 29.1 Managing hypertension in metabolic syndrome. ACE-I, angiotensin-converting enzyme inhibitor; ARB, angiotensin receptor blocker; CCB, calcium channel blocker; DBP, diastolic blood pressure; SBP, systolic blood pressure

favourably influences, other features of the syndrome. Diet, exercise, salt and alcohol restriction are the cornerstones of management in those with prehypertension. Drug treatment should be considered where three or more CV risk factors are present (Figure 29.1). Target BP is 140/90 unless there are multiple risk factors or end-organ damage, in which case 130/85 is a reasonable target. In very high-risk patients 120/80 affords greater protection but may be hard to achieve. Patients with stage 1 hypertension and MetS almost always require drug treatment. Those with stage 2 or above hypertension require two or more drugs generally. Activation of the renin–angiotensin system is emerging as an integral component of MetS, and aldosterone blockers (spironolactone and eplerenone) are increasingly being used in those with resistant hypertension. Because of published evidence, angiotensin-converting enzyme inhibitors or angiotensin receptor blockers are indicated in those with cardiac or renal disease, while calcium channel blockers should be considered in those with CV disease.

Recent Developments

1   The DREAM (Diabetes Reduction Assessment with Ramipril and Rosiglitazone Medication) Study[2] recruited 5269 participants with impaired glucose tolerance or impaired fasting glucose, and without CV disease. Although rosiglitazone had a significant effect on development of diabetes, no such effect was found with ramipril, although it did have a slight beneficial effect on blood glucose levels.

2   There is debate as to whether the concept of MetS is actually useful in clinical practice. The Cardiovascular Health Study[3] involved 4258 adults over 65 years old between 1989 and 2004. MetS was present in 31% of men and 38% of women. Hypertension and increased fasting glucose were highly predictive of mortality but there was no additional predicative value from MetS itself, whether defined by the World Health Organization (WHO) or IDF criteria.

3   A substudy of ALLHAT (Antihypertensive and Lipid-Lowering Treatment to Prevent Heart Attack Trial) compared hypertension in patients with and without MetS.[4] In patients without MetS, diabetes developed in 7.7% of chlorthalidone treated, 4.2% with amlodipine and 4.7% with lisinopril. Comparable figures for those with MetS were 17.1%, 16.0% and 12.6% respectively. In spite of its metabolic disadvantage, chlorthalidone was as effective as the other agents in preventing CV outcomes. Indeed it was superior in preventing heart failure and combined CV disease in patients with MetS.

4   Patients with primary hyperaldosteronism are at increased risk of MetS. Plasma aldosterone is frequently elevated in patients with MetS,[5] and contributes to development of hypertension and also to unfavourable vascular remodelling. Aldosterone-blocking drugs should be considered in patients with MetS and hypertension, which do not respond readily to first-line agents.

5   In a study of 1106 hypertensive subjects aged 45–70 years and with no diagnosed diabetes or CV disease, Korhonen et al.[6] carried out oral glucose tolerance tests. Type 2 diabetes was found in 66 (6%) and impaired glucose tolerance in 220 (20%). The threshold for requesting oral glucose tolerance tests should be low in those with hypertension and other features of MetS.

6   High intake of fructose calories predisposes to hypertension, other features of MetS and renal disease.[7] Fructose-fed rat models have been widely used. Telmisartan, an angiotensin receptor blocker, which has some peroxisome proliferator activated receptor γ agonist properties, had beneficial effects in a rat model with decreased body weight, BP and triglycerides.[8]

Conclusions

The above patient is at high risk. There is scope for lifestyle modifications and this should always be the first line of management. However, the above patient has hypertension, hyperlipidaemia and elevated fasting plasma glucose, which along with hypertension is a major determinant of prognosis. The reasons for hypertension in patients with MetS include activation of renin–angiotensin system and sympathetic nervous system, increased endothelin secretion and action, salt retention and salt sensitivity, as well as dyslipidaemia and adipocytokine secretion from visceral adipose tissue. The approach to managing hypertension in MetS is outlined in Figure 29.1. In spite of the fact that this is a very common clinical scenario, there are no specific published guidelines. It is important to choose agents that control BP and protect end organs but do not have a negative impact on other risk factors such as weight and blood glucose.

References

1   Yanai H, Tomono Y, Ito K, Furutani N, Yoshida H, Tada N. The underlying mechanisms for development of hypertension in the metabolic syndrome. *Nutr J* 2008; **7**: 10–14.

2   The DREAM Trial Investigators. Effect of ramipril on the incidence of diabetes. *N Engl J Med* 2006; **355**: 1551–62.

3   Mozaffarian D, Kamineni A, Prineas RJ, Siscovick DS. Metabolic syndrome and mortality in older adults: the Cardiovascular Health Study. *Arch Intern Med* 2008; **168**: 969–78.

4   Black HR, Davis B, Barzilay J, Nwachuku C, Baimbridge C, Marginean H, *et al.* Metabolic and clinical outcomes in nondiabetic individuals with the metabolic syndrome assigned to chlorthalidone, amlodipine, or lisinopril as initial treatment for hypertension: a report from the Antihypertensive and Lipid-Lowering Treatment to Prevent Heart Attack Trial (ALLHAT). *Diabetes Care* 2008; **31**: 353–60.

5   Chun T-Y, Pratt JH. Hyperaldosteronism: a commonly occurring underlying feature of essential hypertension and the metabolic syndrome? *Curr Opin Endocrinol Diabete Obes* 2007; **14**: 210–12.

6   Korhonen P, Aarnio P, Saaresranta T, Jaatinen P, Kantola I. Glucose homeostasis in hypertensive subjects. *Hypertension* 2008; **51**: 945–9.

7   Johnson RJ, Segal MS, Sautin Y, Nakagawa T, Feig DI, Kang D-H, *et al.* Potential role of sugar (fructose) in the epidemic of hypertension, obesity and the metabolic syndrome, diabetes, kidney disease, and cardiovascular disease. *Am J Clin Nutr* 2007; **86**: 899–906.

8   Kamari Y, Harari A, Shaish A, Peleg E, Sharabi Y, Harats D, *et al.* Effect of telmisartan, angiotensin II receptor antagonist, on metabolic profile in fructose-induced hypertensive, hyperinsulinemic, hyperlipidemic rats. *Hypertens Res* 2008; **31**: 135–40.

30 Antihypertensive Drugs and Risk of Diabetes

Case History

George is 44 years old and has recently been advised that he should commence treatment to lower his blood pressure (BP). He has a strong family history of vascular disease. Also, both his parents suffered from type 2 diabetes (T2D) – mother diagnosed aged 48 and father at age 53. His brother who is two years older has type 2 diabetes. George is not markedly overweight, a non-smoker, and he drinks little alcohol. His cholesterol is 4.2 mmol/l. Electrocardiogram (ECG) and renal function are normal. His fasting blood glucose is 5.7 mmol/l.

Do antihypertensive drugs have a meaningful influence on risk of diabetes?

Should this patient have a glucose tolerance test?

What follow-up should be planned for him?

Background

Age, family history, anthropometric variables and metabolic syndrome components are all highly predictive of T2D and have been combined into risk scores that perform reasonably well. Identifying individuals at high risk of diabetes is important as lifestyle interventions can prevent, or at least retard, the onset of T2D. Also, use of methods to calculate diabetes risk may guide appropriate use of antihypertensive medications. Lifestyle interventions are effective in preventing T2D. Drugs such as metformin and thiazolidinediones are widely used for the treatment of diabetes but hardly used at all for prevention. For both treatment and prevention, there is an argument for considering hypertension and diabetes to be a single entity – treatments for one often influence the risk of the other.

Practitioners should not be deterred from using thiazides or β-blockers where they are indicated. Salt and water retention and salt sensitivity are important aetiological factors in essential hypertension and warrant diuretics, while β-blockers have additional benefits for many patients over and above the ability to lower BP. However, increased surveillance for diabetes is warranted in patients for whom thiazides or β-blockers are prescribed. This should include screening for diabetes at the outset of treatment in high-risk individuals. Although individual trials are statistically powered to, and meta-analyses designed to, identify effects of individual drug classes, the vast majority of patients require multiple drugs to control BP. Risk of diabetes increases in relation to the number of preparations used,[1] although this may partly reflect the strength of the association between hypertension and glucose intolerance in severely affected patients. Any benefits of classes that are apparently protective can be more than offset if diabetogenic classes have to be prescribed in addition.[1]

Figure 30.1 shows that risk of cardiovascular events is not markedly different in patients with recent-onset diabetes compared with those with established diabetes. In both, risk increases with increasing systolic BP, and the risk is markedly increased in patients with left ventricular hypertrophy. When hypertension and diabetes coexist,

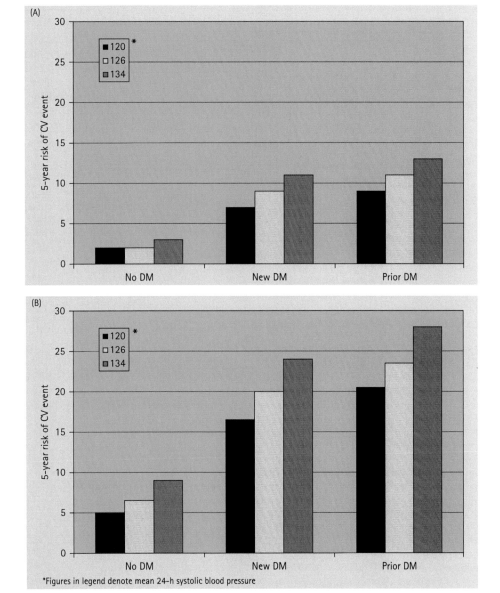

*Figures in legend denote mean 24-h systolic blood pressure

Figure 30.1 Risk of CV events with and without diabetes. (A) Without left ventricular hypertrophy. (B) With left ventricular hypertrophy. CV, cardiovascular; DM, diabetes mellitus. Adapted from Östergren.[2]

strenuous attempts should be made to control both as tightly as possible. The effects of these classes on blood glucose may have offset some of the potential benefits of BP-lowering medications in early trials of β-blockers and diuretics. Onset of T2D in patients treated for hypertension is not a trivial event.

Several large studies in which renin–angiotensin system-blocking drugs have been compared with other classes have shown decreased relative risk (RR) for diabetes:[2]

- 14% RR reduction ($P = 0.034$) in CAPPP (Captopril Prevention Project) (1999) compared with thiazide or β-blocker

- 34% RR reduction ($P < 0.001$) in HOPE (Heart Outcomes Prevention Evaluation) (2000) in which ramipril was compared with placebo

- 30% RR reduction ($P < 0.001$) in ALLHAT (Antihypertensive and Lipid-Lowering Treatment to Prevent Heart Attack Trial) (2002) which compared lisinopril to chlorthalidone

- 25% RR reduction ($P < 0.001$) in LIFE (Losartan Intervention For Endpoint reduction) (2002) comparing losartan and atenolol

- 23% RR reduction ($P < 0.0001$) in VALUE (Valsartan Antihypertensive Long-term Use Evaluation) (2004) in which valsartan was compared with amlodipine

- 22% RR reduction ($P = 0.02$) in CHARM (Candesartan in Heart failure: Assessment of Reduction in Mortality and morbidity) (2005) in which candesartan was compared with placebo in high-risk patients with heart failure

Mechanisms by which renin–angiotensin system inhibition improves glycaemic control and risk of diabetes include increased blood flow to insulin-sensitive tissues thus improving delivery of glucose and insulin, improved insulin action at cellular level, decreased sympathetic activity, and increased insulin secretion from the pancreatic β cell (perhaps through increased islet blood flow). Genetic studies in which the angiotensin (AGT M235T), angiotensin-converting enzyme (ACE) insertion/deletion (I/D), and angiotensin receptor (AGTR1 A1166C) polymorphisms have been studied in relation to insulin resistance have failed to reveal a consistent association between these polymorphisms and risk of diabetes. Numerous short-term studies have been carried out to determine whether renin–angiotensin system blockade improves insulin sensitivity. These have generally, but not universally, showed improved insulin sensitivity with either ACE inhibitors (ACE-Is) or angiotensin receptor blockers (ARBs).

DREAM (Diabetes Reduction Assessment with Ramipril and Rosiglitazone Medication 2006)[2] was a 2×2 factorial study that involved 5269 patients without cardiovascular disease but with impaired fasting glucose or impaired glucose tolerance. Patients were followed for 3 years. Although there was significant regression to normoglycaemia with ramipril, there was no evidence for the prevention of T2D in this study. The major difference to previous ACE-I studies that did show diabetes prevention was that patients were initially free of cardiovascular disease. Also, the period of follow-up was relatively short to demonstrate prevention of diabetes. In spite of DREAM, the balance of evidence favours a preventative role in decreasing risk of new diabetes by about 25%, with ACE-Is and ARBs probably equally effective. The benefits may be especially apparent in high-risk groups – perhaps because of more marked neurohumoral activation.

The increased risk of diabetes with β-blockers has been documented in a recent meta-analysis,[3] which included 12 studies with a total of 94 492 patients followed-up for at least 1 year. When β-blockers were used as a first line treatment, there was a 22% (95% confidence interval [CI]: 1.12 to 1.33) increased risk of T2D compared with other non-diuretic medications. The risk of diabetes was higher with higher baseline fasting glucose, systolic BP and diastolic BP. The risk was greater in those with higher body mass index, in whom BP was not effectively lowered, and with increased duration of β-blocker treatment. Atenolol appeared to pose a particular risk for diabetes in the elderly.

The increased risk of glucose intolerance with thiazides is beyond dispute. However, much of the risk may not be due to the drugs themselves but to the decrease in plasma potassium: Zillich *et al.*[4] examined 59 trials with 83 treatment arms. Not surprisingly, in major trials such as ALLHAT the potassium level is often lower in the diuretic arm. The relationship between low potassium and increased glucose has been long recognized but is not often considered in modern clinical practice. Doses of potassium-lowering drugs should be kept to a minimum and plasma potassium monitored and maintained at ≥4.0 mmol/l – if necessary by using supplements or potassium-sparing diuretics (Figure 30.2). The above observations are in keeping with the known association between low dietary potassium and high BP.

Recent Developments

1   In the Women's Health Study,[5] 38 172 women followed for a mean of 10.2 years were divided into four categories according to baseline BP. Hazard ratios (HR) (with 95% CIs) for the development of diabetes were: 0.66 (0.55–0.80) for patients with low BP, 1.0 with BP in the normal range, 1.45 (1.23–1.71) with prehypertension, and 2.03 (1.77–2.32) with hypertension.

2   BP trials are highly heterogeneous with respect to patient characteristics and interventions, and the major trials have not been, until recently, specifically designed to examine diabetes risk. Elliot and Meyer[6] conducted an analysis that included 22 trials with 143 153 participants free of diabetes at randomization. Accepting that thiazides are associated with risk of diabetes and using this as the referent, adjusted HR for diabetes with β-blockers was 0.90 (95% CI: 0.75 to 1.09, $P = 0.30$), for placebo 0.77 (0.63 to 0.94, $P = 0.009$), for calcium channel blockers 0.75 (0.62 to 0.90, $P = 0.002$), for ACE-Is 0.67 (0.56 to 0.80, $P < 0.0001$), and for ARBs 0.57 (0.46 to 0.72, $P < 0.0001$). The reasons for slight superiority of ARBs over ACE-Is are not clear.

3   Third generation, β-blockers may not have the metabolic disadvantages of older agents. The GEMINI (Glycemic Effects in Diabetes Mellitus: Carvedilol-Metoprolol Comparison in Hypertensives) study compared metoprolol with carvedilol in patients with stage 1/2 hypertension and T2D. Metoprolol was associated with weight gain while carvedilol was not.[7] Diabetes-related symptoms were less frequently reported with carvedilol.

4   The INVEST (INternational VErapamil SR-Trandolapril STudy) study[8] compared a regimen based on verapamil with trandolapril where needed with an atenolol-based strategy. The former was associated with a lower incidence of diabetes in the 16 176 patients who did not have diabetes at baseline (7.0% vs 8.2%, $P < 0.01$). Risk

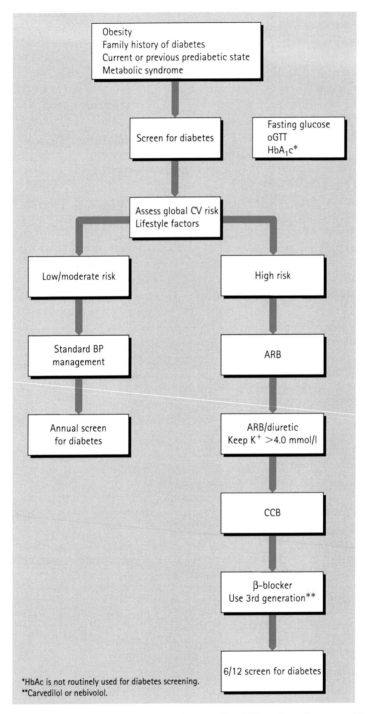

Figure 30.2 Managing diabetes risk in hypertension. ARB, angiotensin receptor blocker; CCB, calcium channel blocker; oGTT, oral glucose tolerance test

factors for diabetes were increased body mass index, left ventricular hypertrophy, previous cerebrovascular event, coronary revascularization, higher BP, increased cholesterol, and being Hispanic.

Conclusions

Patients with hypertension are at increased risk of diabetes and prediabetes irrespective of medications. Numerous studies and meta-analyses confirm that diuretics and β-blockers are associated with increased risk of T2D. The effect of diuretics on diabetes risk is relatively small and may be at least partially nullified by ensuring that the potassium level is maintained. Metabolic side effects, including glucose intolerance, are less likely to occur with the newer vasodilating β-blockers. Concern about the risk of diabetes should not deter us from prescribing diuretics or β-blockers if they are indicated. Some drug classes are neutral with respect to glucose tolerance (calcium channel blockers, α-blockers, and vasodilators). ACE-Is and ARBs have a protective effect. As drugs are most commonly used in combination, we should perhaps not read too much into the documented effects of individual classes or agents. An algorithm for managing the above type of patient is shown in Figure 30.2. As well as carefully managing BP, the possibility of T2D should be borne in mind and appropriate tests carried out where needed, and treatment should be initiated at an early stage should he become glucose intolerant.

References

1   Burke TA, Sturkenboom MC, Ohman-Strickland PA, Wentworth CE, Rhoads GG. The effect of antihypertensive drugs and drug combinations on the incidence of new-onset type-2 diabetes mellitus. *Pharmacoepidemiol Drug Saf* 2007; **16**: 979–87.

2   Ostergren J. Renin-angiotensin-system blockade in the prevention of diabetes. *Diabetes Res Clin Pract* 2007; **76** (Suppl 1): S13–21.

3   Bangalore S, Parkar S, Grossman E, Messerli FH. A meta-analysis of 94 492 patients with hypertension treated with beta blockers to determine the risk of new-onset diabetes mellitus. *Am J Cardiol* 2007; **100**: 1254–62.

4   Zillich AJ, Garg J, Basu S, Bakris GL, Carter BL. Thiazide diuretics, potassium, and the development of diabetes: a quantitative review. *Hypertension* 2006; **48**: 219–24.

5   Conen D, Ridker PM, Mora S, Buring JE, Glynn RJ. Blood pressure and risk of developing type 2 diabetes mellitus: the Women's Health Study. *Eur Heart J* 2007; **28**: 2937–43.

6   Elliott WJ, Meyer PM. Incident diabetes in clinical trials of antihypertensive drugs: a network meta-analysis. *Lancet* 2007; **369**: 201–7.

7   Messerli FH, Bell DSH, Fonseca V, Katholi RE, McGill JB, Phillips RA, *et al.* Body weight changes with beta-blocker use: results from GEMINI. *Am J Med* 2007; **120**: 610–15.

8   Cooper-Dehoff R, Cohen JD, Bakris GL, Messerli FH, Erdine S, Hewkin AC, *et al.* Predictors of development of diabetes mellitus in patients with coronary artery disease taking anti-hypertensive medications (findings from the INternational VErapamil SR-Trandolapril STudy [INVEST]). *Am J Cardiol* 2006; **98**: 890–4.

31 Type 2 Diabetes

Case History

Mary is 57 years old and has been known to have type 2 diabetes (T2D) for 4 years. She weighed 87 kg at diagnosis, but has managed to reduce this to 79.6 kg. As a result, her diabetes has been well controlled with diet and long-acting metformin. Her blood pressure (BP) has been more of a problem. She was initially commenced on an angiotensin-converting enzyme inhibitor (ACE-I), but did not feel well on this. Subsequently, she tried a calcium channel blocker but developed ankle oedema. Her BP is 146/94 and albumin/creatinine ratio is elevated at 6.8 although renal function is normal.

Does tight BP control prevent microvascular and macrovascular complications?

What agent(s) should we choose?

Should we be worried about antihypertensive agents that increase hyperglycaemia?

Background

Hypertension is two to three times more common among patients with T2D compared with the general population. Unlike in type 1 diabetes, it is often present before or at the time of diagnosis. Hypertension is a powerful risk factor for both micro- and macrovascular complications. Even when glycaemic control is suboptimal, the risk of retinopathy and nephropathy is lower if BP is in the recommended range. Hypertension is present in up to 60% of patients with T2D. BP is particularly likely to be high when there is evidence of nephropathy. The aetiology of hypertension in diabetes is complex, although many of the factors are similar to those in essential hypertension: there is activation of the renin–angiotensin system (RAS) and sympathetic nervous system; hyperinsulinaemia contributes to increased salt retention; endothelial dysfunction is associated with impaired vasodilatation. Control of BP is critical in patients with T2D.

Key trials have been reviewed (includes references).[1] The UKPDS (UK Prospective Diabetes Study group) randomized 1148 patients to either tight BP control or standard management. Definition of tight BP control (150/85) was more relaxed than the current definition. Patients were followed for 8.4 years. Those in the tight control group achieved a BP of 144/82 compared with 154/87 in the standard. With tight control, diabetes-related end-points were decreased by 24%, deaths related to diabetes were decreased by 32%, and there was a 37% decrease in microvascular end-points. Overall in UKPDS, there was no difference between captopril and atenolol in preventing complications. A 10 mmHg reduction in systolic BP was associated with relative risk (RR) reductions of:

- 12% for any complication;

- 15% for deaths related to diabetes;

- 11% for myocardial infarction; and

- 13% for microvascular complications.

Many recent key trials on nephropathy have used angiotensin receptor blockers (ARBs) – losartan, irbesartan, telmisartan, eprosartan, valsartan and candesartan have all been shown to be effective options. In RENAAL (Reduction of Endpoints in Non-Insulin Dependent Diabetes Mellitus with the Angiotensin II Antagonist Losartan) (2001),[1] 1513 patients with diabetes and nephropathy were randomized to losartan or placebo and followed for 3.4 years. Patients continued to take other antihypertensives as required. The composite endpoint was doubling of baseline serum creatinine, development of end-stage renal disease or death. A total of 327 patients in the losartan group and 359 in the placebo group ($P = 0.02$), reached the primary end-point – RR reduction of 16%. The RR reduction of increased creatinine was 25% and for end-stage renal disease was 28%. There was no difference in cardiovascular (CV) outcomes. The IDNT (Irbesartan in Diabetic Nephropathy Trial) study (2001)[1] randomized 1715 patients with hypertension and nephropathy due to T2D to irbesartan, amlodipine or placebo. The target BP was 135/85 and the composite end-point identical to that for RENAAL. After a mean follow-up of 2.6 years, the risk of reaching the end-point was 20% lower with losartan compared with placebo ($P = 0.02$) and 23% lower compared with amlodipine ($P = 0.006$). Again, there was no difference in CV outcomes. The IRMA (Irbesartan in Type 2 Diabetics with Microalbuminuria) study (2001) randomized 590 patients with hypertension, T2D and microalbuminuria (MA) to either placebo, or irbesartan at doses of 150 mg or 300 mg (three groups followed for 24 months). The primary end-point was onset of overt albuminuria, and was reached in 5.2% of those taking 300 mg irbesartan, 9.7% of those taking 150 mg irbesartan and in 14.9% of the placebo group. These studies suggest extra value of the ARBs beyond their ability to lower BP.

Three landmark trials examined the effect of antihypertensive drugs on macrovascular complications – UKPDS (1998), the ABCD (Appropriate Blood Pressure Control in Diabetes) study (2000), and the FACET (Fosinopril Versus Amlodipine Cardiovascular Events Randomized Trial) (1998).[1] UKPDS confirmed decrease in death and stroke with BP lowering but found no difference between captopril and atenolol. The ABCD study suggested that, in spite of similar BP lowering, myocardial infarction was less common in those treated with enalapril as opposed to nisoldipine. Further follow-up of this cohort has revealed a strong relationship between left ventricular hypertrophy or microalbumin and risk of CV events. FACET followed patients for a mean of 2.9 years comparing fosinopril with amlodipine. Again, a slightly superior effect of the ACE-I was suggested. Subgroup analyses of the SHEP (Systolic Hypertension in the Elderly Program) and Syst-Eur (Systolic Hypertension in Europe trial) cohorts in the late 1990s confirmed that BP lowering was at least as effective as an intervention in diabetic subjects compared with those without diabetes. In the HOPE (Heart Outcomes Prevention Evaluation) (2000)[1], 3577 patients with diabetes and at least one other risk factor were randomized to ramipril or placebo. In spite of only modest differences in systolic BP and diastolic BP, the ramipril group had lower risk of CV events, death and microvascular complications.

Table 31.1 Effects of antihypertensive agents on diabetes end-points			
Class	Coronary	Renal	Stroke
ACE-I	++ (A)	++ (A)	++ (A)
ARB	?	++ (A)	?
Thiazide	++ (A)	?	++ (A)
Loop diuretic	?	?	?
α-blocker	??	?	?
β-blocker	++ (A)	++ (A)	++ (A)
Dihydropyridine calcium channel blockers	??	??	++ (A)
Non-dihydropyridine	?	+ (C)	?
Calcium channel blockers			
Central adrenergic	?	?	?

ACE-I, angiotensin-converting enzyme inhibitors; ARB, angiotensin receptor blockers. Letters A–C indicate decreasing levels of supporting evidence. Adapted from Arauz-Pacheco et al.[1]

Lifestyle factors are of critical importance in managing the diabetic patient with hypertension. For BP reduction with drugs, the available classes are similar – a reduction of 10 mmHg in systolic BP and 5 mmHg in diastolic BP would typically be expected from addition of each agent. It follows that most people need more than one agent. The effect of antihypertensive drugs on vascular outcomes in patients with T2D has been intensively studied (see Table 31.1).

Two important recent studies are:

1 The BENEDICT (BErgamo NEphrologic DIabetic Complications Trial) study[2] in which 1204 hypertensive patients with T2D and normoalbuminuria were assigned to trandolapril, verapamil, a fixed combination of the two, or placebo. Other antihypertensives were prescribed as required. After 3.6 years follow-up, risk of microalbumin was directly proportional to the lowering of BP achieved. Furthermore, ACE-I had a protective effect independent of BP lowering while verapamil did not. The combination treatment was helpful in achieving target BP.

2 The ADVANCE study[3] recruited 11 140 patients with T2D from 215 centres in 20 countries. They were randomized to perindopril/indapamide combination or placebo and followed for a mean of 4.3 years. Those in the treatment wing had a mean reduction of systolic BP of 5.6 mmHg and diastolic BP of 2.2 mmHg. The hazard ratio for vascular events was 0.91 (95% confidence interval [CI]: 0.83 to 1.00, $P = 0.004$). Similar reductions were noted for micro- and macrovascular events. To avoid one death from vascular disease over 5 years, 79 patients would have to be treated.

Recent Developments

1 The genes of the RAS (angiotensinogen, ACE, and the angiotensin II type 1 receptor) and those that regulate salt sensitivity have variants that are associated with higher

BP.[4] The higher the number of high BP gene variants in an individual, the greater the risk of hypertension. A large study of variants in the β_2-adrenoreceptor gene did not find an association between these variants and risk of either hypertension or T2D.[5]

2   The prevalence of T2D in young people is increasing rapidly. A study of 3259 subjects who had diabetes onset <20 years[6] reported the prevalence of increased albumin/creatinine ratio to be 9.2% in those with type 1 diabetes but 22.2% in those with T2D. Hypertension was an important determinant of albuminuria. Patients with early-onset T2D are at high risk of renal and vascular problems.

3   Masked hypertension is common in patients with T2D, and is associated with increased UAE.[7] Nocturnal non-dipping has been related to an increased risk of retinopathy. A large study has documented that high mean BP is a better predictor for vascular events than office BP, both in patients with and without diabetes.[8]

4   The relationship between thiazolidinedione usage and risk of CV events is currently a controversial area with suggestions that rosiglitazone may increase the event rate. Several recent studies have suggested that pioglitazone may improve BP control as well as decreasing vascular inflammation, and has been documented to improve nocturnal BP control.[9] The PROactive (PROspective PioglitAzone Clinical Trial In MacroVascular Events) study[10] reported that pioglitazone decreased the incidence of myocardial infarction and acute coronary syndrome in patients with T2D. Recent studies have also described renal protective effects of rosiglitazone and the dual α/γ peroxisome proliferator activated receptor agonist tesaglitazar.

5   Resistant hypertension is commonly encountered among patients with diabetes and is associated with the significant prevalence of primary hyperaldosteronism – recently reported at 14%.[11] Where appropriate, renin and aldosterone should be measured and the role of aldosterone blockers should not be forgotten in those in whom BP is difficult to control.

Conclusions

There is overwhelming evidence that controlling hypertension in patients with diabetes lowers the risk of complications. Additionally, there is a strong suggestion that RAS-blocking drugs confer benefits beyond lowering BP. In trials, the risk reduction with hypertension control is substantially greater among patients with diabetes because of their higher baseline risk. Recent studies suggest that RAS-blocking drugs not only slow the advance of diabetic complications, but they also prevent their occurrence. Hypertension is a greater risk factor for macrovascular complications than is hyperglycaemia. An algorithm for BP management in T2D is proposed in Figure 31.1. ACE-I, ARB and thiazides have become regarded as first-line agents, with calcium channel blockers and β-blockers as second-line. Agents that increase hyperglycaemia should not necessarily be avoided but compensatory increases in hypoglycaemic treatment may be required if they are used.

References

1   Arauz-Pacheco C, Parrot MA, Raskin P. The treatment of hypertension in adult patients with diabetes. *Diabetes Care* 2002; **25**: 134–47.

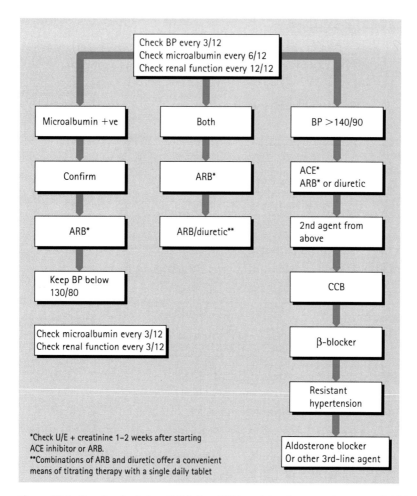

Figure 31.1 Hypertension in type 2 diabetes. ACE-I, angiotensin-converting enzyme inhibitor; ARB, angiotensin receptor blocker; CCB, calcium channel blocker

2   Ruggenenti P, Perna A, Ganeva M, Ene-Iordache B, Remuzzi G, BENEDICT Study Group. Impact of blood pressure control and angiotensin-converting enzyme inhibitor therapy on new-onset microalbuminuria in type 2 diabetes: a post hoc analysis of the BENEDICT trial. *J Am Soc Nephrol* 2006; **17**: 3472–81.

3   Patel A; ADVANCE Collaborative Group, MacMahon S, Chalmers J, Neal B, Woodward M, *et al*. Effects of a fixed combination of perindopril and indapamide on macrovascular and microvascular outcomes in patients with type 2 diabetes mellitus (the ADVANCE trial): a randomised controlled trial. *Lancet* 2007; **370**: 829–40.

4   Yazdanpanah M, Aulchenko YS, Hofman A, Janssen JA, Sayed-Tabatabaei FA, van Schaik RH, *et al*. Effects of the renin-angiotensin system genes and salt sensitivity genes on blood pressure and atherosclerosis in the total population and patients with type 2 diabetes. *Diabetes* 2007; **56**: 1905–12.

5   Gjesing AP, Andersen G, Burgdorf KS, Borch-Johnsen K, Jorgensen T, Hansen T, *et al.* Studies of the associations between functional beta2-adrenergic receptor variants and obesity, hypertension and type 2 diabetes in 7,808 white subjects. *Diabetologia* 2007; **50**: 563–8.

6   Maahs DM, Snively BM, Bell RA, Dolan L, Hirsch I, Imperatore G, *et al.* Higher prevalence of elevated albumin excretion in youth with type 2 than type 1 diabetes: the SEARCH for Diabetes in Youth study. *Diabetes Care* 2007; **30**: 2593–8.

7   Leitao CB, Canani LH, Kramer CK, Moehlecke M, Pinto LC, Ricardo ED, *et al.* Blood pressure means rather than nocturnal dipping pattern are related to complications in Type 2 diabetic patients. *Diabet Med* 2008; **25**: 308–13.

8   Eguchi K, Pickering TG, Hoshide S, Ishikawa J, Ishikawa S, Schwartz JE, *et al.* Ambulatory blood pressure is a better marker than clinic blood pressure in predicting cardiovascular events in patients with/without type 2 diabetes. *Am J Hypertens* 2008; **21**: 443–50.

9   Anan F, Masaki T, Fukunaga N, Teshima Y, Iwao T, Kaneda K, *et al.* Pioglitazone shift circadian rhythm of blood pressure from non-dipper to dipper type in type 2 diabetes mellitus. *Eur J Clin Invest* 2007; **37**: 709–14.

10 Erdmann E, Dormandy JA, Charbonnel B, Massi-Benedetti M, Moules IK, Skene AM, *et al.* The effect of pioglitazone on recurrent myocardial infarction in 2,445 patients with type 2 diabetes and previous myocardial infarction: results from the PROactive (PROactive 05) Study. *J Am Coll Cardiol* 2007; **49**: 1772–80.

11 Umpierrez GE, Cantey P, Smiley D, Palacio A, Temponi D, Luster K, *et al.* Primary aldosteronism in diabetic subjects with resistant hypertension. *Diabetes Care* 2007; **30**: 1699–703.

32 Microalbuminuria

Case History

Mrs BR is a 59-year-old woman with reasonably well controlled hypertension. She takes atenolol 25 mg BD and long-acting diltiazem. There is a strong family history of hypertension, and her mother developed renal failure in her 60s. Mrs BR went through menopause at age 50 and did not take hormone replacement therapy (HRT). She has had a cholecystectomy, and is para 3[+1]. Her GP decided to check her urine for protein. She has microalbuminuria (MA) confirmed on three occasions (albumin/creatinine ratio 12.5, 17.8 and 14.3). She does not have diabetes and her renal function is normal.

How strong is the association between hypertension and MA?

Would current evidence favour her being treated with an angiotensin-converting enzyme inhibitor (ACE-I) or an angiotensin receptor blocker (ARB)?

Does the presence of MA affect prognosis?

Background

MA is urinary protein excretion above that which is regarded as normal or desirable, but below the detection level for standard urine stick testing (300 mg/l) – see Box 32.1. Before it is said to be present, it should be confirmed on three separate occasions within 3 months and in the absence of other factors which increase urinary protein such as urinary tract infection. The prevalence of MA is:

- In diabetes, 25–35%.

- In hypertension, 15–20%.

- With diabetes and hypertension, 30–40%.

- In the normal population, 5–7%.

Macroalbuminuria (urine protein >300 mg/day) occurs in up to 10% of the population. There has been recent interest in what is termed 'low-grade albuminuria' – a level of protein <30 mg/day but in the high range of what was previously regarded as normal and which is also associated with an increased risk of vascular disease. The tendency to higher albumin excretion may be determined from an early stage in life. It is strongly associated with endothelial dysfunction and thus other cardiovascular (CV) risk factors. Numerous studies in diabetes, hypertension and the general population have confirmed that increased albumin excretion is associated with increased risk of CV events (relative risk [RR] = 2–3).[1] These studies (references are given in Weir[1]) include the WHO Monica Study (1999) in which 2085 subjects without ischaemic heart disease, were followed for 10 years. Those with MA had a relative risk of 2.3 for CV events. The HOPE (Heart Outcomes Prevention Evaluation) Study (2001) involved 9297 high-risk patients followed over 5 years. All-cause mortality was 9.4% in those with normal albumin excretion, compared with 18.2% in those with MA. The RR associated with increased protein excretion was 2.09 (95% confidence interval [CI]: 1.84 to 2.38). The PREVEND (Prevention of Renal and Vascular End Stage Disease) study (2002) followed a cohort of 40 458 subjects for a mean of 2.6 years. A two-fold increase in albumin excretion rate was associated with a 29% increase in risk of CV death. The EPIC-Norfolk (European Prospective Investigation into Cancer in Norfolk) study (2004) followed 22 368 subjects who did not have ischaemic heart disease at baseline over 6.4 years. Subjects were divided into tertiles according to albumin excretion when macroalbuminuria was not present. Compared with those in the lowest tertile, those in the second tertile had a hazard ratio (HR) for ischaemic heart disease of 1.30 (95% CI: 0.86 to 1.47), and those in the highest tertile had HR of 1.86 (95% CI: 1.24 to 1.92), while those with macroalbuminuria had HR of 2.84 (95% CI: 1.80 to 2.46).

Box 32.1 Microalbuminuria

- Urinary albumin excretion (UAE) of 30–300 mg/day

- Equivalent to 20–200 µg/min

- As a screen, and to avoid timed collections: albumin/creatinine ratio
  - >2.5 mg/mmol in men
  - >3.5 mg/mmol in women

- The higher normal range in women reflects their lower muscle mass

---

The relationship between urine protein excretion and CV risk is shown in Figure 32.1. These data from the HOPE study are shown by decile of MA with decile 8 corresponding to the normal threshold for MA. The risk increases with increasing albuminuria. There is not much difference in the risk with increasing protein excretion between diabetic and non-diabetic individuals. It is routine to check annually for MA in patients with diabetes, and those who are positive or otherwise at high risk have MA measured every 3–6 months. It is puzzling why MA is measured so infrequently in patients without diagnosed diabetes. In a recent Spanish study[2] the prevalence of MA increased with worsening glycaemia from 39.7% in normoglycaemic subjects, 46.2% and 48.6% in low and high range impaired fasting glucose, and 65.6% in patients with diabetes. There was a strong relationship, as expected, between increased albumin excretion and renal impairment. Poorer glucose or BP control is highly associated with MA, renal abnormalities and risk of vascular events or renal failure. In patients with both diabetes and hypertension, MA is present in at least 40%. Diabetes increases albumin excretion through osmotic diuresis if it is poorly controlled while increased systemic BP leads to glomerular hypertension and thus increased glomerular protein filtration. Both diabetes and hypertension with their

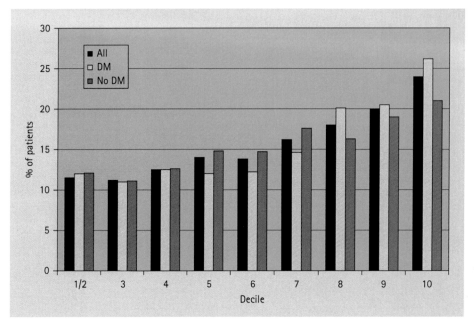

Figure 32.1 Relationship between microalbuminuria and cardiovascular events. DM, diabetes mellitus. Adapted from Weir (2007)1 using data from the HOPE (Heart Outcomes Prevention Evaluation) study.

attendant endothelial dysfunction increase protein leakage across endothelial surfaces. Increased passage of lipoproteins in the vasculature contributes to the development of atherosclerosis. MA correlates with a wide range of CV outcomes including all-cause CV mortality, left ventricular hypertrophy, heart failure, stroke, and peripheral vascular disease. It is also a powerful predictor of renal impairment.

Albumin/creatinine ratio on a first void in the morning or overnight collection is preferred. In reality, it is much easier to screen patients on a random clinic sample. If MA is present, it should be confirmed on at least two further random or early morning samples or on timed collection. A timed overnight collection is usually easier for the patient than a 24-h urine collection. Causes of a false positive screening test include urinary tract infection, exercise, heart failure and menstruation.

In the late 1990s, considerable trial data accumulated showing a protective effect of ACE-Is in high-risk patients, principally those with diabetes. ACE-Is were repeatedly shown to protect against CV events and decline in renal function. These studies culminated in the HOPE study (2000), which demonstrated a protective effect of ramipril.[3] Further support for the hypothesis that renin–angiotensin system (RAS) blockade exerted protective effects beyond simple BP reduction came from studies with ARB – the IDNT (Irbesartan in Diabetic Nephropathy Trial) and IRMA (Irbesartan in Type 2 Diabetics with Microalbuminuria)-2 studies with irbesartan and the RENAAL (Reduction of Endpoints in Non-Insulin Dependent Diabetes Mellitus with Angiotensin II Antagonist Losartan) study with losartan – all three focusing on patients with type 2 diabetes and all published in 2001. These studies were not powered to detect differences in CV events but did show retardation of nephropathy.[3] Two more recent studies with

ACE-Is have provided evidence that targeting MA with RAS blockade significantly reduces CV events: the PREVENT IT study with fosinopril was published in 2004, and the MARPLE study with ramipril followed in 2006.[3] There is a wealth of evidence to show that treatment with RAS-blocking drugs is protective in patients with MA, studies showing a 20% or more decrease in end-point rate. However, other hypotensive drugs (e.g. calcium channel blockers) can also decrease albuminuria and afford protection.

Recent Developments

1   The i-SEARCH study was an observational study involving 21 050 hypertensive patients from 26 countries.[4] Overall, MA was present in 58.4% and was commonest with higher BP, obesity, renal impairment and with proven CV disease. While MA and decreased glomerular filtration rate are strongly associated, each provides independent predictive information regarding future renal function and CV risk.[5]

2   There has been debate as to whether more comprehensive RAS blockade with ACE-I plus ARB is advantageous. Data from the recent IMPROVE (Irbesartan in the Management of PROteinuric patients at high risk of Vascular Events) trial[6] suggest that the combination of ramipril and irbesartan may help patients reach target BP (compared with irbesartan plus placebo). However, there was no evidence that dual blockade was any more effective in protecting renal function or preventing progression of proteinuria.

3   Sympathetic activation not only contributes to increased BP but also to a decline in renal function and increased CV risk with hypertension. β-blockers are effective in preventing renal decline but standard cardioselective agents are not as potent as RAS-blocking drugs. There is emerging evidence that the newer vasodilating β-blockers such as carvedilol and nebivolol are more protective than conventional β-blockers.[7] By decreasing renal vascular resistance, these agents protect against a decrease in glomerular filtration with hypertension.

4   Masked hypertension is emerging as a risk factor for CV disease. One of the major benefits of measuring MA is in picking up patients with suspected masked hypertension who can then be further investigated.[8] Similarly, nocturnal or early morning surges in BP (also missed with office BP measurements) may be suspected if MA is present.[9] Increased nocturnal BP is associated with increased proteinuria and is also predictive of progressive proteinuria.

5   Data from the HyperGEN (Hypertension Genetic Epidemiology Network) and other studies confirm that increased left ventricular mass is frequently found with MA.[10] As with urinary albumin, where changes in excretion within the currently accepted normal range (low-grade albuminuria), increases in left ventricular mass that do not reach the threshold for the diagnosis of left ventricular hypertrophy are also predictive of adverse events. Both increased urinary albumin and increased left ventricular mass can regress with effective treatment of hypertension.

6   Low-grade albuminuria is rapidly emerging as a risk factor for a range of adverse CV outcomes, including cardiac failure.[11,12] These data suggest that, like BP, UAE is a continuous variable with no particular threshold value being associated with increased CV risk.

Conclusions

 Varying rates of MA have been reported in hypertensive patients. MA is a good marker for future risk of renal and cardiac events. MA measurement is grossly underused in practice for patients with hypertension. Management of the patient with increased urinary albumin is summarized in Figure 32.2. There is a wealth of evidence that RAS blockade with either ACE-I or ARB protects the kidneys and decreases CV risk. While much of this evidence has come from studies involving patients with diabetes, there is every reason to believe that the protective effects of these drugs extend to individuals without diabetes. RAS-blocking drugs have a protective effect in addition to their BP-lowering action. Other drugs, including the newer vasodilating β-blockers may also have renal protective effects. While ACE-I and ARB are the logical choice when MA is detected, other drugs are often needed to achieve target BP.

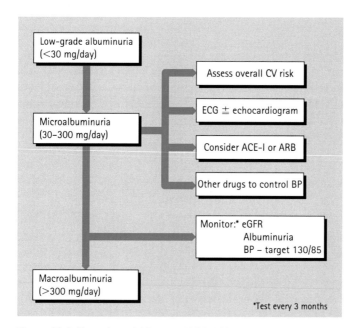

Figure 32.2 The patient with increased UAE. ACE-I, angiotensin-converting enzyme inhibitor; ARB, angiotensin receptor blocker; eGFR, estimated glomerular filtration rate

References

1   Weir MR. Microalbuminuria and cardiovascular disease. *Clin J Am Soc Nephrol* 2007; **2**: 581–90.

2   Redon J, Morales-Olivas F, Galgo F, Brito MA, Mediavilla J, Marin R, *et al.* Urinary albumin excretion and glomerular filtration rate across the spectrum of glucose abnormalities in essential hypertension. *J Am Soc Nephrol* 2006; **17**: S236–45.

3 Schmieder RE, Schrader J, Zidek W, Tebbe U, Paar WD, Bramlage P, *et al.* Low-grade albuminuria and cardiovascular risk. What is the evidence? *Clin Res Cardiol* 2007; **96**: 247–57.

4 Bohm M, Thoenes M, Danchin N, Bramlage P, La Puerta P, Volpe M. Association of cardiovascular risk factors with microalbuminuria in hypertensive individuals: the i-SEARCH global study. *J Hypertens* 2007; **25**: 2317–24.

5 Cirillo M, Lanti MP, Menotti A, Laurenzi M, Mancini M, Zanchetti A, *et al.* Definition of kidney dysfunction as a cardiovascular risk factor: use of urinary albumin excretion and estimated glomerular filtration rate. *Arch Intern Med* 2008; **168**: 617–24.

6 Bakris GL, Ruilope L, Locatelli F, Ptaszynska A, Pieske B, de Champlain J, *et al.* Treatment of microalbuminuria in hypertensive subjects with elevated cardiovascular risk: results of the IMPROVE trial. *Kidney Int* 2007; **72**: 879–85.

7 Hart PD, Bakris GL. Should beta-blockers be used to control hypertension in people with chronic kidney disease? *Semin Nephrol* 2007; **27**: 555–64.

8 Kato T, Horio T, Tomiyama M, Kamide K, Nakamura S, Yoshihara F, *et al.* Reverse white-coat effect as an independent risk for microalbuminuria in treated hypertensive patients. *Nephrol Dial Transplant* 2007; **22**: 911–16.

9 Palmas W, Pickering T, Teresi J, Schwartz JE, Eguchi K, Field L, *et al.* Nocturnal blood pressure elevation predicts progression of albuminuria in elderly people with type 2 diabetes. *J Clin Hypertens* 2008; **10**: 12–20.

10 Djousse L, Kochar J, Hunt SC, North KE, Gu CC, Tang W, *et al.* Relation of albuminuria to left ventricular mass (from the HyperGEN Study). *Am J Cardiol* 2008; **101**: 212–16.

11 Ingelsson E, Sundstrom J, Lind L, Riserus U, Larsson A, Basu S, *et al.* Low-grade albuminuria and the incidence of heart failure in a community-based cohort of elderly men. *Eur Heart J* 2007; **28**: 1739–45.

12 Sung KC, Kim BJ, Ryu S. An association of a variety of cardiovascular risk factors with low grade albuminuria in Korean men. *Atherosclerosis* 2008; **196**: 320–6.

PROBLEM

33 Chronic Kidney Disease

Case History

Mrs JB is a 64-year-old woman who looks after her husband who retired early because of respiratory disease. She has had hypertension for many years and was recently diagnosed with type 2 diabetes. She is concerned about her kidneys as her father died from renal failure and she knows that her kidney tests are abnormal. She has an estimated glomerular filtration rate (eGFR) of 44 ml/min per 1.73m² and her albumin/creatinine ratio (ACR) is increased at 30 mg/mmol. Her diabetes is well controlled on diet (HbA$_1$c 6.5%) and her blood pressure (BP) is about 140/85 typically. She takes a long-acting diltiazem, Moduretic, aspirin and a non-steroidal anti-inflammatory drug for mild osteoarthritis.

What is the relationship between hypertension and renal impairment?

Is this woman's BP control tight enough?

How does the presence of chronic kidney disease (CKD) modify the approach to managing hypertension?

Background

The rising prevalence of diabetes and the ageing population structure mean that CKD is becoming increasingly common. Cardiovascular (CV) risk is markedly increased in patients with CKD, and the effective management of CV risk factors protects against CV events as well as slowing the progress of CKD. It is estimated that CKD (Box 33.1) is present in 1:7 adults. This equates to about 26 million in the USA (10 million with albuminuria but normal eGFR, 15.5 million with eGFR 30–59, and 0.7 million with eGFR 15–29). Many people are unaware that they have renal impairment. CKD is highly prevalent among those with CV disease – 23% of patients with coronary artery disease, 33% with myocardial infarction and 46% of those with heart failure.

Only a minority of patients will develop end-stage renal disease requiring dialysis or transplantation. CV disease represents a much greater risk for a large proportion of patients with CKD, and hypertension is an important component of this risk. Go *et al.*[1] examined data from 1 120 295 adults followed-up over 3 years. In this large, community-based sample there was a graded relationship between decreased eGFR and the risk of death, CV events and hospitalization. The relationship between eGFR and risk of CV events is shown in Figure 33.1. In a study involving 3258 subjects from the Framingham

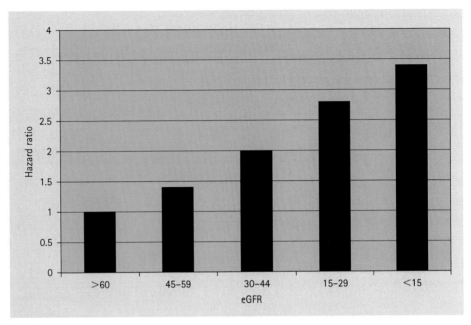

Figure 33.1 Hazard ratio for cardiovascular events. eGFR, estimated glomerular filtration rate. Data from Go *et al.*[1]

Offspring Cohort,[2] those with CKD were more likely to be obese, have diabetes, have high low-density lipoprotein cholesterol and low high-density lipoprotein cholesterol, and to have increased triglyceride levels. Hypertension was present in 71.2% of those with CKD compared with 42.7% of those without CKD. Those with CKD and hypertension were less likely to achieve target BP. GFR declines with age, and this is associated with an increased CV risk as has been demonstrated in a number of studies, including ALLHAT (Antihypertensive and Lipid-Lowering Treatment to Prevent Heart Attack Trial), HOPE (Heart Outcomes Prevention Evaluation), HOT (Hypertension Optimal Treatment), Syst-Eur (Systolic Hypertension in Europe) and VALIANT (VALsartan In Acute myocardial iNfarcTion).[3] Many older patients with renal impairment do not have increased serum creatinine. Even where GFR is relatively preserved, there is an association between albuminuria and CV risk factors.

The kidneys are normally protected from increases in systemic BP by constriction of the afferent and efferent arterioles, limiting glomerular hydrostatic pressure. In those at high risk (diabetes or hypertension), the antiregulatory mechanisms fail due to endothelial dysfunction, and activation of both the sympathetic nervous system and renin–angiotensin system (RAS). The result is increased glomerular hydrostatic pressure with hyperfiltration and proteinuria. Glomerular damage from increased pressure further increases proteinuria. The filtered protein is toxic to the tubules and interstitium, hastening a decline in renal function.[4] The IDNT (Irbesartan in Diabetic Nephropathy Trial) (2005) confirmed the superior effect of angiotensin receptor blockers (ARBs) compared with amlodipine in diabetic nephropathy. Further evidence for the protective effect of ARBs came from the IRMA (Irbesartan in Type 2 Diabetics with

Box 33.1 **Definition of chronic kidney disease**

A:

● Estimated glomerular filtration rate <60 ml/min per 1.73 m^2

● Present for ≥3 months

● With or without evidence of renal damage

Or

B:

● Evidence of renal damage

● Present for ≥3 months

● With or without decreased glomerular filtration rate

● Evidence of renal damage includes:

　　○ Microalbuminuria

　　○ Proteinuria

　　○ Glomerular haematuria

　　○ Abnormal renal biopsy

　　○ Anatomical – polycystic kidney disease, scarring on renal ultrasound, computed tomography or magnetic resonance imaging

Microalbuminuria) and RENAAL (Reduction of Endpoints in Non-Insulin Dependent Diabetes Mellitus with Angiotensin II Antagonist Losartan) trials.[3] Many studies have suggested that RAS blockade is a superior approach to managing BP in those with renal abnormalities. ALLHAT set out to compare chlorthalidone, lisinopril, amlodipine and doxazosin in over 40 000 hypertensive patients with at least one other risk factor followed over 5 years.[4] The α-blocker wing was terminated prematurely because of increased heart failure. There was no superiority of the angiotensin-converting enzyme inhibitors (ACE-Is) over other classes in preventing renal failure, and an increase in stroke was noted with lisinopril. The scale of this study has coloured subsequent analyses, and it remains uncertain to what degree RAS-blocking drugs have a specific renoprotective effect.

Creatinine is not the most useful measure of impaired renal function – it only increases out of the normal range when about 50% of function has been lost and it varies with age, gender and muscle mass. eGFR is now widely reported and is expressed as ml/min per 1.73 m^2. It is calculated using the MDRD (Modification of Diet in Renal Disease) formula, which is now used in place of the previously used Cockroft–Gault formula. The update Schwartz formula is used to calculate eGFR in children. Values between 60 and 90 signal risk of renal deterioration but full investigation is not usually warranted until eGFR falls below 60. eGFR falls by about 10 for every decade above 40 years. For the elderly (>70 years) values of 45–59 are acceptable if there is other evidence of renal damage. Stages of CKD are summarized in Table 33.1. Symptoms of advanced renal failure include nocturia, malaise, shortness of breath, nausea, vomiting and anorexia, pruritus, and restless legs.

Table 33.1 Stages of chronic kidney disease

Stage	Estimated glomerular filtration rate	Description
1	≥90	Renal damage with normal function
2	60–89	Renal damage with mild impairment
3	30–59	Moderate impairment
4	15–29	Severe impairment
5	<15	End-stage kidney disease

Table 33.2 Albuminuria and proteinuria

	Microalbuminuria	Macroalbuminuria	Proteinuria
ACR	♀ 3.6–35	♀ >35	–
	♂ 2.6–25	♂ >25	–
Dipstick	>3 mg/dl	>20 mg/dl	1+ or more
PCR	–	–	>30mg/mmol
24 h protein	–	–	>0.3 g/24 h

ACR, albumin/creatinine ratio expressed as mg/mmol; PCR, protein/creatinine ratio.

In those at risk of CKD (diabetes, hypertension, cardiovascular disease, family history of renal disease and certain racial groups) screening for proteinuria should be undertaken on an annual basis, as it is often the earliest marker. If present, proteinuria should be confirmed on a separate occasion and then quantified. The latter is most simply done on a spot sample, measuring ACR. This ratio is expressed in mg/mmol and daily protein excretion can be calculated by multiplying the ACR figure by 10 – e.g. an ACR of 35 mg/mmol corresponds to a daily protein excretion of 350 mg/24 h. Definitions of proteinuria are given in Table 33.2.

Recent Developments

1 In a recent large study,[5] hypertension was present in 86.2% of over 10 000 patients with CKD. A total of 1:5 patients were not aware of their hypertension, and the majority of patients did not reach the target BP of 130/80. Male gender, black race and high body mass index all correlated with poor BP control. Hypertension was more likely with more advanced CKD. Age is an important influence in the hypertension of CKD, particularly as prevalence of CKD increases with age.[6] Older patients with CKD are more likely to have office hypertension, be nocturnal non-dippers, have isolated systolic hypertension, or to develop diastolic hypotension with treatment.

2 Hypertension is not adequately controlled in the majority of patients with CKD. A Polish study[7] has confirmed that the majority (70%) of patients with CKD are

hypertensive and about 20% of these are on no treatment to lower BP. Of those treated, only 1:5 reached target BP. Being overweight was strongly associated with hypertension in this CKD cohort.

3 Effective BP control is one of the major factors governing progression of CKD. Although multiple CV risk factors including smoking, physical inactivity, being overweight and glucose intolerance contribute to risk of declining renal function, none is as potent a risk factor as hypertension. For example, in the recent study by Obermayr et al.,[8] the odds ratio for the decline in renal function was 1.35 (95% confidence interval [CI]: 1.08 to 1.67) with stage 1 hypertension, compared with 2.01 (95% CI: 1.62 to 2.510 with stage 2.

4 Care has to be taken not to overestimate the benefit of ACE-I and ARB: most patients in trials (as in practice) require multiple drugs to control their BP; in the trial setting, only very small differences in average BP lowering achieved can significantly affect outcome statistics. With that note of caution in mind, early treatment with RAS-blocking drugs is indicated in nearly all patients with hypertension and CKD. An analysis of 25 trials with a combined total of nearly 46 000 patients[9] has also confirmed that the RAS blockade (compared with placebo) protects patients with CKD from total CV outcomes, myocardial infarction and heart failure.

5 Among the recently described associations with CKD and hypertension are obstructive sleep apnoea/hypopnoea syndrome, non-alcoholic fatty liver disease and cerebral white matter intensities. Given the protean nature of complications of CKD/hypertension, early markers would be useful. Cystatin C is a small molecule inhibitor of cysteine proteases and is produced widely in the body. As GFR declines, plasma levels of cystatin C increase and this may be a more sensitive marker than eGFR. The utility of the test in practice has yet to be established, as elevated levels are common in high-risk groups including African American men and the elderly,[10] and those with the metabolic syndrome.[11]

Conclusions

More than 80% of patients with CKD have hypertension, many are unaware of the risk associated with their increased BP, and only a minority achieves the currently agreed BP target of 130/80. The above patient does not have tight enough BP control. The management of hypertension and CKD is considered in Figure 33.2. RAS blockade with either ACE-Is or ARBs should be considered early. An early small increase in serum creatinine after starting an RAS-blocking drug should not cause concern, and is actually predictive of good long-term response. Creatinine increase beyond this should lead to consideration of renal artery stenosis. Dual blockade with ACE-I plus ARB is controversial as there is not a dramatic decrease in BP when the two are combined (compared with one agent only), but there may be an additional renoprotective effect. Diuretics are an important component of a regimen and patients with CKD often require loop diuretics. The vasodilating β-blockers (carvedilol and nebivolol) have favourable effects on renal haemodynamics and should be considered (especially in patients with cardiac disease). BP control is not only important to slow the rate of declining renal function but also to protect these high-risk patients from CV events.

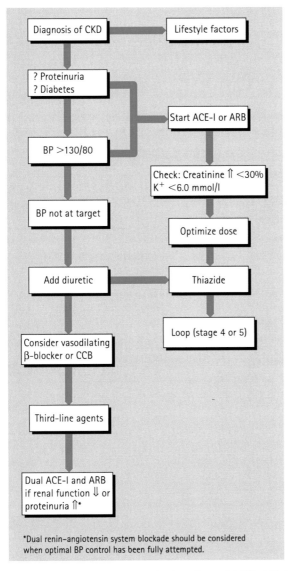

Figure 33.2 Managing hypertension in patients with CKD. ACE-I, angiotensin-converting enzyme inhibitor; ARB, angiotensin receptor blocker; CCB, calcium channel blocker; CKD, chronic kidney disease

References

1   Go AS, Cherlow GM, Fan D, McCulloch CE, Hsu C. Chronic kidney disease and the risk of death, cardiovascular events and hospitalization. *N Engl J Med* 2004; **351**: 1296–305.

2   Parikh NI, Hwang S-J, Larson MG, Meigs JB, Levy D, Fox CS. Cardiovascular disease risk factors in chronic kidney disease: overall burden and rates of treatment and control. *Arch Intern Med* 2006; **166**: 1884–91.

3 Dukkipati R, Adler S, Mehrotra R. Cardiovascular implications of chronic kidney disease in older adults. *Drugs Aging* 2008; **25**: 241–53.

4 Lindeman RD. Hypertension and kidney protection in the elderly: what is the evidence in 2007? *Int Urol Nephrol* 2007; **39**: 669–78.

5 Sarafidis PA, Li S, Chen S-C, Collins AJ, Brown WW, Klag MJ, *et al.* Hypertension awareness, treatment, and control in chronic kidney disease. *Am J Med* 2008; **121**: 332–40.

6 Minutolo R, Borrelli S, Chiodini P, Scigliano R, Bellizzi V, Cianciaruso B, *et al.* Effects of age on hypertensive status in patients with chronic kidney disease. *J Hypertens* 2007; **25**: 2325–33.

7 Krol E, Czarniak P, Rutkowski B. Effectiveness of antihypertensive treatment in patients with chronic kidney disease. *J Renal Nutr* 2008; **18**: 134–9.

8 Obermayr RP, Temml C, Knechtelsdorfer M, Gutjahr G, Kletzmayr J, Heiss S, *et al.* Predictors of new-onset decline in kidney function in a general middle-European population. *Nephrol Dial Transplant* 2008; **23**: 1265–73.

9 Balamuthusamy S, Srinivasan L, Verma M, Adigopula S, Jalandara N, Hathiwala S, *et al.* Renin angiotensin system blockade and cardiovascular outcomes in patients with chronic kidney disease and proteinuria: a meta-analysis. *Am Heart J* 2008; **155**: 791–805.

10 Kottgen A, Selvin E, Stevens LA, Levey AS, Van Lente F, Coresh J. Serum cystatin C in the United States: the Third National Health and Nutrition Examination Survey (NHANES III). *Am J Kidney Dis* 2008; **51**: 385–94.

11 Servais A, Giral P, Bernard M, Bruckert E, Deray G, Isnard Bagnis C. Is serum cystatin-C a reliable marker for metabolic syndrome? *Am J Med* 2008; **121**: 426–32.

34 Obstructive Sleep Apnoea/Hypopnoea Syndrome

Case History

Mr GM is 58 years old and complains of feeling constantly tired by day, and tends to fall asleep readily. His wife confirms that he sleeps fitfully and snores loudly. He has been overweight most of his adult life (body mass index 34 kg/m²) but remains very active. He is a moderately heavy drinker and smokes 10 cigarettes per day. Until recently, his blood pressure (BP) has been well controlled with a single agent. However, his systolic BP (SBP) is now consistently about 145 and his diastolic BP about 100.

Why is there an association between hypertension and sleep apnoea?

How should an individual with this combination be investigated?

What are the important features of management?

Background

Obstructive sleep apnoea/hypopnoea syndrome (OSAHS) occurs in 3–7% of adult men and in 2–5% of women. It is intrinsically important as it affects quality of life. It is also associated with increased risk of hypertension, glucose intolerance, stroke and other cardiovascular (CV) events.[1] Features include:

- Frequent nocturnal awakenings with excessive urination (nocturia)

- Severe snoring

- Morning asthenia ± headaches

- Daytime somnolence

Precipitating factors include upper respiratory tract abnormalities, obesity, age, smoking and alcohol consumption. Diagnosis is by polysomnography, which simultaneously records electroencephalogram (EEG), sleep and nasal pressure, along with thoracic and abdominal respiratory movements. The apnoeic episodes may be due to obstruction (in which case respiratory effort continues), to central causes (where there is no respiratory effort), or a mixed picture may present. Polysomnography allows the measurement of the number of apnoeic or hypopnoeic episodes. In the latter, there is either a 50% reduction in inspiratory flow or a 30% reduction with >3% desaturation. Respiratory polygraphy (with no sleep record) is useful where polysomnography is not available. The

Box 34.1 **Epworth Sleepiness Scale**

Patients score 0–3 according to how likely they are to fall asleep in certain situations: the total score is out of 24. Score 11–16 indicates a high likelihood of obstructive sleep apnoea/hypopnoea syndrome. >16 indicates severe sleepiness.

Score:
- 0 Would never doze
- 1 Slight chance of dozing
- 2 Moderate chance of dozing
- 3 High chance of dozing

Situations:
1 Sitting and reading
2 Watching television
3 Sitting inactive in a public place (e.g. cinema or a meeting)
4 Passenger in a car for an hour without a break
5 Lying down to rest in the afternoon (circumstances permitting)
6 Sitting and talking with someone
7 Sitting quietly after lunch (with no alcohol)
8 In a car when stopped for a few minutes in traffic

presence of 15 or more episodes per hour is consistent with OSAHS. The severity of the syndrome is expressed as the apnoea–hypopnoea index (AHI), which is defined as the number of episodes per hour. The Epworth Sleepiness Scale (Box 34.1) is a useful screening tool.

Increased prevalence of obesity, along with increased awareness of OSAHS has led to increasing diagnosis of this condition. It is commoner in men, but women are less likely to be investigated. Obesity is a powerful risk factor, and independent associations with waist and neck circumference have been noted. OSAHS is present in 40% of obese individuals and about 70% of those with OSAHS are obese, many of the remainder being overweight. Not only does obesity predispose to the occurrence of OSAHS, but also to its progression. It is estimated that a 10% increase in body weight increases AHI by up to 30%.[1] There is a genetic influence with first-degree relatives of sufferers being more likely to develop OSAHS. Racial differences also exist – Asian subjects develop the syndrome at a much lower body weight than Caucasians, and there is a high prevalence in older African Americans.

Hypertension is a common association with OSAHS, and up to 30% of hypertensive subjects have OSAHS. On the other hand, about 60% of patients with OSAHS are hypertensive. There appears to be a continuous relationship between AHI and risk of hypertension – compared with those who have AHI of 0, those with AHI 0–5 have an odds ratio (OR) for hypertension of about 1.4, those with AHI 5–15 have an OR of 2 and those with AHI >15 have an OR of about 3. The relative risk (RR) of hypertension in men who snore has been reported at 1.94 for men and 3.19 for women. There is a continuous increase in prevalent BP with increasing severity of sleep symptoms. Often, daytime SBP is normal but there is isolated diastolic hypertension or nocturnal BP disturbance with lack of the normal night-time dip. BP typically falls during the apnoeic/hypopnoeic episodes but increases as the episode progresses and arousal begins. Stimuli to increased BP include hypoxia, carbon dioxide retention, increased respiratory effort and changes in arousal. The repeated episodes lead to an increase in average nocturnal BP, as well as decreased baroreflex sensitivity and sympathetic nervous system activation. Also, there is increased plasma endothelin, endothelial dysfunction, and renin–angiotensin system (RAS) activation.

Treatments for OSAHS include postural changes in sleeping (avoid sleeping on the back), avoid alcohol and sedatives, weight loss, and upper airways surgery. The cornerstone of modern management is continuous positive airway pressure (CPAP), which prevents collapse of airways during inspiration. In addition to its positive effect on sleep symptoms, CPAP lowers BP – typically a 5–10 mmHg drop in SBP. As OSAHS symptoms can increase markedly with modest increases in body weight, weight loss is an important goal. There is a reciprocal relationship between body weight and OSAHS symptoms – improvement in the latter can make it easier for the patient to lose weight. Left ventricular hypertrophy is common in OSAHS, and its prevalence increases with severity, and with the severity of hypertension. The occurrence of left ventricular hypertrophy is a marker for increased risk of CV events, and should prompt vigorous hypertension management. Because of the role of the sympathetic nervous system in OSAHS-associated hypertension, β-blockers are often considered the first line of treatment. Lipid-soluble β-blockers (oxprenolol, pindolol and propranolol) cross the blood–brain barrier and are thus more likely to cause central nervous system (CNS) side effects, including sleep disturbances, and are perhaps best avoided. RAS is also activated in OSAHS and angiotensin-converting enzyme inhibitors or angiotensin receptor blockers should be considered.

Recent Developments

1   The beneficial effect of CPAP in reducing BP has been questioned. A meta-analysis of 10 studies (three crossover, seven parallel) with a total of 587 patients[2] reported only modest effect. SBP was decreased by only 1.38 (95% CI: 3.6 to −0.88, $P = 0.23$) and diastolic BP by 1.52 (95% CI: 3.1 to −0.07, $P = 0.06$). This contrasts with a recent study[3] that involved patients with a mean BP of 154.9/90 at baseline, and in which mean SBP was decreased by 5.2 mmHg and nocturnal SBP by 6.1 mmHg. There was no change in diastolic BP. The beneficial effect of CPAP was even greater when analysis only included those who complied well with CPAP.

2   The presence of OSAHS may account, in large part, for the association between obesity and resistant hypertension. Activation of RAS occurs in many patients with resistant hypertension, and is reflected in an increased plasma aldosterone or increased aldosterone/renin ratio. A correlation between the severity of OSAHS and plasma aldosterone concentration has been documented.[4] The aldosterone/renin ratio should be checked in patients with both OSAHS and hypertension, and RAS-blocking drugs, including aldosterone antagonists, should be considered in those with elevated aldosterone/renin ratio.

3   Patients with hypertension and OSAHS have increased fractional clearance of sodium at night and increased levels of ambulatory venous pressure.[5] The latter almost certainly contribute to plasma volume expansion and increased pressor

effects. Urinary symptoms (nocturia) are very common in OSAHS and probably relate to altered nocturnal handling of salt and water. A clearer understanding of the endocrine changes that occur will lead to effective management of urinary symptoms as well as hypertension associated with OSAHS.

4   There is a correlation between OSAHS and features of the metabolic syndrome, including hypertension.[6,7] This association exists even in non-obese patients with OSAHS. Patients with sleep-related symptoms should have assessment of their overall CV risk, and multifactor intervention where indicated. The relationship

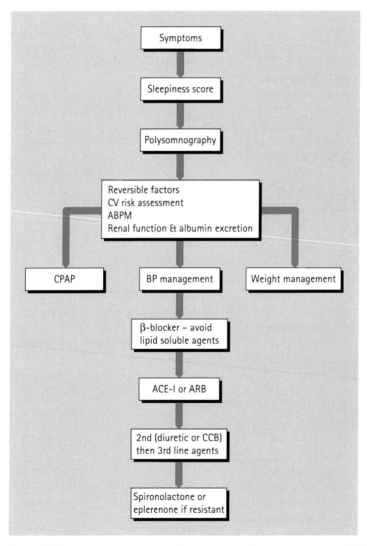

Figure 34.1 Hypertension and obstructive sleep apnoea/hypopnoea syndrome. ABPM, ambulatory BP monitoring; ACE-I, angiotensin-converting enzyme inhibitor; ARB, angiotensin receptor blocker; CCB, calcium channel blocker; CPAP, continuous positive airways pressure

between BP and what appears to be sleep disturbance may not be so strong in very elderly subjects.[8]

5   There is a high prevalence of chronic kidney disease in patients who have hypertension and concurrent sleep disorders.[9] It is possible that obesity actually has a protective effect, and that chronic kidney disease is particularly likely in lean patients with hypertension and OSAHS. Regular screening (including urinary albumin excretion [UAE]) is indicated in this high-risk group.

6   Patients with sleep disorders are at increased risk of stroke, coronary artery disease, heart failure, atrial fibrillation and sudden cardiac death.[10] A recent small 10-year follow-up study[11] of patients who had suffered stroke demonstrated that those with high AHI were at increased risk of death.

Conclusions

Sleep-related disturbances occur in up to 50% of those aged 65 or above. OSAHS has been increasingly diagnosed over the past decade but 70% or more remain undiagnosed. It is unclear to what extent effective management of sleep symptoms contributes to BP lowering and decreased cardiac risk. Improvement in sleep symptoms may improve patients' engagement with weight loss and exercise programmes. Hypertension may not be apparent in office BP measurements, and there should be a low threshold for requesting ambulatory BP monitoring. Various mechanisms have been implicated, including sympathetic nervous system activation, nocturnal changes in salt and water handling, and RAS activation. Investigation and management are summarized in Figure 34.1. Because of the increased risk of CV events and chronic kidney disease, and doubt as to whether managing the OSAHS *per se* is beneficial, effective management of BP is essential and requires consideration of the pattern of BP abnormalities seen.

References

1   Punjabi NM. The epidemiology of adult obstructive sleep apnea. *Proc Am Thorac Soc* 2008; **5**: 136–43.

2   Alajmi M, Mulgrew AT, Fox J, Davidson W, Schulzer M, Mak E, *et al*. Impact of continuous positive airway pressure therapy on blood pressure in patients with obstructive sleep apnea hypopnea: a meta-analysis of randomized controlled trials. *Lung* 2007; **185**: 67–72.

3   Martinez-Garcia MA, Gomez-Aldaravi R, Soler-Cataluna JJ, Martinez TG, Bernacer-Alpera B, Roman-Sanchez P. Positive effect of CPAP treatment on the control of difficult-to-treat hypertension. *Eur Respir J* 2007; **29**: 951–7.

4   Pratt-Ubunama MN, Nishizaka MK, Boedefeld RL, Cofield SS, Harding SM, Calhoun DA. Plasma aldosterone is related to severity of obstructive sleep apnea in subjects with resistant hypertension. *Chest* 2007; **131**: 453–9.

5   Gjorup PH, Sadauskiene L, Wessels J, Nyvad O, Strunge B, Pedersen EB. Increased nocturnal sodium excretion in obstructive sleep apnoea. Relation to nocturnal change in diastolic blood pressure. *Scand J Clin Lab Invest* 2008; **68**: 11–21.

6   McArdle N, Hillman D, Beilin L, Watts G. Metabolic risk factors for vascular disease in obstructive sleep apnea: a matched controlled study. *Am J Respir Crit Care Med* 2007; **175**: 190–5.

7   Kono M, Tatsumi K, Saibara T, Nakamura A, Tanabe N, Takiguchi Y, *et al.* Obstructive sleep apnea syndrome is associated with some components of metabolic syndrome. *Chest* 2007; **131**: 1387–92.

8   van den Berg JF, Tulen JHM, Neven AK, Hofman A, Miedema HME, Witteman JCM, *et al.* Sleep duration and hypertension are not associated in the elderly. *Hypertension* 2007; **50**: 585–9.

9   Iseki K, Tohyama K, Matsumoto T, Nakamura H. High prevalence of chronic kidney disease among patients with sleep related breathing disorder (SRBD). *Hypertens Res* 2008; **31**: 249–55.

10 McNicholas WT, Bonsigore MR, Management Committee of EU COST ACTION B26. Sleep apnoea as an independent risk factor for cardiovascular disease: current evidence, basic mechanisms and research priorities. *Eur Respir J* 2007; **29**: 156–78.

11 Sahlin C, Sandberg O, Gustafson Y, Bucht G, Carlberg B, Stenlund H, *et al.* Obstructive sleep apnea is a risk factor for death in patients with stroke: a 10-year follow-up. *Arch Intern Med* 2008; **168**: 297–301.

Secondary Causes of Hypertension

PROBLEM

35 Catecholamines and Phaeochromocytoma

Case History

Mr JT is 42 years old. He is generally healthy with no past medical history of note. He gives a 5-year history of episodes during which he experiences palpitations, a feeling of fear and panic, and headache. His blood pressure (BP) has been noted to be high but the measurements are very variable, often being normal. There is no strong family history of hypertension or vascular disease. Electrocardiogram (ECG) and plasma electrolytes are normal.

When should investigations for phaeochromocytoma (PH) be undertaken?

How should a suspected PH be investigated?

How should PH be managed?

Background

PH is rare, but should be considered in cases of refractory or variable hypertension, and when other possible clinical features are present (Box 35.1): Remember the 4 Ps: pressure, palpitation, pallor and perspiration. It is present in 1:200 patients referred to specialist centres for hypertension but in less than 1:2000 hypertensive patients in the general population. Up to 25% are diagnosed when adrenal adenomas are incidentally discovered although less than 1:20 adrenal adenomas are PHs. Hypertension and hyperglycaemia become sustained with time, other symptoms are usually intermittent. Episodes can be precipitated by food, exercise or drugs (e.g. tricyclics or metoclopramide), and last from seconds to an hour typically. Diagnosis is often delayed and patients, all too often, present with vascular events. Investigations should be undertaken whenever the syndrome is suspected.

Box 35.1 **Features of phaeochromocytoma**

- Sustained or paroxysmal hypertension
- Episodes of fear or panic
- Anxiety
- Dyspnoea
- Nausea
- Headache
- Sweating
- Palpitations
- Weakness
- Hyperglycaemia

The tumours arise from chromaffin cells in the adrenal medulla. Annual incidence is 2–8 per million, and they typically present in the third to fifth decades. Men and women are equally affected. About half of PHs are sporadic, while the remainder have a genetic cause. About 10% occur in patients with MEN-2 (medullary carcinoma of the thyroid, primary hyperparathyroidism and phaeochromocytoma). A total 40% of MEN-2 patients have PH. Other conditions in which PH is inherited include neurofibromatosis type 1 (multiple skin and tongue fibromas and café au lait spots) and von Hippel–Lindau syndrome (pancreatic and renal cysts or neoplasms, retinal and central nervous system (CNS) haemangioblastomas, epidydimal cystadenoma). They are also present in the Carney triad (gastric leiomyosarcoma, pulmonary chondroma and paraganglionoma). Patients with mutations of the succinate dehydrogenase (SDH) *SDHB*, *SDHC* or *SDHD* genes may present with PH, which can be large, metabolically silent, extra-adrenal and malignant. These familial tumours can produce catecholamines – about 5% of head and neck tumours compared with about 50% of abdominal tumours. The 'rule of 10' is still useful – around 10% of tumours are bilateral, 10% extra-adrenal (actually more), and 10% are malignant. Extra-adrenal tumours are usually termed paraganglionomas (functional paraganglioma [FGPL]). Malignancy is more common in large tumours, those that are extra-adrenal and with SDH (especially *SDHB*) mutations.

The screening test of choice is measurement of fractionated urinary metanephrines (metadrenaline and normetadrenaline).[1] This has sensitivity of 97% and a specificity of 70%. Plasma measurements are more sensitive and specific. Urinary vanillylmandelic acid is less specific. Fractionated plasma catecholamine measurements are now widely available. Dopamine-secreting tumours are described, but their clinical significance unclear. Plasma catecholamines should be measured in the resting state through an indwelling cannula. A variety of drugs can produce false positive results – phenoxybenzamine, L-DOPA, methyldopa, metoclopramide, tricyclics and labetalol. β-blockers and calcium channel blockers should also be stopped wherever possible before the measurement of catecholamines. The majority of patients with high plasma catecholamine levels turn out not to have PH. The clonidine suppression test is required less frequently now – in normal subjects following 0.3 mg clonidine orally plasma catecholamines suppress to <50% of baseline within 3 hours.

Once the diagnosis is confirmed biochemically, the next stage is to localize the tumour. It is important to remember that, although they may be extra-adrenal, 98% are located in the abdomen or pelvis. It is preferable to use computed tomography or magnetic resonance imaging scanning to identify adrenal or extra-adrenal lesions prior to nuclear medicine scanning. The radiopharmaceutical ^{131}I-meta-iodobenzylguanidine (MIBG), is used for functional radionuclide scanning and is 75–90% sensitive but very specific. Positive results may occur with other tumours – small cell lung cancer, carcinoid, medullary carcinoma of thyroid, or neuroblastoma. Adrenergic drugs (especially labetalol), tricyclics, calcium channel blockers and cocaine interfere with the uptake of the agent, and should be omitted in the week before the scan.

The logical medical treatment is adrenergic blockade, but other agents may be required to control severe hypertension. The α-blocker phenoxybenzamine is generally used initially – at a dose of 10 mg BD increasing to 20–40 mg BD or TDS. Titration can be stopped once BP is controlled – target systolic BP is 120 mmHg sitting and 90 mmHg standing. Patients may find the postural drop in BP difficult to tolerate but adequate preparation is essential prior to surgery. Doxazosin or prazosin can be used in place of phenoxybenzamine. When the patient is α-blocked it is time to start β-blockers. The aim is to control the tachycardia associated with α-blockade and excess catecholamines rather than to directly lower BP. If additional treatment is required to lower BP, calcium channel blockers should be considered first. Operative and peri-operative care should be undertaken by a surgeon, physician and anaesthetist with experience of managing PH. Careful follow-up should be undertaken in each case as 10% of adrenal tumours and one-third of extra-adrenal tumours will recur. Malignant tumours are treated surgically, with chemotherapy, and with therapeutic doses of ^{131}I-MIBG. All cases should be carefully followed up with regular screening for recurrent disease.

Recent Developments

1   Understanding of the genetics of PH has increased in recent years.[2] Traditionally, 10% have been considered to be familial but it now appears that as many as 20–25% are genetic in origin – the most common genes involved being the *RET*, *SDHB* and *SDHD*, *VHL*, and *NF1* genes. The SDH genes are part of the mitochondrial complex and act as tumour suppressors. Inactivating mutations lead to enhanced activity of the hypoxia-induced angiogenesis pathways. Genetic screening and counselling should now be considered for all patients with PH and FPGL.

2   There is now consensus[3] that fractionated metanephrines (urine or plasma) is a more effective screening test. Chromogranin A (CgA) is a useful marker for neuroendocrine tumours and is elevated in 90% of patients with PH or FPGL. The CgA fragment catestatin (CgA 352–372) is a naturally occurring inhibitor of catecholamine secretion, and decreases hypertension in some animal models.[4] A variant form of catestatin (genetically determined) has recently been shown to alter human autonomic reactivity and susceptibility to hypertension.[5] These developments have elevated the CgA pathway from simple marker status to a mechanism that may be involved in the aetiology of hypertension and a possible therapeutic target.

3   The prevailing BP in patients with PH does not correlate directly with circulating catecholamine levels. Very high levels of the latter may lead to receptor desensitization,[6] the result of which may be paroxysms of very high BP with episodes of hypotension (sometimes severe),[7] and alteration of the normal diurnal pattern of BP regulation.

4   Genetic differences in the catecholamine pathway may account for the susceptibility of black populations to hypertension and renal disease. Recent studies have focused on common polymorphisms – the deletion polymorphism in the α_{2C}-adrenergic receptor gene[8] and a common variation in the CgA gene.[9] The latter determines the level of catestatin, which, when low, increases the effect of catecholamines on the progression of end-stage renal disease.

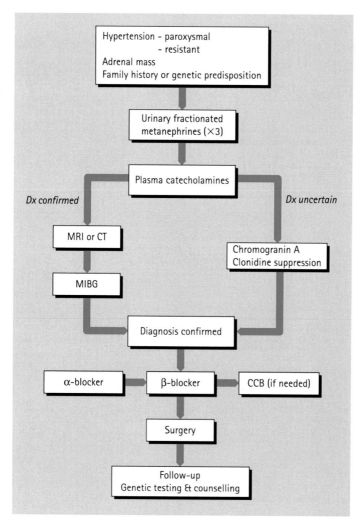

Figure 35.1 Investigation of suspected phaeochromocytoma. CCB, calcium channel blocker; CT, computed tomography; MIBG, meta-iodobenzylguanidine; MRI, magnetic resonance imaging

Conclusions

Although rare, PH frequently has to be excluded in practice. It should be considered when there is a family history of the condition, with adrenal tumours, and when hypertension is either severe or resistant. Advances in biochemical measurements and imaging have made the diagnosis much easier (Figure 35.1). However, after initial screening, investigation and management should be undertaken by clinicians that have experience of the condition. The role of genetic factors has come to the fore recently and all patients should be considered for genetic screening and counselling. Finally, study of these rare tumours has led to increased understanding of catecholamine secretion in common forms of hypertension and will possibly lead to novel treatments.

References

1   Young WF, Jr. Adrenal causes of hypertension: pheochromocytoma and primary aldosteronism. *Rev Endocr Metab Disord* 2007; **8**: 309–20.

2   Gimenez-Roqueplo A-P, Burnichon N, Amar L, Favier J, Jeunemaitre X, Plouin P-F. Recent advances in the genetics of phaeochromocytoma and functional paraganglioma. *Clin Exp Pharmacol Physiol* 2008; **35**: 376–9.

3   Peaston RT, Ball S. Biochemical detection of phaeochromocytoma: why are we continuing to ignore the evidence? *Ann Clin Biochem* 2008; **45**: 6–10.

4   Mahapatra NR, Mahata M, Mahata SK, O'Connor DT. The chromogranin A fragment catestatin: specificity, potency and mechanism to inhibit exocytotic secretion of multiple catecholamine storage vesicle co-transmitters. *J Hypertens* 2006; **24**: 895–904.

5   Rao F, Wen G, Gayen JR, Das M, Vaingankar SM, Rana BK, *et al.* Catecholamine release-inhibitory peptide catestatin (chromogranin A(352-372)): naturally occurring amino acid variant Gly364Ser causes profound changes in human autonomic activity and alters risk for hypertension. *Circulation* 2007; **115** (17): 2271–81.

6   Zelinka T, Pacak K, Widimsky J, Jr. Characteristics of blood pressure in pheochromocytoma. *Ann N Y Acad Sci* 2006; **1073**: 86–93.

7   Kobal SL, Paran E, Jamali A, Mizrahi S, Siegel RJ, Leor J. Pheochromocytoma: cyclic attacks of hypertension alternating with hypotension. *Nat Clin Pract Cardiovasc Med* 2008; **5**: 53–7.

8   Kurnik D, Muszkat M, Friedman EA, Sofowora GG, Diedrich A, Xie H-G, *et al.* Effect of the alpha2C-adrenoreceptor deletion322-325 variant on sympathetic activity and cardiovascular measures in healthy subjects. *J Hypertens* 2007; **25**: 763–71.

9   Salem RM, Cadman PE, Chen Y, Rao F, Wen G, Hamilton BA, *et al.* Chromogranin A polymorphisms are associated with hypertensive renal disease. *J Am Soc Nephrol* 2008; **19**: 600–14.

36 Aldosterone and Conn's Syndrome

Case History

GB is 53 years old and his hypertension is difficult to control. He takes three agents (angiotensin-converting enzyme inhibitor [ACE-I], diuretic and β-blocker), yet systolic blood pressure (BP) is consistently above 145 mmHg. He has normal renal function but the albumin/creatinine ratio is increased. Electrocardiogram (ECG) shows voltage criteria for left ventricular hypertrophy although there is no strain pattern. Renal ultrasound shows normal sized kidneys and no suggestion of renovascular abnormalities. A random clinic aldosterone measurement is 920 pmol/l (normal 340–800 pmol/l for an ambulant sample). He has been hypokalaemic on a number of occasions, although his electrolytes are generally normal.

How likely is he to have primary hyperaldosteronism (PA)?

How should he be investigated further?

What is likely to be the optimal management of his condition?

Background

The role of aldosterone excess and the benefits of aldosterone blockade have come to prominence in recent years. Amongst patients with apparently 'essential' hypertension, PA has been reported in 8–13%. A further 20% or so have an elevated aldosterone/renin ratio (ARR) but aldosterone level within the normal range. Furthermore, up to 20% of patients with resistant hypertension are responsive to aldosterone blockade. Although the true prevalence of PA is debated, it should be remembered that it is the commonest remediable cause of hypertension. PA most commonly occurs in the 4th to 7th decades and is twice as common in men. Sixty per cent of cases are due to aldosterone producing adenoma (APA), 30 % to bilateral adrenal hyperplasia and 10% to multiple adrenal nodules, with carcinoma being very rare. Increased aldosterone from the zona glomerulosa leads to increased sodium retention in the distal convoluted tubule, with loss of hydrogen ions, potassium and magnesium. Table 36.1 summarizes the consequences of increased aldosterone. The association between high aldosterone and metabolic syndrome/glucose intolerance has now been well documented. Secondary aldosteronism occurs in heart failure, nephrotic syndrome and cirrhosis. In these conditions, high levels of aldosterone contribute to end-organ damage.

Table 36.1 Effects of excess aldosterone

Cardiovascular	Renal	Metabolic
Left ventricular hypertrophy	Glomerular damage	Hypokalaemia
Left ventricular dysfunction	Interstitial damage	Impaired glucose
Stroke	Vascular damage	tolerance
Myocardial infarction	Glomerular hyperfiltration	Metabolic syndrome
Atrial fibrillation	Increased albumin excretion rates	

Table 36.2 Effects of antihypertensive drugs

Lower renin, increase ARR	Increase renin, lower ARR	Drugs with minimal effects
β-blockers	Diuretics	Slow-release verapamil
Clonidine	Angiotensin-converting enzyme inhibitors	Hydralazine
Methyldopa	Angiotensin receptor blockers	Doxazosin
Non-steroidal anti-inflammatory drugs	DCCBs	Prazosin

ARR, aldosterone/renin ratio; DCCB, dihydropyridine calcium channel blocker.

There has been controversy surrounding aldosterone measurement as there is no universally agreed upper limit of normal and many factors influence the plasma concentration, including drugs (Table 36.2). Typical reference ranges are:

- Aldosterone
  - Supine: 30–450 pmol/l
  - Ambulant: 100–900 pmol/l

- Renin (mass)
  - Supine: 2–30 mU/l
  - Ambulant: 3–40 mU/l
  - ARR: normal <70.0

Measurements should be taken after overnight recumbence, and then following 4 hours of being ambulatory. In patients with APA, values are uniformly high. In those with bilateral adrenal hyperplasia (BAH), the levels are high but may increase with posture. The test should be performed in the morning, and in the normal non-stressed individual cortisol should decrease during the test. Renin has been measured traditionally as enzyme activity – leading to difficulty in standardization between laboratories and difficulty with transporting samples. ARR has now been adopted as the screening measurement of choice. The ratio can be disproportionately affected by relatively small changes in renin. Measurement of renin concentration (mass) is being increasingly used and overcomes many of the technical problems with enzyme activity measurements. A cut-off value of

70 pmol/mU for ARR using mass measurements should diagnose most with aldosterone excess. Hypokalaemia should be corrected before aldosterone measurements and dynamic tests are performed.

When screening tests suggest aldosterone excess, at least one confirmatory test should be carried out. These are:

- *IV saline suppression.* The recumbent patient is given 2 litres of saline IV over 4 hours. This suppresses mineralocorticoid production in normal people. This test does not require prolonged preparation or the patient to be admitted.

- *Fludrocortisone suppression.* Although time-consuming and demanding, this remains the gold standard. The patient is loaded with sodium (slow release sodium 30 mmol [1.75 g] TDS) and, if needed, then supplemented with potassium. Fludrocortisone is administered (0.1 mg every 6 hours for 4 days), following which ambulant aldosterone is measured. Failure to suppress the latter suggests PA. The test should not be carried out in patients with heart failure or other serious cardiac states.

- *Oral sodium loading.* Aim for an intake of >200 mmol/day with potassium supplementation if needed. This is widely used in North America as an outpatient screening test.

- Captopril challenge. ARR is measured 2 h after 25–50 mg captopril. The ACE-I decreases aldosterone in patients with essential hypertension but not in those with PA.

When PA is confirmed, investigations (Figure 36.1) should then define the subtype. Magnetic resonance imaging or high-resolution computed tomography identify adrenal nodules and may identify micronodular disease. There is no functional scan to identify aldosterone-secreting lesions. Adrenal vein sampling should be carried out where possible when a nodule is identified. This is technically demanding, and not universally available. Cortisol in the adrenal vein should be at least twice that in a peripheral vein. The side with the adenoma should have adrenal vein aldosterone at least twice that in a peripheral vein. The contralateral side should be suppressed, although suppression is not always complete. Patients with a strong family history of mineralocorticoid hypertension in early life should have genetic testing for glucocorticoid-remediable aldosteronism (GRA). In this rare genetic disorder, the glucocorticoid promoter regulates the aldosterone gene, and mineralocorticoid excess can be suppressed with glucocorticoid. The effect of drugs on renin, aldosterone, and ARR should not be forgotten (Table 36.1). Where possible, investigations should be carried out with the patient taking no, or minimal, treatment. Admission may be necessary and BP can be controlled for a short spell with drugs, which do not have major effects on the renin–angiotensin system. Clearly, tests should not be carried out with the patient taking aldosterone blockers.

Recent Developments

1   In a recent Greek study,[1] 1616 patients with resistant hypertension were screened. Increased ARR was found in 338 patients and, on the basis of salt suppression tests, 182 (11.3%) had PA. Diagnosis was confirmed by a BP-lowering effect of

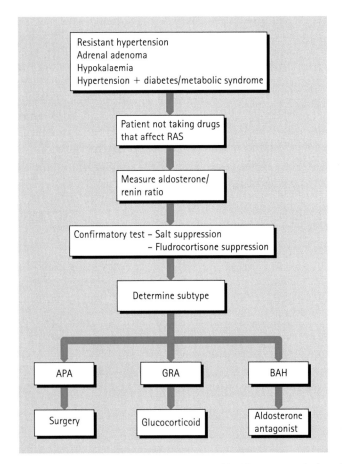

Figure 36.1 Suspected hyperaldosteronism. APA, aldosterone producing adenoma; BAH, bilateral adrenal hyperplasia; GRA, glucocorticoid-remediable aldosteronism; RAS, renin–angiotensin system

spironolactone. Hypokalaemia was present in only 83 (45.6%) patients with PA. Although this study confirmed a high prevalence of PA with resistant hypertension, the prevalence was not as high as that reported in some studies.

2   The widespread use of ARR for screening has increased the diagnosis of PA by up to 15-fold.[2] There has also been a shift from hypokalaemia to resistant hypertension as the major trigger for investigation. Hypokalaemia is only present in 9–37% of PA. The Italian PAPY (Primary Aldosteronism Prevalence in Italy) study[3] investigated 1180 patients referred to one of 14 centres. APA was diagnosed in 54 (4.8%) and bilateral adrenal hyperplasia in 72 (6.4%). In both of these studies,[2,3] the pick-up rate for adenomas was increased where adrenal vein sampling was available. This is important because APA is surgically remediable, although up to 70% of cases still require some antihypertensive treatment after operation. The PAPY study also confirmed that patients with excess aldosterone are at increased risk of early and more marked renal damage.

3 Increased aldosterone contributes directly to renal damage. While not routinely recommended at present, the addition of mineralocorticoid blockers to ACE-I or ARB may increase renal protection and diminish proteinuria.[4] These data add to the growing evidence that increased aldosterone is a major contributor to end-organ damage in patients with severe hypertension.[5,6]

4 Aldosterone breakthrough has been recognized in patients taking either ACE-I or ARB.[7] With time, in spite of RAS blockade, the increased mineralocorticoid may contribute to end-organ damage, offsetting the potential benefits of ACE-I or ARB. There are no widespread recommendations for screening for aldosterone excess in patients treated with RAS-blocking drugs, but growing evidence of benefit from dual blockade with aldosterone antagonist plus ACE-I/ARB.

5 A direct relationship has been documented in hypertensive patients between the level of aldosterone and insulin resistance.[8] The mechanism for this association is beginning to be understood. Aldosterone has been reported[9] to decrease expression of the insulin receptor substrate-1, which is involved in insulin signalling. This effect is attenuated by eplerenone.

Conclusions

Whatever the precise prevalence of PA, which may vary between populations, it is not as common as was once thought. Hypokalaemia occurs in only a minority of cases. There is a strong association of PA with resistant hypertension, and its recognition is critical as diagnosis may lead to surgery, or more rational medical treatment. There is also a growing body of evidence for the association between PA and insulin-resistant states. The threshold for investigation should be low in those with family or personal history of metabolic syndrome or type 2 diabetes. Investigations are now much more streamlined with screening using ARR, followed by confirmatory tests (saline or fludrocortisone suppression), and followed by imaging and venous sampling. For those in whom medical therapy for PA is indicated, eplerenone has become available and has a lower incidence of side effects (gynaecomastia and menstrual disturbance) than spironolactone.

References

1 Douma S, Petidis K, Doumas M, Papaefthimiou P, Triantafyllou A, Kartali N, *et al.* Prevalence of primary hyperaldosteronism in resistant hypertension: a retrospective observational study. *Lancet* 2008; **371**: 1921–6.

2 Mulatero P, Stowasser M, Loh K-C, Fardella CE, Gordon RD, Mosso L, *et al.* Increased diagnosis of primary aldosteronism, including surgically correctable forms, in centers from five continents. *J Clin Endocrinol Metab* 2004; **89**: 1045–50.

3 Rossi GP, Bernini G, Caliumi C, Desideri G, Fabris B, Ferri C, *et al.* A prospective study of the prevalence of primary aldosteronism in 1,125 hypertensive patients. *J Am Coll Cardiol* 2006; **48**: 2293–300.

4 Bomback AS, Kshirsagar AV, Amamoo MA, Klemmer PJ. Change in proteinuria after adding aldosterone blockers to ACE inhibitors or angiotensin receptor blockers in CKD: a systematic review. *Am J Kidney Dis* 2008; **51**: 199–211.

5 Yoshimoto T, Hirata Y. Aldosterone as a cardiovascular risk hormone. *Endocr J* 2007; **54**: 359–70.

6 Connell JMC, MacKenzie SM, Freel EM, Fraser R, Davies E. A lifetime of aldosterone excess: long-term consequences of altered regulation of aldosterone production for cardiovascular function. *Endocr Rev* 2008; **29**: 133–54.

7 Yoneda T, Takeda Y, Usukura M, Oda N, Takata H, Yamamoto Y, *et al.* Aldosterone breakthrough during angiotensin II receptor blockade in hypertensive patients with diabetes mellitus. *Am J Hypertens* 2007; **20**: 1329–33.

8 Colussi G, Catena C, Lapenna R, Nadalini E, Chiuch A, Sechi LA. Insulin resistance and hyperinsulinemia are related to plasma aldosterone levels in hypertensive patients. *Diabetes Care* 2007; **30**: 2349–54.

9 Hitomi H, Kiyomoto H, Nishiyama A, Hara T, Moriwaki K, Kaifu K, *et al.* Aldosterone suppresses insulin signaling via the downregulation of insulin receptor substrate-1 in vascular smooth muscle cells. *Hypertension* 2007; **50**: 750–5.

37 Cortisol and Cushing's Syndrome

Case History

Catherine is 48 years old and complains that her health is deteriorating. Although she is not particularly active and her diet could be better, she has gained an undue amount of weight in the past 5 years. She was noted to be hypertensive 2 years ago (although is still not taking treatment). A recent oral glucose tolerance test shows her to have impaired glucose tolerance. One or two second-degree relatives have been hypertensive, but there is no family history of diabetes. She has been researching on the internet and feels that she may have Cushing's.

How should the diagnosis of Cushing's be excluded or confirmed?

What is the relationship between cortisol excess and hypertension?

How should hypertension be managed in a patient with suspected Cushing's?

Background

Features of Cushing's syndrome are common in patients who are taking glucocorticoids. Non-iatrogenic Cushing's is rare, occurring in 2–3 per million per year. Clinical features are summarized in Box 37.1. Apart from Cushing's due to exogenous steroids, the following causes should be considered:

- Pituitary adenoma (80% of cases). Adenoma usually small (<10 mm). Female/male = 4:1

- Adrenal adenoma (5%) or carcinoma (4%) – commoner in females

- Ectopic adrenocorticotrophic hormone (ACTH) secretion (10%) – most commonly from small cell lung tumours, commoner in men

- Rare causes – ectopic corticotrophin-releasing hormone (CRH) secretion, micronodular and macronodular adrenal hyperplasia

- Pseudo-Cushing's – clinical and mild biochemical features of the syndrome are often present in patients who are obese, severely depressed, or who are consuming large amounts of alcohol

The first step is to confirm the presence of Cushing's (Figure 37.1). Random cortisol measurements are of little value. Cortisol levels are usually high in those using oral contraceptive pills due to high levels of cortisol-binding globulin being induced by oestrogen. Patients with Cushing's lack diurnal variation in their cortisol levels but it is not usually convenient to use this as a screening test in outpatients. If Cushing's is not

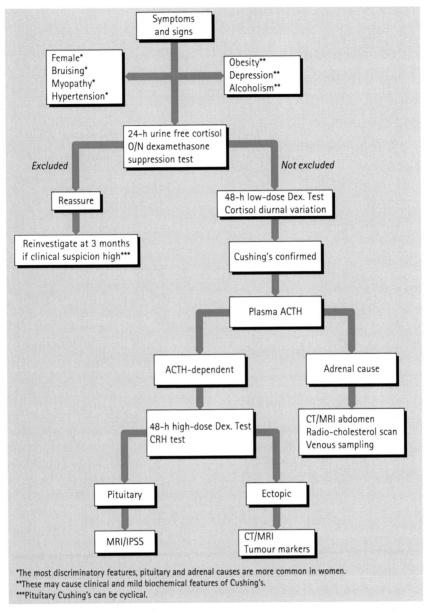

Figure 37.1 Investigation of suspected Cushing's. ACTH, adrenocorticotrophic hormone; CRH, corticotrophin-releasing hormone; Dex., dexamethasone; IPSS, inferior petrosal sinus sampling

excluded by the above, the next step is a 48-h, low-dose dexamethasone suppression test: 0.5 mg dexamethasone is given 6-hourly for 48 h. Cushing's is excluded if plasma cortisol suppresses to <60 nmol/l and urine-free cortisol is <100 nmol/24 h.

Having confirmed that Cushing's is present, the next step is to determine the source with biochemical tests. ACTH measurement is most useful: if undetectable, an adrenal source is highly likely and the patient should be further investigated by imaging the

Box 37.1 Features of Cushing's syndrome

- Cataracts
- Centripetal obesity
- Facial plethora
- Frontal baldness
- Glucose intolerance/diabetes
- Height loss (vertebral fracture)
- Hirsutism
- Hypertension*
- Low bone density
- Menstrual disturbance
- Moon face
- Other osteoporotic fracture
- Proximal myopathy*
- Psychosis
- Striae
- Tendency to bruise*
- Thinning of skin

*The most discriminatory features.

adrenals (computed tomography or magnetic resonance imaging [MRI]); a radio-cholesterol scan will give a functional image of an adrenal adenoma; and in specialist centres selective venous sampling should be considered. If plasma ACTH is normal or high (>3 pmol/l), a pituitary source or ectopic ACTH secretion is likely. The 48-h high-dose dexamethasone suppression test is usually carried out immediately following the low-dose test so that investigations can be conveniently completed in 1 week: 2 mg dexamethasone is given 6-hourly for 48 h. Suppression of urinary free cortisol to <50% of basal strongly suggests pituitary-driven Cushing's. No suppression is obtained in ectopic ACTH secretion. The CRH test may be useful: 100 μg ovine or human CRH is given IV and blood is sampled every 15 min for 2 h. If plasma cortisol rises to >120% of basal or ACTH rises to >150% of basal, pituitary Cushing's is likely. At this stage, MRI scan of the pituitary is indicated if pituitary Cushing's seems likely. Only 70–80% of Cushing's adenomas are visible, while 5% of the normal population have lesions suggestive of an adenoma on pituitary MRI. This cautions against over-reliance on the radiology before the biochemical diagnosis is confirmed. Inferior petrosal sinus sampling is a useful further investigation: following placement of the catheters in the inferior petrosal sinuses, peripheral IV CRH is given. ACTH >300% of peripheral value confirms pituitary Cushing's. Inferior petrosal sinus sampling is also useful (but not invariably) for lateralizing the adenoma. For ectopic ACTH syndrome, computed tomography or MRI of the thorax and abdomen is the next stage. Further investigations depend on the source of ACTH – the commonest are small cell lung tumour, pancreatic carcinoma and carcinoid tumours.

Treatment of choice for pituitary Cushing's is transsphenoidal removal of the adenoma. This leads to a cure in 70–80%. In specialized centres, re-operation should be considered in those not cured. Failing that, radiotherapy can be used – the onset of benefit is slow and panhypopituitarism frequently results. Medical treatment is useful leading up to surgery or following failed surgery, particularly pending benefit from radiation. Metyrapone and ketoconazole are the most commonly used agents. Laparoscopic removal of adrenal lesions leads to cure in most cases of adenoma. Adrenal carcinomas are usually aggressive and surgery is followed by irradiation ± drug treatment with mitotane or aminoglutethimide. Treatment of ectopic ACTH depends on the underlying lesion and medical treatment for Cushing's may be needed if this is not curable.

Hypertension occurs in up to 80% of adult patients with Cushing's and in 50% of children or adolescents with the disorder. Pathogenesis is complex and includes:[1] glucocorticoids having intrinsic mineralocorticoid activity; activation of renin–angiotensin system; enhanced vasoconstrictor effect of catecholamines, vasopressin and angiotensin II; decreased vasodilatation through decreased nitric oxide and prostacyclin; insulin resistance and sleep apnoea.

The enzyme 11β-hydroxysteroid dehydrogenase (11β-HSD) inter-converts cortisol and the inactive cortisone, and exists in two isoforms. 11β-HSD1 is predominantly expressed in liver and adipose and predominantly converts cortisone to the active cortisol. 11β-HSD2 is expressed mainly in mineralocorticoid target tissues and mainly converts cortisol to cortisone. This is important because, even without Cushing's, the levels of cortisol are at least 100 times those of aldosterone while both molecules have a similar affinity for the mineralocorticoid receptor. Liquorice and carbenoxolone are competitive inhibitors of 11β-HSD2, and mutation of the gene leads to apparent mineralocorticoid excess (AME) – a rare genetic form of hypertension. With excess cortisol the capacity of 11β-HSD2 to inactivate cortisol is exceeded. Treatment of the underlying Cushing's, even if successful, does not always cure hypertension – particularly if the condition has been present for a long time before treatment. Renin–angiotensin system-blocking drugs including aldosterone antagonists are logical choices. Loop diuretics are calciuretic and should be used with caution as they may worsen osteoporosis. Calcium channel blockers and α- or β-blockers are relatively ineffective.

Recent Developments

1. No test is 100% sensitive and specific for Cushing's.[2] Late night salivary cortisol measurements are increasingly being used as a screening test and have sensitivity and specificity of 92–100%.[3] Loss of the normal night-time nadir in cortisol occurs in stressed or depressed patients, those with sleep disturbance and those with intercurrent illness.

2. Levels of cortisol are increased in obese subjects partly due to increased 11β-HSD1 expression in adipose tissue. This is responsible for some of the phenotypic features of obesity and contributes to hypertension and glucose intolerance. Inhibitors of 11β-HSD1 may be beneficial in metabolic syndrome, and have shown promise in early studies on animal models of obesity.[4]

3. Patients with diabetes have a higher than expected prevalence of abnormalities of the pituitary–adrenal axis. This may relate to the effects of underlying obesity, and to the stress of chronic disease. However, pituitary or adrenal adenomas are

not rare in patients with diabetes. While routine screening for Cushing's is not recommended in diabetic clinics,[5] the threshold for carrying out tests should be relatively low. Activation of the pituitary–adrenal axis, in effect subclinical Cushing's, correlates with the presence and number of diabetic complications.[6]

4 Even in lean normotensive subjects with a family history of hypertension, cortisol levels are higher than in those with no family history.[7] Variations in salt sensitivity appear to be partly determined by cortisol status in those at risk of hypertension,[8] and part of this variation may be mediated through variable expression of 11β-HSD – inherited through polymorphisms in the gene or acquired through changes in body weight.

Conclusions

Although Cushing's syndrome is rare, it is often suspected in clinical practice. When there is a clinical suspicion, the patient should always be investigated (Figure 37.1). Hypertension occurs in the majority of patients with Cushing's and is due to multiple aetiologies, including altered salt sensitivity and the mineralocorticoid actions of cortisol. Because the syndrome is rare, there are no extensive trial data on the management of associated hypertension. Obviously, treatment of the underlying Cushing's is essential – left untreated, the syndrome has 50% 5-year mortality. Renin–angiotensin system-blocking drugs, including aldosterone antagonists are the most logical choice for first-line agents. Less florid degrees of pituitary adrenal activation are being increasingly recognized in those at risk of hypertension, those with metabolic syndrome, and in patients with type 2 diabetes. In these circumstances, the threshold for screening for Cushing's should be low.

References

1 Magiakou MA, Smyrnaki P, Chrousos GP. Hypertension in Cushing's syndrome. *Best Pract Res Clin Endocrinol Metab* 2006; **20**: 467–82.

2 Elamin MB, Murad MH, Mullan R, Erickson D, Harris K, Nadeem S, *et al.* Accuracy of diagnostic tests for Cushing's syndrome: a systematic review and metaanalyses. *J Clin Endocrinol Metab* 2008; **93**: 1553–62.

3 Carroll T, Raff H, Findling JW. Late-night salivary cortisol measurement in the diagnosis of Cushing's syndrome. *Nat Clin Pract Endocrinol Metab* 2008; **4**: 344–50.

4 Stimson RH, Walker BR. Glucocorticoids and 11beta-hydroxysteroid dehydrogenase type 1 in obesity and the metabolic syndrome. *Minerva Endocrinol* 2007; **32**: 141–59.

5 Newsome S, Chen K, Hoang J, Wilson JD, Potter JM, Hickman PE. Cushing's syndrome in a clinic population with diabetes. *Intern Med J* 2008; **38**: 178–82.

6 Chiodini I, Adda G, Scillitani A, Coletti F, Morelli V, Di Lembo S, *et al.* Cortisol secretion in patients with type 2 diabetes: relationship with chronic complications. *Diabetes Care* 2007; **30**: 83–8.

7 Matuszek MA, Boutcher SH. Elevated levels of circulating cortisol in young normotensive adult men with a family history of hypertension. *Clin Exp Pharmacol Physiol* 2008; **35**: 280–6.

8 Chamarthi B, Kolatkar NS, Hunt SC, Williams JS, Seely EW, Brown NJ, *et al.* Urinary free cortisol: an intermediate phenotype and a potential genetic marker for a salt-resistant subset of essential hypertension. *J Clin Endocrinol Metab* 2007; **92**: 1340–6.

38 Renovascular Hypertension

Case History

George is a 72-year-old man with widespread vascular disease. He suffers from angina and intermittent claudication, and has had at least one previous transient ischaemic attack/accident. He has recently undergone coronary angiography because of worsening of angina, and was incidentally noted to have greater than 50% stenosis of his left renal artery. His hypertension was not perfectly controlled on a diuretic/angiotensin receptor blocker combination plus amlodipine – typical blood pressure (BP) is 146/78. His renal function is marginally impaired (estimated glomerular filtration rate is 45). His cardiologist has suggested that he may benefit from angioplasty or stenting of his renal artery stenosis.

What are the common causes of renovascular hypertension (RVH)?

How useful is the measurement of renin in routine clinical practice?

When should endovascular treatment be recommended to patients with RVH?

Should such patients be treated with angiotensin–converting enzyme inhibitors or angiotensin receptor blockers?

Background

Renin is an aspartic protease that is synthesized as a preprohormone in the juxta-glomerular (JG) cells of the kidney. The JG apparatus is a baroreceptor that responds to decreased perfusion with increased renin secretion. Decreased sodium and chloride in the macula densa also increases renin secretion. The latter is inhibited when the plasma volume or salt concentrations are restored. Renin is a specific protease that cleaves angiotensinogen to angiotensin I, which is the precursor for the biologically active angiotensin II. The signal peptide directs the molecule to the endoplasmic reticulum for secretion. The N-terminal propeptide renders the molecule biologically inactive as it sterically hinders the catalytic cleft in the renin molecule. Prorenin, the secreted product, actually circulates in much higher concentration than that of active renin. Proteolytic activation of renin (removal of the propeptide) is effected by kallikrein or other prote-olytic enzymes, and much of this takes place in the kidney.

Plasma renin can now be quantified in two ways. Until recently, plasma renin activity was almost universally used: this is determined by the levels of both renin and angiotensinogen. The latter is increased in women who are either pregnant or taking the combined contraceptive pill. Exogenous angiotensinogen can be added to defray differences in angiotensin I but there are no readily available human sources. Serum from nephrectomized sheep is sometimes used and the resulting measurement is termed plasma renin concentration. Recently, several immunoassays have become available to measure the concentration of the renin molecule directly – renin mass assays. Renin measurements have been underused in clinical practice because the assay has been available only in reference laboratories, and because of sample transport difficulties. Levels of renin are particularly low in patients who are anephric, those with Conn's syndrome and those with low-renin essential hypertension.

Causes of high renin are summarized in Figure 38.1. Particularly high levels are seen in patients with RVH or cirrhosis. Rare causes of very high levels are Bartter syndrome and renin-secreting tumours. Bartter's is an autosomal recessive condition where there is excessive sodium loss in the thick ascending limb of the loop of Henle, with hypokalaemic alkalosis. A variety of underlying genetic disorders has been identified, allowing subtyping of the disease. Characteristically, there is JG hypertrophy and high circulating aldosterone. BP is normal or low. JG tumours are rare (haemangiopericytomas) and typically present in the 2nd to 4th decade. The tumours are small (<4 mm) and are benign or very low-grade malignant. The effects of drugs should not be forgotten and results of renin measurements must be interpreted with caution in patients who are taking drugs that are known to affect the renin–angiotensin system (RAS). Direct renin inhibitors (e.g. aliskiren) are an important advance in treatment. However, available agents do not completely inhibit renin (80–90% inhibition) and their use is associated with a compensatory increase in renin secretion.

RVH tends to occur in the young or in the old – but for different reasons. It accounts for up to 10% of childhood hypertension, with cases clustered at the more severe end of the spectrum. The rising prevalence of obesity has meant that more childhood hypertension is attributable to this cause now, and thus a relatively smaller proportion is due to secondary causes, including renovascular causes. Fibromuscular dysplasia (FMD) is the commonest cause of RVH in children. There is proliferation of mainly medial tissue leading to arterial narrowing and the typical 'string of beads' appearance on angiography. Its cause is unknown but there is a genetic contribution. Indeed, whatever the underlying condition, genetic influences account for up to 60% of RVH in children. FMD may be associated with intra-renal disease, and is frequently associated with other vascular disorders, including coarctation of the aorta, stenosis of other vessels (coeliac axis, superior and inferior mesenteric vessels etc.), and cerebrovascular disorders.

The diagnosis of RVH is often delayed in children as BP is not often checked. Childhood RVH is frequently associated with systolic BP >200 mmHg. Fundoscopy and echocardiography should be carried out in all cases. Sixty per cent have retinopathy, a similar proportion have left ventricular hypertrophy, and about 10% have renal impairment. Other presenting features may include a cerebrovascular event, cardiac failure, Bell's palsy, polyuria, hypokalaemia and hyponatraemia. Investigation follows the same principles as for adults (see below). Endovascular treatment, with or without stenting, cures 50% of all cases of FMD. For the remainder, reconstructive surgery is required and is usually delayed until the child is fully-grown.

RVH has been reported variously to occur in <1–4% of hypertensive adults, and in 2–5% of those referred to specialist centres. The differential diagnosis is similar to that in children, except for the overwhelming prevalence of atherosclerotic disease (Box 38.2).

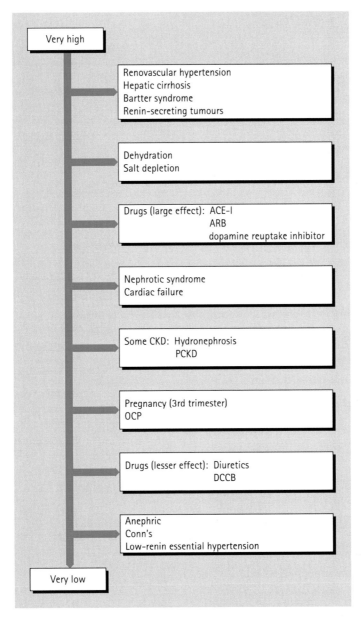

Figure 38.1 Causes of increased plasma renin. ACE-I, angiotensin-converting enzyme inhibitor; ARB, angiotensin receptor blocker; CKD, chronic kidney disease; DCCB, dihydropyridine calcium channel blocker; OCP, oral contraceptive pill; PCKD, polycystic kidney disease

While diabetes is the commonest cause of end-stage renal disease, hypertension and vascular disease are also very common. Renal replacement therapy is very costly and a potentially reversible cause should be sought. Atherosclerotic renal artery stenosis is frequently discovered incidentally during cardiac catheterization procedures, and there is a

> **Box 38.1 Renovascular hypertension in children**
>
> 1 FMD.
>
> 2 Syndromes: neurofibromatosis type 1, tuberous sclerosis, Marfan's syndrome, William's syndrome, etc.
>
> 3 Vasculitis: Takayasu's, polyarteritis nodosa, Kawasaki disease, etc.
>
> 4 External compression: neuroblastoma, Wilm's tumour, etc.
>
> 5 Other causes: radiation, trauma, congenital rubella, transplant renal artery stenosis, etc.
>
> FMD, fibromuscular dysplasia. Adapted from Tullus *et al.*[1]

very strong association with abdominal aortic aneurysm and peripheral vascular disease. Patients are frequently hypertensive, and there is an increased risk of cardiovascular (CV) events and progressive renal impairment. Atherosclerotic renal artery stenosis is present when there is 50% or more narrowing of the renal artery. It is present in 15–30% of patients with angiographically proven coronary artery disease. Ischaemic nephropathy secondary to atherosclerotic renal artery stenosis accounts for up to 5% of cases of end-stage renal disease, and this proportion is probably increasing. While atherosclerotic lesions of the renal artery are amenable to improvement or cure with endovascular procedures, their correlation with hypertension and renal impairment is not consistent. To date, randomized trials have not provided convincing evidence that intervention improves BP control, preserves renal function, or protects against vascular events.[2] While techniques and stents for surgical management have improved, so too has medical treatment. Given the uncertainties about long-term benefit of surgical intervention, it is not routinely recommended when the lesion is discovered incidentally. Intervention should

> **Box 38.2 Differential diagnosis of renovascular hypertension in adults**
>
> - Atherosclerotic renal artery stenosis: 80%
> - FMD: 5%
> - Dissecting aortic aneurysm
> - Renal artery aneurysm or intimal tear
> - Renal thrombosis or embolism
> - Coarctation
> - Arteriovenous fistulas, malformations or angiomas
> - Arteritis
> - Trauma
> - Irradiation
> - Following renal transplant
> - Extrinsic compression – tumour

be considered in those with rapidly declining renal function or where hypertension control is unsatisfactory with drugs.

Clues to the presence of RVH include: accelerated or refractory hypertension; widespread atherosclerosis; hypertension of moderate or greater severity before the age of 30 and after 50; sudden worsening of hypertension or renal function; flash pulmonary oedema; unexplained renal impairment or small kidneys with hypertension; and abdominal bruits. The measurement of renin and angiotensin is being more frequently requested in non-specialist settings. Results are hard to interpret if patients are taking certain drugs (Figure 38.1). Patients may need admission to temporarily stop drugs, or change to agents that do not affect RAS if BP control is needed during investigation. Non-invasive radiological investigations include: Doppler ultrasound (which may not identify renal artery narrowing); renal scintigraphy with 99m-Tc-DMSA or 99m-Tc-MAG3, which may be carried out before and after angiotensin-converting enzyme inhibitor administration; computed tomography angiography; magnetic resonance angiography. Catheter-based digital subtraction angiography remains the gold standard test. In specialist centres, tests using captopril or saralasin (angiotensin II receptor antagonist) may be useful to show that BP and renal function are dependent on RAS activation. Renal vein sampling may also be useful. Endovascular treatments include angioplasty, renal artery stenting, and alcohol ablation of an occluded branch artery. For selected cases, vascular reconstruction or unilateral nephrectomy may be beneficial.

Recent Developments

1 RVH accounts for up to 10% of childhood hypertension,[3] but a lower proportion of adult patients with hypertension. Although FMD and atherosclerosis are by far the commonest diagnoses in children and adults respectively, the broad range of diagnostic possibilities should always be considered. In older patients, the prevalence of atherosclerotic renovascular disease is increasing, and is now present in over 10% of elderly patients with end-stage renal disease.[4]

2 The association of renovascular disease with abdominal aortic and peripheral vascular disease is not surprising. The association with coronary artery disease is also well documented. It is often forgotten that patients with severe carotid artery disease are at increased risk of, and have a higher prevalence of, renovascular disease.[5]

3 Hypertensive patients with increased plasma renin have a worse prognosis than those with normal renin. This is assumed to be because of the adverse effects of RAS activation on remodelling of heart, kidneys and vasculature. A follow-up study of 3408 subjects from the Framingham cohort has confirmed the association of high plasma renin with increased short-term mortality risk. There was no relationship between renin and overall CV disease incidence. Renin measurement should be considered more frequently in clinical practice.

4 Accelerated atherosclerosis can both arise from and be the root cause of renal artery stenosis. The prevalence of CV risk factors in patients with renal artery stenosis is high.[6,7] In addition to vigorous management of their hypertension, other risk factors need to be considered in these patients, their global CV risk considered, and multifactor intervention initiated.

5   Dipeptidyl peptidase IV (DPP-IV) inhibitors (e.g. sitagliptin) are finding increased use in the management of type 2 diabetes. DPP-IV has a number of endogenous substrates, including peptide YY (1–36). *In vitro*, the use of a DPP-IV inhibitor decreases conversion of PYY (1–36) to PYY (3–36).[8] The former peptide, but not the

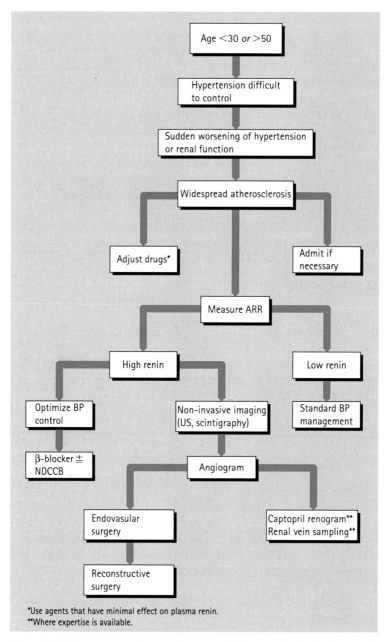

*Use agents that have minimal effect on plasma renin.
**Where expertise is available.

Figure 38.2 Management of suspected renovascular hypertension. ARR, aldosterone/renin ratio; NDCCB, non-dihydropyridine calcium channel blocker; US, ultrasound

latter, enhances the hypertensive effect of angiotensin II in the kidney. There is currently no evidence that DPP-IV inhibitors worsen hypertension in the clinical situation, but the above *in vitro* evidence should be borne in mind as this group of drugs is increasingly prescribed.

Conclusions

Renin, and its downstream pathway, plays a crucial part in maintaining BP. In some individuals with high sodium intake, the levels of renin are inappropriately high leading to a combination of plasma volume expansion and vasoconstriction – thus hypertension. For such people, treatment to offload sodium (dietary restriction, diuretics) and to block the RAS is a logical approach. However, the use of angiotensin-converting enzyme inhibitors or angiotensin receptor blockers may lead to an exaggerated hypotensive effect and worsening of renal function. In patients with renal artery stenosis, use of these drugs should perhaps be confined to specialist centres. Atherosclerotic renal artery stenosis is increasingly being diagnosed as a cause for hypertension. While endovascular and reconstructive treatment is effective in restoring perfusion and, to an extent, restoring BP, its role in protecting from declining renal function and CV outcomes remains to be established. Management of the patient with suspected renal artery stenosis is outlined in Figure 38.2. Renin measurement is a useful screening tool, but the patient should not be using drugs that influence circulating renin levels. Apart from its role in diagnosing RVH, there is increasing evidence that high renin is itself a marker for poorer prognosis in those at risk of CV events.

References

1   Tullus K, Brennan E, Hamilton G, Lord R, McLaren CA, Marks SD, *et al.* Renovascular hypertension in children. *Lancet* 2008; **371**: 1453–63.

2   Levin A, Linas S, Luft FC, Chapman AB, Textor S, ASH HTN Advisory Group. Controversies in renal artery stenosis: a review by the American Society of Nephrology Advisory Group on Hypertension. *Am J Nephrol* 2007; **27**: 212–20.

3   Bayazit AK, Yalcinkaya F, Cakar N, Duzova A, Bircan Z, Bakkaloglu A, *et al.* Reno-vascular hypertension in childhood: a nationwide survey. *Pediatr Nephrol* 2007; **22**: 1327–33.

4   Guo H, Kalra PA, Gilbertson DT, Liu J, Chen S-C, Collins AJ, *et al.* Atherosclerotic renovascular disease in older US patients starting dialysis, 1996 to 2001. *Circulation* 2007; **115**: 50–8.

5   Nakamura S, Iihara K, Matayoshi T, Yasuda H, Yoshihara F, Kamide K, *et al.* The incidence and risk factors of renal artery stenosis in patients with severe carotid artery stenosis. *Hypertens Res* 2007; **30**: 839–44.

6   Dzielinska Z, Januszewicz A, Demkow M, Makowiecka-Ciesla M, Prejbisz A, Naruszewicz M, *et al.* Cardiovascular risk factors in hypertensive patients with coronary artery disease and coexisting renal artery stenosis. *J Hypertens* 2007; **25**: 663–70.

7   Paraskevas KI, Hamilton G, Cross JM, Mikhailidis DP. Atherosclerotic renal artery stenosis: association with emerging vascular risk factors. *Nephron* 2008; **108**: c56–66.

8   Jackson EK, Mi Z. Sitagliptin augments sympathetic enhancement of the renovascular effects of angiotensin II in genetic hypertension. *Hypertension* 2008; **51**: 1637–42.

Drugs to Treat Hypertension

PROBLEM

39 Diuretics

Case History

 JT is a 72-year-old woman who has fallen and fractured her neck of femur. After emergency surgery, she initially makes a good recovery but 2 days after surgery her blood pressure (BP) is elevated at 200/114. She has a long history of hypertension treated with chlorthalidone 25 mg OD and atenolol 50 mg OD. Renal function is normal. She is restarted on her antihypertensive medications but 2 days later, her BP is still not controlled. A physician is called to see her. Her blood test shows plasma sodium of 116 mmol/l and potassium of 2.4 mmol/l. The corresponding values prior to surgery were modestly decreased at 130 and 3.0 mmol/l respectively.

Are diuretics safe for treatment of hypertension in the elderly?

Should we still regard them as first-line treatment in this age group?

Which agents are the most suitable for uncomplicated hypertension?

Background

For most patients with hypertension, particularly the elderly, diuretics are the first-line treatment. Thiazides have been the most widely used, and are effective in preventing stroke and cardiac events. Included in this class is chlorthalidone, a thiazide-like diuretic, which was used in two major trials – SHEP (Systolic Hypertension in the Elderly Program) and ALLHAT (Antihypertensive and Lipid-Lowering Treatment to Prevent Heart Attack Trial). These two trials respectively confirmed that thiazides are appropriate as initial treatment for elderly patients with isolated systolic hypertension and for African Americans with hypertension. Thiazides can be effectively used in combination with other major classes, including calcium channel blockers, angiotensin-converting enzyme inhibitor or angiotensin receptor blocker, and β-blockers. Three classes of diuretics are available: loop diuretics, thiazides, and potassium-sparing diuretics, including aldosterone antagonists.

Loop diuretics act at the apical membrane in the thick ascending limb of the loop of Henle. They complete with chloride for binding to the $Na^+/K^+/2Cl^-$ cotransporter. They are actively secreted by probenecid-sensitive anion transporters in the proximal tubule and need to be secreted to gain access to their luminal site of action. This explains why higher doses are needed when the glomerular filtration rate is decreased. In addition to increasing sodium and water excretion, loop diuretics increase fractional clearance of calcium by 30%, magnesium excretion and they decrease uric acid excretion. Frusemide (furosemide) is by far the most widely used drug in this class in spite of the fact that it has very variable absorption and bioavailability. Bumetanide and torsemide are more predictable, and the latter has the advantage of a longer duration of action.

Thiazides act in the early distal convoluted tubule where they block the Na^+/Cl^- cotransporter. This transporter is mutated in Gitelman's syndrome, an autosomal recessive disorder, in which patients are usually normotensive but have metabolic alkalosis, hypocalcaemia and hypomagnesaemia. They decrease excretion of calcium and uric acid, but increase magnesium excretion. Hydrochlorthiazide has been the most widely used thiazide. It is of fairly short duration (Table 39.1) and also variably absorbed. The drug has, therefore, limited use in treatment of heart failure. Chlorthalidone is much more potent and of longer duration. Metolazone is a quinazoline diuretic, which is also long-acting and potent, particularly when used with loop diuretics. Its oral absorption is slow and unpredictable. Its main action is in the distal convoluted tubule but it also has some action in decreasing sodium reabsorption in the proximal convoluting tubule. Side effects of thiazides occur commonly. Hyponatraemia is usually asymptomatic if mild (plasma sodium 130–134 mmol/l). Metabolic alkalosis occurs because of contraction of the extracellular fluid with retention of bicarbonate. It is corrected with potassium or chloride administration or, in extreme cases, carbonic anhydrase inhibitors. Hypokalaemia is common but usually in the 'safe' range (3.0–3.5 mmol/l). However, ventricular ectopics are increased in this range and potassium supplementation or potassium-sparing diuretic should be considered for all hypokalaemic patients, particularly with what is now known about the relationship between low potassium status and hypertension.

The potassium-sparing diuretics amiloride and triamterene act by blocking the epithelial sodium channel in the distal convoluted tubule and collecting duct.

Activating mutations of the epithelial sodium channel lead to the autosomal dominant inherited Liddle's syndrome where excessive sodium resorption leads to hypertension. As the two potassium-sparing diuretics have limited ability to influence overall sodium excretion, their effect in treating hypertension *per se* is limited. They are, however, highly effective in conserving potassium. The aldosterone antagonists, spironolactone and eplerenone, are now widely used in the treatment of heart failure. They inhibit sodium reabsorption in the late distal tubule and collecting duct. They have a mild diuretic effect but help preserve potassium and magnesium. They may precipitate hyperkalaemia, particularly in those with chronic kidney disease and in those concurrently taking angiotensin-converting enzyme inhibitors or angiotensin receptor blockers. Spironolactone commonly causes gynaecomastia in men and menstrual irregularity in premenopausal women. It is, therefore, most suitably used in postmenopausal women while eplerenone is finding increasing usage in men and in premenopausal women.

Table 39.1 Diuretics in common use

	Brand name	Half–life (h)	Dose (mg)
A: Loop diuretics			
Frusemide	Frusid, Frusehexal	1.5	20–40 BD
	Lasix, Uremide		
Bumetanide	Burinex	1–1.5	1–2
Torsemide	Demadex	4	5–20
Ethacrynic acid	Edecrin	4	25–100*
B: Thiazides			
Bendroflumethiazide	Aprinox	3–4	2.5–5
Hydrochlorthiazide	Dithiazide	8	12.5–25
Chlorthalidone	Hygroton	48–72	25–50
Xipamide	Diurexan	7	20
C: Non-thiazide sulphonamide			
Indapamide	Napamide, Natrilix	14–18	2.5
	Natrilix SR		1.5
D: Potassium-sparing			
Amiloride	Midamor, Kaluril**	6–9	2.5–5
Triamterene	Dyrenium**	2–4	50–100
E: Aldosterone antagonist			
Spironolactone	Aldactone	1.5	50–100*
Eplerenone	Inspra	4–6	25–50

*Use divided doses for higher dosing.
**Usually used in combination preparations.

There are a number of reasons for resistance to diuretics, the most obvious of which is high intake of sodium. Without dietary sodium restriction, the benefit of mild diuretics, such as once daily hydrochlorthiazide, might easily be lost (Figure 39.1). Salt and water are best resorbed with the patient recumbent, while diuretic is typically given before the most ambulant part of the day to avoid the inconvenience of the patient having to wake up to pass urine. Non-steroidal anti-inflammatory drugs antagonize the sodium-losing effects of loop diuretics in particular. Short-acting loop diuretics are often associated

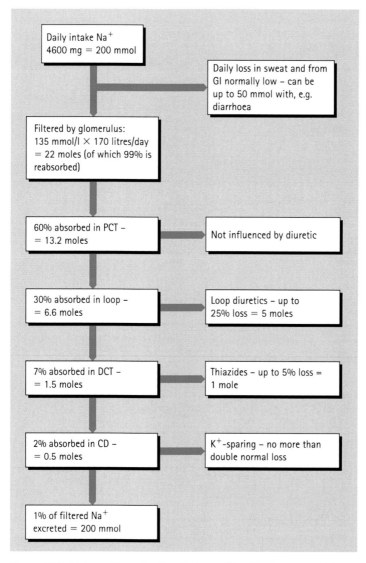

Figure 39.1 Actions of the major diuretic classes. CD, collecting duct; DCT, distal convoluted tubule; GI, gastrointestinal; PCT, proximal convoluted tubule

with a compensatory increase in sodium resorption once their effect has worn off (the braking phenomenon). This is avoided by multiple dosing or by combining agents that act at multiple sites. For BP control, potent diuretics used alone are associated with a neurohumoral response with activation of the renin–angiotensin system and sympathetic nervous system in response to volume depletion. This helps explain why diuretics are usefully combined with renin–angiotensin system-blockers or β-blockers.

It can be seen from Figure 39.1 that intake of sodium (up to 4600 mg = 200 mmol) is normally balanced by output. Their relatively low absorption and bioavailability, coupled with a short duration, which means that they only influence sodium excretion for part of the day, determine the actions of many diuretics in practice. Compared with mild diuretics of short duration of action, dietary sodium restriction can achieve the same effect. Conversely, to make a major impact on sodium excretion requires a more potent or longer-acting diuretic. The recently documented benefits of aldosterone-blocking drugs in resistant hypertension are not just due to their effect in promoting potassium excretion. Measurement of plasma renin is useful – high levels suggest RVH, while low levels suggest that the hypertension is more likely to be salt-sensitive and, therefore, amenable to diuretic treatment. It can also be useful to measure urinary sodium excretion in steady state before initiating drug treatment. This may give an indication of sodium intake, and thus the potential for dietary restriction. Diuretics are commonly used in combination preparations, use of which is encouraged (assuming that the individual drugs are indicated) as compliance is enhanced – Table 39.2.

Although other classes of drugs (renin–angiotensin system blockers and calcium channel blockers) have the potential to influence development of vascular complications of hypertension, none has proved superior to thiazides.[1] This suggests that lowering the

Table 39.2 Combination preparations with diuretics

	Brand name
A: Diuretic combinations	
HCT + amiloride	Amizide, Hydrene, Moduretic
Frusemide + amiloride	Frumil
B: Diuretic + angiotensin-converting enzyme inhibitor	
HCT + quinapril	Accuretic
Indapamide + perindopril	Coversyl Plus
HCT + fosinopril	Monoplus
HCT + lisinopril	Zestoretic
C: Diuretic + angiotensin receptor blocker	
HCT + candesartan	Atacand Plus
HCT + irbesartan	Avapro HCT, Karvezide
HCT + telmisartan	Micardis Plus
HCT + olmesartan	Olmetec Plus

BP is the single most important factor. Early studies, including MRFIT (Multiple Risk Factor Intervention Trial) and ALLHAT (Antihypertensive and Lipid-Lowering Treatment to Prevent Heart Attack Trial), suggested that chlorthalidone might be a superior agent to other thiazides, but this was refuted by subsequent analyses.[1] Data with thiazides suggest that there is an optimal dose for BP lowering and stroke prevention. A low dose should be used to start with in the elderly and the optimal (not maximal) dose should not be exceeded because of the risk of metabolic and other side effects.[2] For chlorthalidone, the starting dose in the elderly should be 6.25 mg and the maximum 25 mg. For hydrochlorthiazide, a 12.5-mg starting dose may be increased up to 50 mg. The use of lower doses minimizes metabolic side effects, particularly the development of diabetes, dyslipidaemia and hypokalaemia. The former two may offset any benefit accrued from lowering BP, while hypokalaemia predisposes to sudden death.

One important aspect that is not widely recognized is the relationship between hypokalaemia with thiazides and risk of hyperglycaemia. Zillich *et al.*[3] reviewed 59 trials with 83 thiazide study arms. Thiazides significantly increased incidence of new diabetes. For example, in ALLHAT, 11.6% of patients treated with thiazides developed diabetes compared with 9.8% taking amlodipine and 8.1% taking lisinopril. There was no difference between the treatments in the incidence of fatal and non-fatal myocardial infarction (MI). The benefits of modest BP reduction may be offset by the increase in hyperglycaemia, including risk of new diabetes. The mechanism for worsening glucose tolerance with thiazides is not absolutely known but it is thought that low potassium status decreases insulin secretion in response to a glycaemic stimulus.

Indapamide is a low potency thiazide-type diuretic whose major BP-lowering effect may be through direct vasodilatation.[4] The slow release preparation (1.5 mg OD) is now widely used. Favourable effects on vascular hypertrophy and left ventricular hypertrophy have been reported. It has minimal effect on blood glucose and a lower incidence of hypokalaemia or hyperuricaemia. Studies have variously reported reductions in systolic BP of 7–24 mmHg and reductions in diastolic BP of 4–13 mmHg.

Recent Developments

1   In a population-based cohort study involving 194 761 elderly patients,[5] thiazides were prescribed as first-line antihypertensive treatment in 35%. Factors associated with the use of a thiazide were advanced age and presence of comorbidities. Not surprisingly, thiazides were less used in men (risk of erectile dysfunction) and in patients with diabetes. These prescription patterns appear to be in line with recent trials and guidelines, but the study suggests that thiazides are still underprescribed given their proven efficacy and cost.

2   ALLHAT[6] reported an incidence of diabetes over 4 years of 17.1, 16.0 and 12.6% for patients with the metabolic syndrome who were treated respectively with chlorthalidone, amlodipine and lisinopril. These differences may well reflect a protective effect of the angiotensin-converting enzyme inhibitor rather than increased risk with the other two agents. Corresponding figures for those without the metabolic syndrome were 7.7, 4.2 and 4.7%. The slight metabolic disadvantage with thiazides does not diminish their protective effect – they are at

least as effective as other classes, including in African American patients who are at increased risk.[7]

3 Renin–angiotensin system-blocking drugs and calcium channel blockers may have benefits beyond simple BP reduction. It is doubtful whether diuretics have any such additional advantages. One recent study[8] reported improved arterial elasticity with low-dose thiazide, an effect that was lost if the patient developed diabetes. Older subjects do have decreased vascular compliance and enhanced salt sensitivity contributes to this. Thiazides probably do not influence other processes that contribute to atherosclerosis, such as oxidative stress and endothelial

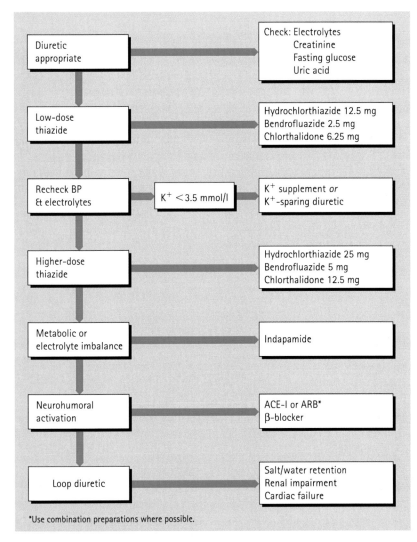

*Use combination preparations where possible.

Figure 39.2 Diuretics in treatment of hypertension. ACE-I, angiotensin-converting enzyme inhibitor; ARB, angiotensin receptor blocker

dysfunction.[9] Diuretics have a relatively pure action in lowering BP by offloading sodium and water.

4 A sustained protective effect of thiazides on bone loss in the elderly has been confirmed.[10] This is largely due to the reduction of renal calcium loss, although direct effects of thiazides on bone cells have been described *in vitro*. By contrast, loop diuretics increase calcium excretion and may thus contribute to bone loss. Lower urinary calcium excretion make thiazides the logical choice for hypertension treatment in those predisposed to osteoporosis and in those with renal stones.

Conclusions

A schema for the use of diuretics is proposed in Figure 39.2. Given the central role of salt and water balance in hypertension, diuretics are a logical first-line treatment for many patients. They are safe and protect from vascular events at least as much as other classes. Hypokalaemia is a risk and predisposes to arrhythmias and sudden cardiac death. Hyponatraemia may occur when fluid balance is perturbed by other factors. Electrolytes should be monitored and consideration given to stopping the drugs where there is inter-current illness. Hypokalaemia may also be a major link between thiazides and risk of diabetes. Potassium should be maintained at least above 3.5 mmol/l, and a target of 4.0 mmol/l is reasonable. Low potassium status also predisposes to hypertension and may offset the BP-lowering effects of diuretics. Loop diuretics are generally not required for uncomplicated hypertension. Indapamide is a useful agent with some thiazide-like activity but also vasodilatory actions and a low incidence of metabolic side effects. Thiazides remain the drugs of first choice for the management of hypertension, particularly in the elderly.

References

1 Salvetti A, Ghiadoni L. Thiazide diuretics in the treatment of hypertension: an update. *J Am Soc Nephrol* 2006; **17** (Suppl 2): S25–9.

2 Papadopoulos DP, Papademetriou V. Metabolic side effects and cardiovascular events of diuretics: should a diuretic remain the first choice therapy in hypertension treatment? The case of yes. *Clin Exp Hypertens* 2007; **29**: 503–16.

3 Zillich AJ, Garg J, Basu S, Bakris GL, Carter BL. Thiazide diuretics, potassium, and the development of diabetes: a quantitative review.[See comment.] *Hypertension* 2006; **48**: 219–24.

4 Robinson DM, Wellington K. Indapamide sustained release: a review of its use in the treatment of hypertension. *Drugs* 2006; **66**: 257–71.

5 Tu K, Campbell NRC, Chen Z, McAlister FA. Thiazide diuretics for hypertension: prescribing practices and predictors of use in 194,761 elderly patients with hypertension. *Am J Geriatr Pharmacother* 2006; **4**: 161–7.

6   Black HR, Davis B, Barzilay J, Nwachuku C, Baimbridge C, Marginean H, *et al.* Metabolic and clinical outcomes in nondiabetic individuals with the metabolic syndrome assigned to chlorthalidone, amlodipine, or lisinopril as initial treatment for hypertension: a report from the Antihypertensive and Lipid-Lowering Treatment to Prevent Heart Attack Trial (ALLHAT). *Diabetes Care* 2008; **31**: 353–60.

7   Wright JT, Jr, Harris-Haywood S, Pressel S, Barzilay J, Baimbridge C, Bareis CJ, *et al.* Clinical outcomes by race in hypertensive patients with and without the metabolic syndrome: Antihypertensive and Lipid-Lowering Treatment to Prevent Heart Attack Trial (ALLHAT). *Arch Intern Med* 2008; **168**: 207–17.

8   Shargorodsky M, Boaz M, Davidovitz I, Asherov J, Gavish D, Zimlichman R. Treatment of hypertension with thiazides: benefit or damage-effect of low- and high-dose thiazide diuretics on arterial elasticity and metabolic parameters in hypertensive patients with and without glucose intolerance. *J Cardiometab Syndr* 2007; **2**: 16–23.

9   Zhou M-S, Schulman IH, Jaimes EA, Raij L. Thiazide diuretics, endothelial function, and vascular oxidative stress. *J Hypertens* 2008; **26**: 494–500.

10   Bolland MJ, Ames RW, Horne AM, Orr-Walker BJ, Gamble GD, Reid IR. The effect of treatment with a thiazide diuretic for 4 years on bone density in normal postmenopausal women. *Osteoporosis Int* 2007; **18**: 479–86.

40 β-blockers: If and When

Case History

Mr GM is 62 years old, and has had hypertension for 10 years. He uses a combination of diuretic and angiotensin-converting enzyme inhibitors, as well as aspirin and inhalers (salbutamol and beclomethasone). His blood pressure (BP) is not well controlled (164/98) and the time has come to consider adding another agent. He was a heavy smoker until 3 years ago. He is quite active but his walking is limited by intermittent claudication (IC) at 400 yards and he also gets breathless on exertion. Resting pulse rate is 84 beats per minute.

What is the current place of β-blockers in hypertension management?

Do they worsen IC?

Should they be avoided in patients with obstructive airways disease?

When should a β-blocker be chosen and when should it be avoided?

Background

Adrenergic receptors mediate the effects of catecholamines (adrenaline and noradrenaline), and are thus responsible for the actions of the sympathetic nervous system – 'fight or flight'. Adrenoreceptors are divided into two classes (α and β) based on their specificity for catecholamines. Adrenaline and noradrenaline are much more potent than isoprenaline as agonists for α receptors, while isoprenaline is the most potent agonist for β receptors. Adrenoreceptors are further divided:

- α_1 adrenoreceptors
  - G protein: G_q, activates phospholipase C, increases calcium and inositol triphosphate (IP_3)
  - Distribution: ureter, vas deferens, hairs (erector pili), urethral sphincter
  - Effect: smooth muscle contraction
  - Agonist: phenylephrine
  - Antagonist: phenoxybenzamine, phentolamine, prazosin, doxazosin, tamsulosin

- α_2 adrenoreceptors
  - G protein: G_i, inactivates adenylate cyclase, decreases cyclic adenosine monophosphate (cAMP)
  - Distribution: smooth muscle, brain, pancreas
  - Effect: contraction of gastrointestinal sphincters, decreases neurotransmitter effects, decreases insulin release

- Agonist: clonidine
- Antagonist: yohimbine
- β₁ adrenoreceptors
  - G protein: G_s, activates adenylate cyclase, increases cyclic AMP
  - Distribution: cardiac muscle, juxtaglomerular (JG) cells, adipocytes
  - Effect: increases heart rate and stroke volume, increases renin release, lipolysis
  - Agonist: adrenaline, noradrenaline, dobutamine
  - Antagonist: metoprolol, atenolol
- β₂ adrenoreceptors
  - G protein: G_s, activates adenylate cyclase, increases cyclic AMP
  - Distribution: bronchi, blood vessels, JG cells, liver, bladder
  - Effect: smooth muscle relaxation, increases renin, increases glucose
  - Agonist: salbutamol, salmeterol, terbutaline, ritodrine
  - Antagonist: propranolol
- β₃ adrenoreceptors
  - G protein: G_s, activates adenylate cyclase, increases cyclic AMP
  - Distribution: adipocytes
  - Effect: lipolysis
  - Agonist: experimental compounds

Overactivity of the sympathetic nervous system is an important mechanism in the pathogenesis of hypertension. Agents that block the effect of circulating or locally produced catecholamines have been used in treatment for many years. The predominant effect of β-agonists on blood vessels is vasodilatation, e.g. in the vessels to skeletal muscle. It follows that blockade of these receptors does not contribute to the antihypertensive effect of β-blockers – these arise indirectly by decreasing central sympathetic tone (agents that cross the blood–brain barrier such as propranolol), by negative inotropic and chronotropic effects on the heart leading to decreased carbon monoxide, and by decreased renal renin release. Indications for β-blockers are summarized in Box 40.1.

Opinion has become divided about the role of β-blockers in hypertension management. In spite of their well-proven effects in those who have myocardial infarction, in hypertrophic cardiomyopathy, and in heart failure (HF) as well as their antiarrhythmic effect, the balance of evidence is that, in patients with uncomplicated hypertension, they do not decrease the incidence of coronary artery disease or overall mortality.[1] Furthermore, they may increase the incidence of stroke. Compared with other antihypertensives, they are less likely to favourably impact on surrogate end-points such as endothelial dysfunction and left ventricular hypertrophy. Doubts about whether β-blockers should be used as first-line agents largely arose from two meta-analyses:

1 Lindholm et al.[2] analysed 13 randomized controlled trials involving a total of nearly 106 000 patients. Compared with other agents, atenolol (the most widely used β-blocker) was found to be relatively ineffective. β-blockers did not protect against myocardial infarction and, compared with other agents, there was a 16% increase in stroke. β-blockers did decrease stroke incidence when compared with no treatment or placebo.

2 Khan and McAlister[3] examined 21 trials with a total of 146 000 participants. In younger patients, β-blockers decreased major cardiovascular outcomes – RR 0.86

(95% CI: 0.74 to 0.99). There was no such apparent protection in older subjects – RR 0.89 (95% CI: 0.75 to 1.05). Again, there was an excess risk for stroke compared with other agents.

While the above do not exclude benefit from β-blockers in uncomplicated hypertension, they do not support use as first-line agents. The pathogenesis of hypertension is different in younger and older subjects. In younger patients, central sympathetic tone is increased and this is favourably impacted by β-blockade. In older patients, decreased vascular compliance is more important, and is not affected by β-blockade. Atenolol is a useful drug, but when given in a single daily dose may not provide round the clock coverage. Central aortic pressure strongly correlates with stroke risk and is not decreased to the same extent as brachial artery pressure with β-blockers. Angiotensin-converting enzyme inhibitors are more effective agents in this regard.

Clinical trials in the past 10 years have completely reversed our thinking about the use of β-blockers with HF. Ten years ago this class of drug was thought to be contraindicated if HF was present. Now it is strongly indicated for treatment of the HF itself. β-blockers decrease sympathetic drive, decreasing heart rate and improving ejection fraction (EF). They also improve cardiac remodelling, partly indirectly by decreasing activity of the renin–angiotensin system. For this indication, to avoid side effects and maximize benefit, β-blockers should be started at a low dose and increased gradually. The agents that are specifically indicated (based on trial evidence) for the treatment of HF are carvedilol, bisoprolol, sustained-release metoprolol and nebivolol.

Bearing in mind the altered thinking about β-blockers and HF, we need to think critically about their use in other conditions in which they have traditionally been contraindicated. For example, the balance of evidence now suggests that β-blockers do not affect severity of intermittent claudication or the pain-free walking distance in patients with peripheral vascu-

---

Box 40.1 Indications for β-blockers

- Strong indication
  - Secondary prevention after myocardial infarction
  - Angina pectoris
  - Hyperthyroidism
  - Phaeochromocytoma (with α-blocker)
- Moderately strong indication (other agents may be more useful)
  - Hypertension
  - Tachyarrhythmia
  - Congestive cardiac failure
  - Glaucoma
  - Migraine prophylaxis
  - Hypertrophic cardiomyopathy
  - Acute aortic dissection
- Sometimes used or useful
  - Portal hypertension
  - Anxiety disorders – tremor, hyperhydrosis
  - Benign essential tremor
  - Non-medical, e.g. anxiety related to public performances

lar disease (PVD). Hypertension is an important risk factor for PVD with a two- to four-fold increase in hypertensive subjects. Many patients with PVD have coexisting coronary artery disease and should not be denied the protective effects of β-blockers. Patients with severe PVD and those with Raynaud's phenomenon should not be given β-blockers.

β-blockers have been associated with an increase in the incidence of type 2 diabetes. In the meta-analysis by Bangalore et al.,[4] involving over 94 000 subjects, the incidence of new-onset diabetes was increased by 22%. Diabetes was particularly increased with atenolol, in older subjects and with longer duration of treatment. β-blockers can also worsen control of pre-existing diabetes and treatment leads to a modest weight gain in many subjects. Use of thiazides together with β-blockers is particularly likely to worsen glycaemic control. Newer agents (carvedilol, nebivolol) appear to be less likely to worsen glycaemic control. β-blockers are associated with a range of adverse effects (Box 40.2), which should be considered before and during treatment.

Recent Developments

1   Published data on the efficacy of β-blockers usually examines their effects in isolation. Data from a large US database[5] examined the effect when other agents were added to β-blockers. The greatest benefit was with combination of β-blocker and dihydropyridine calcium channel blockers, followed by angiotensin-converting enzyme inhibitors and then angiotensin receptor blockers.

2   We have had cause to rethink the effect of β-blockers in patients with PVD. Ubbink et al.[6] studied the skin microcirculation using non-invasive methods in patients with IC after withdrawal, and following reintroduction, of β-blockers. There was no difference in skin circulation with or without the drugs, confirming that it is safe to use β-blockers in patients with IC and those with ischaemic rest pain.

3   Brooks et al.[7] examined rates of hospitalization and emergency department attendance in patients on cardioselective and non-cardioselective β-blockers. Compared with controls, patients with asthma on cardioselective β-blockers had RR of hospitalization of 0.89 (95% CI: 0.53 to 1.50) and for emergency department attendance of 1.40 (1.20 to 1.62). Corresponding figures for non-cardioselective β-blockers were 2.47 (1.37 to 4.48) for hospitalization and 1.21 (0.91 to 1.62) for emergency department visits. In those with chronic obstructive pulmonary disease (COPD), the RR on cardioselective agents was 0.64 (0.43 to 0.96) for hospitalization and 1.19 (1.02 to 1.39) for emergency department visits. On non-cardioselective agents, the corresponding figures were 1.02 (0.152 to 2.02) for hospitalization and 0.51 (0.33 to 0.80) for emergency department visits. If patients with asthma have to be treated with β-blockers, a cardioselective agent should be used. β-blockers appear to be safe and perhaps even protective in patients with pure COPD. Another recent study[8] has suggested a protective effect of β-blockers in patients with acute exacerbations of COPD.

4   Trials question the efficacy of β-blockers as first-line agents and their ability to protect against cardiovascular end-points, including stroke. There is no suggestion that atenolol or other β-blockers actually cause stroke. Indeed recent studies[9,10] have suggested that they may be neuroprotective in patients with acute stroke, decreasing the severity of stroke and improving outlook. This is

Box 40.2 **Adverse effects of β-blockers**

- Cardiovascular: hypotension, bradycardia, heart block, worsening heart failure
- Respiratory: bronchospasm
- Gastrointestinal: nausea, diarrhoea
- Reproductive: decreased libido, erectile dysfunction
- Peripheral: cold extremities, worsening of Raynaud's
- Central nervous system: impaired concentration, hallucinations, nightmares, depression
- Metabolic: new-onset diabetes, worsening glycaemic control
- General: weight gain, decreased maximal exercise tolerance

presumably due to decreased sympathetic activity and is akin to the cardioprotective effects of β-blockers in patients with myocardial infarction.

5   Data from the UK General Practice Research Database[11] confirm that β-blockers do increase the incidence of type 2 diabetes, particularly when combined with thiazides. Calcium channel blockers also increased the incidence of diabetes, while regimens that included angiotensin-converting enzyme inhibitors were protective. Cardioselective β-blockers may lower BP without worsening insulin sensitivity. Extended release metoprolol was effective in lowering BP but did not affect insulin sensitivity in an insulin clamp study.[12]

6   Although β-blockers are now widely used in patients with HF, they still need to be used cautiously. Overdosing may precipitate decompensation of cardiac function. Patients often have β-blockers withdrawn or the dose reduced when they present with an exacerbation of their HF. Data from the COMET (Carvedilol Or METoprolol European) Study[13] suggest that it is not only safe but desirable for them to continue with β-blockers unless specifically contraindicated.

Conclusions

β-blockers have been the mainstay of treatment for many patients in recent years, and should not be stopped if they are providing cardioprotection and hypertension control with no adverse effects. Much of the published data on adverse effects of β-blockers relate to atenolol. Newer vasodilatory agents such as nebivolol have a much cleaner side effect profile, including fewer metabolic side effects. β-blockers are now less used as first-line agents for hypertension, particularly for older patients. This probably reflects advances that have been made with other classes more than problems with β-blockers (Figure 40.1). They are now considered safe to use in patients with IC and those with pure COPD (with no asthma). β-blockers are most useful for younger patients where resting pulse rate is increased (reflecting increased sympathetic tone). Increased resting pulse rate has been associated with higher mortality. There is no direct evidence that decreasing pulse rate with drugs improves outlook. β-blockers should also be considered for hypertension where there is comorbidity such as angina or HF.

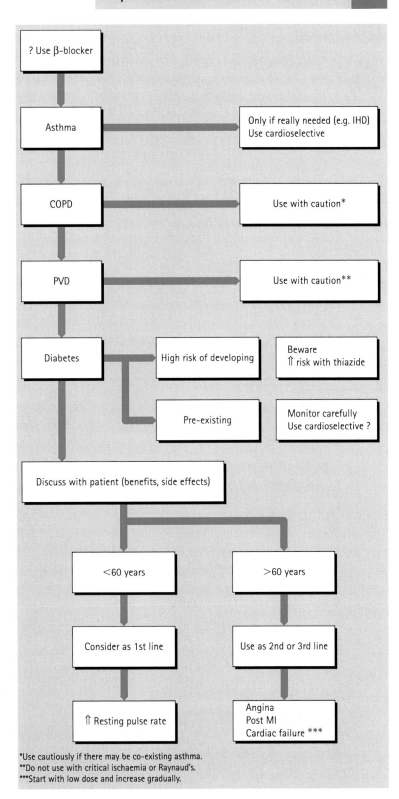

Figure 40.1 β-blockers as treatment for hypertension. COPD, chronic obstructive pulmonary disease; IHD, ischaemic heart disease; PVD, peripheral vascular disease

*Use cautiously if there may be co-existing asthma.
**Do not use with critical ischaemia or Raynaud's.
***Start with low dose and increase gradually.

References

1 Bangalore S, Messerli FH, Kostis JB, Pepine CJ. Cardiovascular protection using beta-blockers. A critical review of the evidence. *J Am Coll Cardiol* 2007; **50**: 563–72.

2 Lindholm LH, Carlberg B, Samuelsson O. Should beta blockers remain first choice in the treatment of primary hypertension? A meta-analysis. *Lancet* 2005; **366**: 1545–53.

3 Khan N, McAlister FA. Re-examining the efficacy of beta-blockers for the treatment of hypertension: a meta-analysis. *Can Med Assoc J* 2006; **174**: 1737–42.

4 Bangalore S, Parkar S, Grossman E, Messerli FH. A meta-analysis of 94,492 patients with hypertension treated with beta blockers to determine the risk of new-onset diabetes mellitus. *Am J Cardiol* 2007; **100**: 1254–62.

5 Bisognano JD, McLaughlin T, Roberts CS, Tang SSK. Calcium channel blockers, angiotensin receptor blockers, and angiotensin-converting enzyme inhibitors: effectiveness in combination with diuretics or beta-blockers for treating hypertension. *Vasc Health Risk Manage* 2007; **3**: 579–85.

6 Ubbink DT, Verhaar EE, Lie HKI, Legemate DA. Effect of beta-blockers on peripheral skin microcirculation in hypertension and peripheral vascular disease. *J Vasc Surg* 2003; **38**: 535–40.

7 Brooks TWA, Creekmore FM, Young DC, Asche CV, Oberg B, Samuelson WM. Rates of hospitalizations and emergency department visits in patients with asthma and chronic obstructive pulmonary disease taking beta-blockers. *Pharmacotherapy* 2007; **27**: 684–90.

8 Dransfield MT, Rowe SM, Johnson JE, Bailey WC, Gerald LB. Use of beta blockers and the risk of death in hospitalised patients with acute exacerbations of COPD. *Thorax* 2008; **63**: 301–5.

9 Laowattana S, Oppenheimer SM. Protective effects of beta-blockers in cerebrovascular disease. *Neurology* 2007; **68**: 509–14.

10 Dziedzic T, Slowik A, Pera J, Szczudlik A. Beta-blockers reduce the risk of early death in ischemic stroke. *J Neurol Sci* 2007; **252**: 53–6.

11 Burke TA, Sturkenboom MC, Ohman-Strickland PA, Wentworth CE, Rhoads GG. The effect of antihypertensive drugs and drug combinations on the incidence of new-onset type-2 diabetes mellitus. *Pharmacoepidemiol Drug Saf* 2007; **16**: 979–87.

12 Falkner B, Kushner H. Treatment with metoprolol succinate, a selective beta adrenergic blocker, lowers blood pressure without altering insulin sensitivity in diabetic patients. *J Clin Hypertens* 2008; **10**: 51–7.

13 Metra M, Torp-Pedersen C, Cleland JGF, Di Lenarda A, Komajda M, Remme WJ, *et al.* Should beta-blocker therapy be reduced or withdrawn after an episode of decompensated heart failure? Results from COMET. *Eur J Heart Fail* 2007; **9**: 901–9.

41 β-blockers: Efficacy and Choice of Agent

Case History

Alice aged 58 years, is a slightly anxious lady who has had trouble controlling her blood pressure (BP) in recent years. She tried diuretics and also two different angiotensin-converting enzyme inhibitors but did not feel well while taking them. She takes aspirin but no other medications. Three years ago, she began to suffer from angina, attacks of which have been more frequent. The attacks respond to nitrate spray. A coronary angiogram last year confirmed triple vessel disease but she did not require stenting or coronary artery bypass graft. Her BP is 164/96.

Would a regimen based on a β-blocker be an effective way of controlling her BP?

How would you choose the most appropriate agent?

Is there much difference between the available agents?

Background

Despite the controversy over their role as first-line agents, β-blockers continue to occupy an important place in management of hypertensive patients. Development of angiotensin-converting enzyme inhibitors and angiotensin receptor blockers (ARBs) in particular, and trials showing their benefit in end-point reduction have relegated the place of β-blockers. End-point trials are critical and inform development of guidelines, most of which still advocate β-blockers as agents that should be considered first-line, or at least second-line, for BP control. However, in clinical practice, we are not in a position to make a judgement generally about whether an agent is effective in preventing a long-term outcome. We have to rely on surrogate end-points including BP control, and assume that if we control BP effectively we are doing what is required.

A recent Cochrane review[1] considered data from 13 trials with a total of 91 561 subjects. Four studies compared β-blocker with placebo or no treatment, five with diuretic, four with calcium channel blockers, and four with renin–angiotensin system blockade. With β-blockers, the risk for mortality was no greater than for placebo, diuretics or renin–angiotensin system blockade but was higher than for calcium channel blockers. Risk for total cardiovascular (CV) diagnoses was lower with β-blockers than with placebo. Discontinuation of treatment with β-blockers was greater than that with diuretics or with renin–angiotensin system blockade, but similar to calcium channel blockers. There is a striking lack of head-to-head comparisons between β-blockers. The vast majority of patients in published studies have been treated with atenolol – 30 150 out of the total of 40 243 β-blocker-treated patients in the Cochrane review. Also, the vast majority of patients in published trials are of Caucasian descent.

Considerations around the efficacy of β-blockers in hypertension are complex. In many trials, they are used as part of a regimen since most patients are not controlled with a single agent. Trials have tended to focus on CV end-points rather than BP control. Often, clinical trial papers have to be studied quite carefully to gain an idea as to how well BP was controlled. The more recent studies in the Cochrane review of β-blockers in hypertension were (references are given in the review):

1. ELSA (European Lacidipine Study on Atherosclerosis) 1996. 2334 patients with hypertension followed for 4 years, comparison between lacidipine (calcium channel blocker) and atenolol. Lacidipine was more effective in decreasing carotid intima-media thickness. BP control was similar with the two agents.

2. UKPDS-39 (UK Prospective Diabetes Study group, 1998). 1148 patients with hypertension and type 2 diabetes followed for 10 years. Tight BP control with either captopril or atenolol decreased microvascular and macrovascular complications to a similar degree. Fewer people withdrew from taking angiotensin-converting enzyme inhibitors. There was no difference in the number of people who required other agents or in BP control.

3. LIFE (Losartan Intervention For Endpoint reduction) 2002. 9193 patients with essential hypertension (baseline systolic BP 160–200 mmHg, diastolic BP 95–115 mmHg) and left ventricular hypertrophy were followed for 4 years on either losartan- or atenolol- based regimen. It was found that CV morbidity and mortality were lower on losartan and there was a lower incidence of type 2 diabetes. There was no difference in BP control.

4. AASK (African American Study of Kidney Disease and Hypertension) 2002. 1094 black Americans with hypertensive renal disease were followed for 4 years. The study was a comparison of ramipril, amlodipine and metoprolol. There was no difference in BP control but ramipril was found to be the most effective agent for slowing the progression of renal disease.

5. INVEST (INternational VErapamil SR-Trandolapril Study) 2003. 22 576 patients with hypertension and coronary artery disease (CAD), aged 50+, followed for 2.7 years. Comparison of regimen based on sustained release verapamil with trandolapril added if needed with regimen based on atenolol with hydrochlorthiazide as needed. Other agents were added if required. There was no difference with the two regimens in death from any cause, non-fatal myocardial (MI) stroke, or new-onset angina. Patients on the β-blocker-based regimen were more likely to develop wheezing, bradycardia or constipation. There was no difference in BP control.

6. ASCOT (Anglo-Scandinavian Cardiac Outcomes Trial) 2005. 19 255 patients with hypertension and at least one other risk factor. Comparison of regimens based on amlodipine ± perindopril or atenolol ± bendrofluazide. The trial was stopped after 5 years because there were fewer CV events in the amlodipine group. There was more diabetes in the atenolol group and no difference in BP control.

Figures 41.1 and 41.2 show the changes in systolic BP and diastolic BP with β-blocker respectively in these six trials. Note that the changes are with regimens based on β-blocker, with other drugs added as needed. There is a consistent and marked reduction in BP.

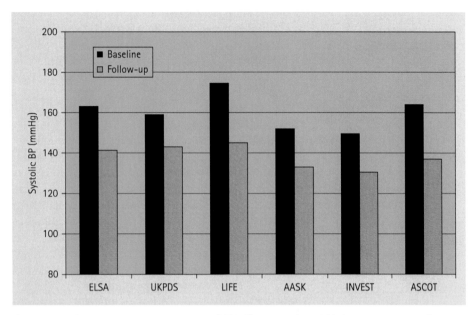

Figure 41.1 Change in systolic blood pressure (BP) in β-blocker trials. ELSA, European Lacidipine Study on Atherosclerosis; UKPDS, UK Prospective Diabetes Study group; LIFE, Losartan Intervention For Endpoint reduction; AASK, African American Study of Kidney Disease and Hypertension; INVEST, INternational VErapamil SR-Trandolapril Study; and ASCOT, (Anglo-Scandinavian Cardiac Outcomes Trial)

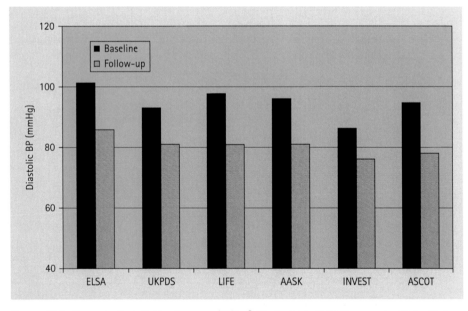

Figure 41.2 Change in diastolic blood pressure (BP) in β-blocker trials. ELSA, European Lacidipine Study on Atherosclerosis; UKPDS, UK Prospective Diabetes Study group; LIFE, Losartan Intervention For Endpoint reduction; AASK, African American Study of Kidney Disease and Hypertension; INVEST, INternational VErapamil SR-Trandolapril Study; and ASCOT, (Anglo-Scandinavian Cardiac Outcomes Trial)

There is a wide choice of preparations (Table 41.1). Usage of these varies from country to country and the list is not an exhaustive one. It does not include agents that are generally used for glaucoma only. Also not included is esmolol (Brevibloc), a cardioselective agent used intravenously for the control of supraventricular tachycardia (SVT). In general, once daily preparations lead to better compliance. Several other properties should inform the choice of β-blocker (Table 41.2).

Cardioselectivity

β-blockers that are cardioselective block mainly β_1-receptors, although the degree of selectivity is variable and may be lost at higher doses. Clearly, selective agents are most useful for purely cardiac indications such as rhythm and angina control. It is not entirely clear what the predominant modes of action are for BP control with β-blockers. As non-cardiac actions are important (decreased central sympathetic tone and renin release), non-cardioselective agents should intuitively be more effective. This turns out not to be the case – cardioselective agents are slightly more effective for BP control. This is because β_2 stimulation leads to vasodilatation, particularly in muscle beds. Blocking this effect leaves the pressor effects of α-adrenoreceptor stimulation unopposed. This consideration is particularly important in high catecholamine states (stress and phaeochromocytoma). β-receptor blockade may provoke bronchospasm in patients with asthma who should have cardioselective agents if they need β-blockers.

The receptors responsible for metabolic effects of catecholamines are also β_2. Blockade of these predisposes to insulin resistance and dyslipidaemia. The changes in total-, low-density lipoprotein-, and high-density lipoprotein-cholesterol are usually modest but non-cardioselective β-blockers can increase triglycerides by 25–50%, while cardioselective agents increase triglycerides by only 15–25%. Paradoxically, cardiac protection following MI may be better with non-cardioselective agents, e.g. decreasing central sympathetic tone may protect from sudden death. Other means may be needed to control the hyperglycaemia and dyslipidaemia, which may worsen with non-cardioselective β-blockers.

Intrinsic sympathomimetic activity

Some β-blockers are partial agonists – they exert some agonist activity while the overall effect is inhibitory. These agents may be better tolerated with lower incidence of some side effects such as fatigue. Such agents may have fewer metabolic side effects such as increased triglycerides. However, they may be less cardioprotective following MI, and less useful in the management of angina and tachyarrhythmia. They may have a tendency to promote left ventricular hypertrophy.

Membrane stabilizing activity

Some agents have activity like sodium channel blockers and may thus have enhanced effect in protecting against arrhythmias. Such agents may have the potential to reduce seizure threshold.

Lipid-soluble agents

These may be better absorbed and thus have greater bioavailability. They tend to be eliminated by the liver. Because they cross the blood–brain barrier, they have a greater volume of distribution, and are more likely to cause central nervous system side effects.

Table 41.1 Commonly used β-blockers

Generic name	Brand names	Daily dose (mg)
Acebutolol	Sectral	200–1200*
Atenolol	Anselol, Atehexal, Noten,Tenormin, Tensig	50–100*
Bisoprolol	Bicor	1.25–10
Carvedilol	Dilatrend, Kredex	12.5–50**
Labetalol	Presolol, Trandate	200–1200**
Metoprolol	Betaloc, Lopressor, Metohexal, Metolol, Metral, Minax	50–200***
Metoprolol (extended release)	Toprol-XL	23.75–190
Nadolol	Corgard	40–160
Oxprenolol	Corbeton	80–320
Pindolol	Barbloc, Visken	10–30**
Propranolol	Deralin, Inderal	120–320***
Sotalol	Cardol, Sotab, Solavert, Sotacor, Sotahexal	80–320***

*Consider divided dose for higher doses.
**Divided dose for higher doses.
***Divided dose generally applies.

Table 41.2 Properties of β-blockers

Agent	$t_{1/2}$	β_1	ISA	MSA	Lipo
Acebutolol	3–4	+	+	+	+
Atenolol	6–9	++	–	–	±
Bisoprolol	9–12	+++	–	–	–
Carvedilol	5–7	–	–	+	+
Esmolol	9 min	+++	–	–	±
Labetalol	3–6	–	–	–	+
Metoprolol	3–4	++	–	–	+
Nadolol	10–20	– –	–	–	±
Oxprenolol	1–2	–	+	+	++
Pindolol	3–4	–	++	+	++
Propranolol	3–4	–	–	++	++
Sotalol	9–10	–	–	–	–

β_1, cardioselectivity; ISA, intrinsic sympathomimetic activity; Lipo, lipid soluble; MSA, membrane stabilizing activity; $t_{1/2}$, half-life (h).

They have shorter half-lives. Lipophilic agents may be more effective in cardioprotection after a MI.

Other properties

Sotalol has class III antiarrhythmic activity (prolongs duration of the action potential), and is thus useful in tachyarrhythmias. Vasodilatory agents may have specific benefit in heart failure and hypertension. Labetalol and carvedilol are non-cardioselective β-blockers with α_1-blocking action. Nebivolol is cardioselective and causes vasodilatation by acting as a nitric oxide donor. Vasodilatory β-blockers may be more neutral with respect to metabolic effects.

Recent developments

1   Nebivolol has recently become available. By acting as a nitric oxide donor, this agent improves endothelial function and can thus decrease arterial stiffness and central aortic pressure.[2] The agent has no intrinsic sympathomimetic activity and appears to be neutral as far as metabolic side effects are concerned.[3] In a recent trial,[4] systolic BP was reduced by 4.4–9.5 mmHg, and diastolic BP by 8.0–11.2 mmHg, with nebivolol. Its effect is comparable with that of atenolol, but it has greater effect on central aortic pressure.[5]

2   The BEST (Beta-blocker Evaluation of Survival) study was first published in 2001, and followed 2708 patients with advanced heart failure, randomized to bucindolol or placebo. The drug produced no beneficial neurohormonal responses and no clinical benefit overall,[6] and was not marketed further. Further analysis from this trial revealed heterogeneity with respect to response due to a common polymorphism in the β_1-adrenergic gene. At position 389 in the gene, 50% of individuals are homozygous for arginine, 20 homozygous for glycine, and 20% are heterozygous. Survival was increased by 38% in arginine homozygotes.[7] This drug is the first example from a major clinical trial of a drug that clearly acts on individuals with a particular genotype, but is ineffective on others.

3   From animal studies, it appears that bone remodelling is under β-adrenergic control. β-blockers have been shown to have beneficial effects on bone architecture in humans.[8] In a cohort from the MONICA Augsburg Study,[9] 1793 patients were followed-up >10 years. The relative risk of fracture was 0.57 (95% CI: 0.36 to 0.90) in those taking β-blocker. This was only slightly attenuated when figures were adjusted for possible confounding factors such as body mass index. Improved bone health may be an additional bonus for patients who need β-blockers.

Conclusions

The pharmacology of β-blockers is complex, making the choice of agent not always easy. Most of the long-term trial data is with atenolol, which is still useful. For many patients, once the decision to use a β-blocker has been taken, the choice of agent is not critical. However, informed choice will help the patient derive maximum benefit with the low

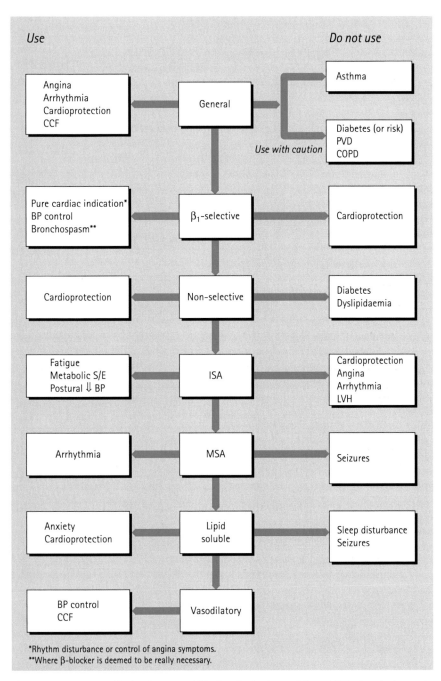

Figure 41.1 Choice of β-blocking agent. CCF, chronic circulatory failure; COPD, chronic obstructive pulmonary disease; ISA, intrinsic sympathomimetic activity; LVH, left ventricular hypertrophy; MSA, membrane stabilizing activity; PVD, peripheral vascular disease

chance of adverse effects. This is important as β-blockers are frequently discontinued because of side effects. Although they are now used less frequently as first-line agents, regimens based on a β-blocker are generally highly effective in reducing BP. A schema to assist with choice of agent is proposed in Figure 41.3. Optimizing the choice of agent will not only maximize the benefit and decrease risk of side effects, but will also improve patient concordance.

References

1   Wiysonge CS, Bradley H, Mayosi BM, Maroney R, Mbewu A, Opie LH, Volminck J. Beta-blockers for hypertension. *Cochrane Database of Systemic Rev* 2007; Issue 1.

2   Cockcroft J. A review of the safety and efficacy of nebivolol in the mildly hypertensive patient. *Vasc Health Risk Manage* 2007; **3**: 909–17.

3   Karter Y. Nebivolol: more than a highly selective Beta blocker. *Recent Patents Cardiovasc Drug Discov* 2007; **2**: 152–5.

4   Weiss RJ, Weber MA, Carr AA, Sullivan WA. A randomized, double-blind, placebo-controlled parallel-group study to assess the efficacy and safety of nebivolol, a novel beta-blocker, in patients with mild to moderate hypertension. *J Clin Hypertens* 2007; **9**: 667–76.

5   Dhakam Z, Yasmin, McEniery CM, Burton T, Brown MJ, Wilkinson IB. A comparison of atenolol and nebivolol in isolated systolic hypertension. *J Hypertens* 2008; **26**: 351–6.

6   Frantz RP, Lowes BD, Grayburn PA, White M, Krause-Steinrauf H, Krishnan V, *et al.* Baseline and serial neurohormones in patients with congestive heart failure treated with and without bucindolol: results of the neurohumoral substudy of the Beta-Blocker Evaluation of Survival Study (BEST). *J Cardiac Fail* 2007; **13**: 437–44.

7   Liggett SB, Mialet-Perez J, Thaneemit-Chen S, Weber SA, Greene SM, Hodne D, *et al.* A polymorphism within a conserved beta(1)-adrenergic receptor motif alters cardiac function and beta-blocker response in human heart failure. *Proc Natl Acad Sci USA* 2006; **103**: 11288–93.

8   Bonnet N, Gadois C, McCloskey E, Lemineur G, Lespessailles E, Courteix D, *et al.* Protective effect of beta blockers in postmenopausal women: influence on fractures, bone density, micro and macroarchitecture. *Bone* 2007; **40**: 1209–16.

9   Meisinger C, Heier M, Lang O, Doring A. Beta-blocker use and risk of fractures in men and women from the general population: the MONICA/KORA Augsburg cohort study. *Osteoporosis Int* 2007; **18**: 1189–95.

42 Calcium Channel Blockers

Case History

Joanna is 65 years old, and has had hypertension for many years. Until recently, her blood pressure (BP) has been well controlled on a combined diuretic and angiotensin-converting enzyme inhibitor (ACE-I) preparation. She has mild renal impairment (creatinine 128 µmol/l), and also suffers from mild asthma. The time has come to step up her BP treatment. You discuss the various options with her and decide that a calcium channel blocker (CCB) would be the most appropriate agent.

What are dihydropyridine CCBs (DCCBs) and non–dihydropyridine CCBs (NDCCBs)?

Is there much to choose between available agents in this class?

Do they protect against cardiovascular (CV) events?

Will a CCB help prevent this woman's renal function deteriorating further?

Background

Voltage-dependent calcium channels are present in the membrane of excitable cells. They are closed at rest, when the membrane is polarized. On depolarization, the channels open allowing the calcium influx. This leads to excitation–contraction coupling in muscle cells or to neuronal stimulation in cells of the central nervous system. Different classes of calcium channels are distinguished by their response to inhibitors:

- L-type: inhibited by dihydropyridines
- N-type: inhibited by conotoxin
- P/Q-type: inhibited by agatoxin
- R-type: resistant to standard inhibitors
- T-type: transient, low voltage activated (LVA)

CCBs (Table 42.1) have now been used clinically for about 30 years. Those currently used act mainly on L-type calcium channels. This membrane channel consists of α_1, α_2, β, δ, and γ subunits. L-type channels are present in cardiac, skeletal and vascular smooth muscle. CCBs acting on vascular smooth muscle cause vasodilatation and thus lower BP. The most commonly used CCBs are based on the dihydropyridine moiety (Figure 42.1). Notable exceptions are verapamil and diltiazem. Agents vary in their selectivity for

Table 42.1 Calcium channel blockers for hypertension

Drug	Brand name	$t_{1/2}$ (h)	Daily dose (mg)
1. Dihydropyridines			
Amlodipine	Istin, Norvasc, Perivasc, Sandoz	30–50	2.5–10
Felodipine	Plendil ER, Felodur ER, Triasyn (with Ramipril)	15–20*	2.5–20
Lacidipine	Lacipil, Motens	12–18	2–6
Lercanidipine	Zanidip	4–7**	10–20
Nicardipine	Cardene, Cardene SR*	2	20–40 TDS
Nifedipine	Adalat, Procardia, Nifehexal, Nyefax Adalat Oros,	2	10–40 BD
	Addos XR, Adefin XL	–*	30–120
Nisoldipine	Sular	7–12	20–40
2. Phenylalkylamine			
Verapamil	Anpec, Isoptin	8–12	80–160 TDS
	Anpec SR, Cordilox SR, Isoptin SR, Veracaps SR, Tarka (240 mg with trandolapril)	–*	180–240
3. Benzothiazepine			
Diltiazem	Cardizem, Diltahexal	3–5	80–160 BD
	Dilzem, Vasocardol	–*	180–360
	CD versions of above		

*Extended release designed to provide round the clock cover.
**Long effective half-life.

Figure 42.1 Dihydropyridine

peripheral and cardiac actions. With the exception of amlodipine, dihydropyridines are not used in patients with angina because they tend to cause reflex tachycardia. Verapamil has a predominantly cardiac action (decreasing heart rate and negatively inotropic) with relatively little peripheral vasodilatation. It should not be used with β-blockers generally.

By the early 1990s, CCBs were the most widely used agents for hypertension. However, several trials in the mid-1990s reported increased mortality from cardiac events.[1] Concerns were mainly over short-acting agents, use of which was associated with a reflex increase in sympathetic tone. Increased heart rate and force of ventricular contraction in the face of peripheral vasodilatation has the potential to predispose to myocardial ischaemia. Furthermore, many of the agents used in early trials would have had to be given several times a day to provide 24-h calcium channel blockade. This consideration also applies to verapamil and diltiazem, although concerns from trials in the 1990s did not relate to NDCCBs. Studies in patients without established renal disease suggest that, in common with other classes of agent, lowering BP with CCBs protects against renal disease. This is probably purely related to BP lowering – there is no suggestion that CCBs have a specific direct renal protective action. In patients with established renal abnormalities, CCBs also protect from decline in glomerular filtration rate and increase in proteinuria but they are less effective than ACE-Is or angiotensin receptor blockers (ARBS). The latter two classes should, therefore, be considered first-line antihypertensives in those at risk of renal failure, but DCCBs are very useful as second-line agents to augment the hypotensive effect of ACE-is or ARBs.

More recent trials (summarized by Epstein *et al.*[2] which includes references) have provided reassurance that CCBs are safe and effective. The following studies should be considered:

1 ALLHAT (Antihypertensive and Lipid-Lowering Treatment to Prevent Heart Attack Trial) (2002). 33 357 subjects aged ≥55 years with hypertension and at least one other risk factor. The trial compared amlodipine, lisinopril, clorthalidone and doxazosin. The doxazosin wing was terminated early because of increased incidence of heart failure. Over 4.9 years, the other three agents were comparable in preventing CV outcomes, and there was no increase in malignant disease with amlodipine.

2 VALUE (Valsartan Antihypertensive Long-term Use Evaluation) (2004). 15 245 subjects were randomized to either amlodipine or valsartan and followed for 4.2 years. There was no difference in overall mortality and CV events, but BP control was better in the amlodipine wing. Surprisingly, valsartan was more frequently associated with myocardial infarction, but appeared to have a protective effect with respect to development of new diabetes.

3 CAMELOT (Comparison of Amlodipine Versus Enalapril to Limit Occurrences of Thrombosis trial) (2004). This involved 1997 subjects with ischaemic heart disease but who were normotensive, and it compared the effect of amlodipine with enalapril. Amlodipine decreased overall event rate by 31% while enalapril was not different to placebo. In a substudy, progression of atherosclerosis was assessed using intravascular ultrasound. There was a tendency for less progression with CCB, confirming the results of the ELSA (European Lacidipine Study on Atherosclerosis) study (2002), in which lacidipine decreased the progression and number of plaques compared with atenolol.

4 ASCOT-BPLA (Anglo-Scandinavian Cardiac Outcomes Trial – Blood Pressure Lowering Arm) (2005). This compared an amlodipine-based regimen with an atenolol-based regimen. It included 19 257 subjects with hypertension plus other risk factors who were followed for 5.5 years. The amlodipine-based regimen (which included perindopril where required) was superior in preventing CV events, and was associated with a lower incidence of diabetes. BP control was identical in the two groups – baseline BP was 164.0/94.7, decreasing to 136.9/78.3 with treatment.

5 FEVER (Felodipine Event Reduction) (2005). This study randomized 9800 Chinese patients whose primary treatment was diuretic to either felodipine or placebo, and followed them for 3.3 years. Stroke and overall CV events were

significantly lower in the felodipine group, which also had a lower incidence of cancer.

Results of these, and other studies, confirm that DCCBs are not only effective at lowering BP, but also protect against stroke, myocardial infarction and other vascular events. The recent INVEST (INternational VErapamil SR-Trandolapril) study,[3] which used a verapamil-based regimen with trandolapril as required, confirms that the benefits of CCBs are likely to extend to NDCCBs. There is a suggestion that they are more protective than renin–angiotensin system blockers, although the latter are more effective in retarding progression of renal disease. CCBs may have a direct beneficial effect on atherosclerosis, which extends beyond their BP-lowering effect. Possible mechanisms include antioxidant effects, increasing nitric oxide generation and decreasing vascular smooth muscle cell proliferation. CCBs are safe with no increase in cardiac events or gastrointestinal bleeding. A haemorrhagic tendency with CCBs has been attributed to effects on platelets along with loss of protective vasoconstriction. Data on cancer with CCBs have been conflicting, and the general consensus is now that there is no increased risk.

CCBs may protect against stroke by mechanisms not directly related to BP lowering. Compared with diuretics and β-blockers, CCBs are neutral with respect to glucose and lipids. They are generally well tolerated (for side effects see Box 42.1). The beneficial effects of CCBs appear to be irrespective of race. African American patients not only have increased prevalence and earlier incidence of hypertension, but also respond relatively less satisfactorily to ACE-Is, ARBs and β-blockers.

Amlodipine is the most widely used CCB for hypertension, and is particularly indicated for those with concomitant angina (although β-blockers should also be considered). Most preparations use the besylate salt of amlodipine. The maleate salt is used in some and has identical efficacy and tolerability. The long half-life makes it ideal for once-daily dosage and it provides round the clock cover. Because of the wealth of trial and clinical experience with the drug, it is suitable for use in combinations. For example, Caduet (Pfizer) combines amlodipine (5 or 10 mg) with atorvastatin (10, 20, 40 or 80 mg).

Box 42.1 Side effects of calcium channel blockers

- Dizziness
- Headache
- Facial flushing
- Peripheral oedema
- Gingival hyperplasia
- Muscle cramps
- Gastro-oesophageal reflux
- Constipation
- Heart rate
  - reflex tachycardia
  - bradycardia (especially with β-blockers)

Lercanidipine, although it has a relatively short half-life in plasma, has a much longer duration of action because it is a highly lipophilic compound. It should be taken before meals and especially not eaten with high fat meals. Some CCBs, including lercanidipine and felodipine, are metabolized by the enzyme CYP3A4. This enzyme is inhibited by grapefruit juice, which may thus increase plasma levels of CCBs. Although there is not much evidence of teratogenicity from CCBs, there has been a suggestion of increased limb bud abnormalities and the drugs are not recommended in early pregnancy. Some CCBs are excreted in breast milk, and the drugs are best avoided in breast-feeding mothers.

Recent Developments

1   Available CCBs block mainly L-type calcium channels. There is potential for benefit from drugs that block other types of calcium channel. Benidipine (Coniel) is used in Japan and other Far Eastern countries, and is a long-acting blocker of both L- and N-type channels. It may have particular benefits compared with other CCBs in renal protection. By protecting from glomerular hypertension, it may specifically decrease hypertension-induced renal damage and diminish proteinuria.[4] It is both clinically effective and cost effective when used with an ARB, helping to keep down the dose of the latter.[5] A T-type channel blocker, mibefradil, was developed and withdrawn. T-type channels are present in cardiac muscle cells, Purkinje cells, the sino-atrial node, and in the central nervous system. They are involved in biological pacemakers and rhythms and may also be important in the pathogenesis of epilepsy. Blockage of T-type channels may be useful in angina, in tachyarrhythmias where they can decrease heart rate without negative inotropic action, and in renal protection.

2   Many commonly used antidepressants inhibit L-type calcium channels.[6] This action appears to be mediated by a mechanism distinct from that of diltiazem. This may help explain why antidepressant treatment tends to lower BP.

3   Recent data from the Leiden 85-plus study[7] suggests that use of a CCB is associated with a decreased risk of dementia. The fact that a similar effect is not seen with other antihypertensive drugs suggests that any benefit may be mediated directly through calcium channel blockade rather than through BP reduction. The Syst-Eur (Systolic Hypertension in Europe) trial also suggested a decreased risk of dementia with the CCB nitrendipine. Work with a diabetic mouse model[8] has confirmed that CCB treatment has the potential to be neuroprotective, perhaps through decreasing vascular disease, decreasing free radicals, and improving neural differentiation.

4   Secretion of aldosterone from the adrenal cortex is partly regulated through T-type calcium channels. Efonidipine is a novel L/T-type CCB that has been shown to decrease aldosterone levels in hypertensive subjects compared with treatment with amlodipine.[9] Furthermore, it is possible that some of the vascular protective effects of CCBs are mediated by inhibition of the mineralocorticoid receptor.[10] Nimodipine and felodipine are the most potent of the available CCBs in this respect, while amlodipine is relatively impotent. NDCCBs are devoid of mineralocorticoid blocking activity.

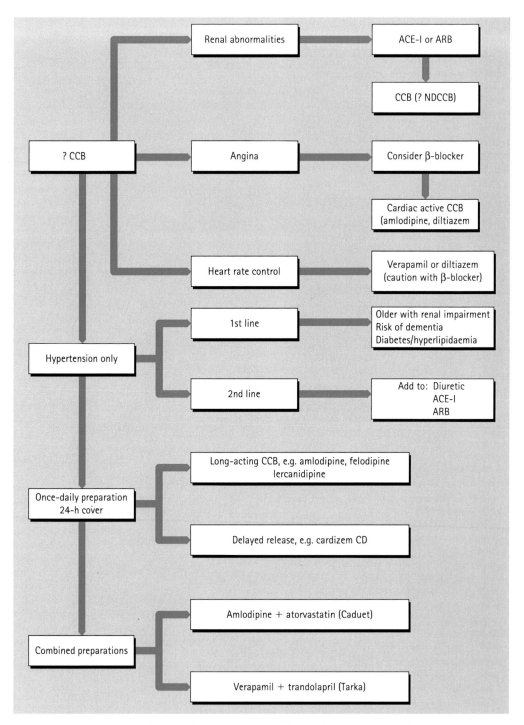

Figure 42.2 Use of CCBs. ACE-I, angiotensin-converting enzyme inhibitor; ARB, angiotensin receptor blocker; CCB, calcium channel blocker; NDCCB, non-dihydropyridine calcium channel blocker

5 When added to diuretic therapy, DCCBs are more potent than either ACE-Is or ARBs in reducing BP.[11] Adding the dual L/N-type CCB cilnidipine to ARBs leads to improved BP control with no reflex increase in heart rate.[12] For elderly people, the combination of CCB and ACE-I not only provides effective BP control for many but the relative lack of postural and metabolic side effects is also an advantage.[13] CCBs have a good safety and benefit profile when combined with other agents.

Conclusions

CCBs are among the most widely used drugs for hypertension. Recent trials have confirmed that they are both safe and effective in protecting against CV outcomes. They are useful across different age groups and in different racial groups, as well as being very effective in combination – particularly with diuretics, ACE-Is or ARBs. A schema to guide the use of CCBs is proposed in Figure 42.2. DCCBs are most widely used, largely because of the wealth of trial data supporting amlodipine. Of NDCCBs, verapamil is particularly used when cardiac rate or rhythm control is an issue. NDCCBs are as effective as DCCBs in providing BP control, but may be slightly more effective in renal protection. In combination with ACE-I or ARB, CCBs provide additional BP control that protects the kidneys. There is considerable interest in agents that block other classes of calcium channel than the L-type.

References

1 Furberg CD, Psaty BM, Meyer JV. Dose-related increase in mortality in patients with coronary heart disease. *Circulation* 1995; **92**: 1326–31.

2 Epstein BJ, Vogel K, Palmer BF. Dihydropyridine calcium channel antagonists in the management of hypertension. *Drugs* 2007; **67**: 1309–27.

3 Brunner M, Cooper–Dehoff RM, Gong Y, Karnes JH, Langaee TY, Pepine CJ, Johnson JA. Factors influencing blood pressure response to trandolapril add-on therapy in patients taking verapamil SR/trandolapril (INVEST) Study. *J Am Coll Cardiol* 2007; **99**: 1549–54.

4 Uzu T, Nishimura M, Fujii T, Sakaguchi M, Kanasaki M, Isshiki K, *et al.* Benidipine attenuates glomerular hypertension and reduces albuminuria in patients with metabolic syndrome. *Hypertens Res* 2007; **30**: 161–5.

5 Saito F, Fujita H, Takahashi A, Ichiyama I, Harasawa S, Oiwa K, *et al.* Renoprotective effect and cost-effectiveness of using benidipine, a calcium channel blocker, to lower the dose of angiotensin receptor blocker in hypertensive patients with albuminuria. *Hypertension Res* 2007; **30**: 39–47.

6 Zahradnik I, Minarovic I, Zahradnikova A. Inhibition of the cardiac L-type calcium channel current by antidepressant drugs. *J Pharmacol Exp Ther* 2008; **324**: 977–84.

7 Trompet S, Westendorp RGJ, Kamper AM, de Craen AJM. Use of calcium antagonists and cognitive decline in old age. The Leiden 85-plus study. *Neurobiol Aging* 2008; **29**(2): 306–8.

8 Tsukuda K, Mogi M, Li J-M, Iwanami J, Min L-J, Sakata A, *et al.* Diabetes-associated cognitive impairment is improved by a calcium channel blocker, nifedipine. *Hypertension* 2008; **51**: 528–33.

9 Tanaka T, Tsutamoto T, Sakai H, Fujii M, Yamamoto T, Horie M. Comparison of the effects of efonidipine and amlodipine on aldosterone in patients with hypertension. *Hypertension Res* 2007; **30**: 691–7.

10 Dietz JD, Du S, Bolten CW, Payne MA, Xia C, Blinn JR, *et al.* A number of marketed dihydropyridine calcium channel blockers have mineralocorticoid receptor antagonist activity. *Hypertension* 2008; **51**: 742–8.

11 Bisognano JD, McLaughlin T, Roberts CS, Tang SSK. Calcium channel blockers, angiotensin receptor blockers, and angiotensin-converting enzyme inhibitors: effectiveness in combination with diuretics or beta-blockers for treating hypertension. *Vasc Health Risk Manage* 2007; **3**: 579–85.

12 Nagahama S, Norimatsu T, Maki T, Yasuda M, Tanaka S. The effect of combination therapy with an L/N-Type Ca(2+) channel blocker, cilnidipine, and an angiotensin II receptor blocker on the blood pressure and heart rate in Japanese hypertensive patients: an observational study conducted in Japan. *Hypertens Res* 2007; **30**: 815–22.

13 Fogari R, Derosa G, Zoppi A, Rinaldi A, Preti P, Lazzari P, *et al.* Effects of manidipine/delapril versus olmesartan/hydrochlorothiazide combination therapy in elderly hypertensive patients with type 2 diabetes mellitus. *Hypertension Res* 2008; **31**: 43–50.

43 α-blockers, Combined α- and β-blockers, and Vasodilating β-blockers

Case History

Harry is 66 years old and has had treatment for hypertension for 10 years. His blood pressure (BP) was initially well controlled with a diuretic and a calcium channel blocker. Five years ago, his BP was less than ideally controlled. He also had mild prostatic symptoms, and his GP decided that an α-blocker would be a logical choice. Again, his hypertension came under control but in recent years he has complained of fatigue and dizziness. He thought that his tablets were responsible and stopped them. His symptoms improved but, predictably, his BP increased.

What is the current place of α-blockers in the management of hypertension?

Do combined α- and β-blockers offer an advantage?

Are the latter drugs useful in patients with hypertension and prostatic symptoms?

Are drugs that combine β-blockade with other properties useful?

Background

The drugs considered in this chapter are summarized in Table 43.1. α_1-receptor blockade has been used for around two decades as a means of controlling high BP. There are three subtypes: α_{1a}, α_{1b} and α_{1d}. The α_{1a}-receptor is highly expressed in the prostate, while the latter two subtypes are responsible for some of the side effects (Box 43.1) as well as beneficial effect of α-blockers. α_2-blockers, of which yohimbine is the best-known example, are not widely used in clinical practice. The fatigue and dizziness experienced by some patients taking α-blockers is not necessarily directly related to BP lowering. Prazosin was the first selective α_1-blocker to be developed – utility is limited by its very short half-life. Terazosin was the next, but was mainly used to control prostatic symptoms. Doxazosin, with its longer half-life, found wide usage in hypertension. However, ALLHAT (Antihypertensive and Lipid-Lowering Treatment to Prevent Heart Attack Trial)[1] published in 2000 suggested that it was a less than ideal first-line agent: over 24 000 patients were randomized either to doxazosin or chlorthalidone. The α-blocker wing was terminated early after a mean follow-up of 3.3 years. There was no difference in total mortality, fatal coronary heart disease or non-fatal myocardial infarction. Patients treated with doxazosin had a higher risk of stroke – RR 1.19 (95% CI: 1.01 to 1.40) – and higher risk of combined cardiovascular disease – RR 1.25 (95% CI: 1.17 to 1.33). Most importantly, the

Table 43.1 Available drugs

Drug	Brand names	Half–life (h)	Usual daily dose (mg)
Prazosin	Hypovase	2–3	2–20*
Terazosin	Hytrin	12	2–10
Doxazosin	Cardura Cardura XL**	22	2–8
Labetalol	Presolol Trandate	6–8	200–2400*
Carvedilol	Coreg, Dilasig Dilatrend, Eucardic Kredex Coreg CR**	7–9	12.5–25
Nebivolol	Bystolic Nebicip Nebilet	10	2.5–5

*In up to three divided doses.
**Long-acting formulations.
CR, controlled release.

risk of heart failure (HF) was doubled in the doxazosin group – RR 2.04 (95% CI: 1.79 to 2.32). This very large study led to the conclusion that α-blockers should not be used as first-line agents. The difference in chronic circulatory failure in ALLHAT may have been due to an adverse effect of doxazosin (slight fluid retention) or to a beneficial effect of the diuretic offloading salt and water.

Interest in the α-blockers increased dramatically in the mid-1970s when the non-selective α-blocker phenoxybenzamine was introduced for the management of prostatic symptoms. This drug group is still most useful when lower urinary tract symptoms are present in the male hypertensive patient. In the ageing male, proliferation of the prostatic stroma and epithelial components leads to bladder outlet obstruction. Smooth muscle cells make up about half of the stroma, and their contraction is inhibited by α-blockers. Lower urinary tract symptoms include poor stream, difficulty voiding and dribbling. Prostatic hypertrophy may also lead to urinary retention (acute and chronic), urinary tract infections, renal impairment and haematuria. For this usage, phenoxybenzamine and prazosin gave way to the long-acting agents, terazosin and doxazosin. Hypotensive symptoms were minimized and benefits on nocturnal urinary symptoms maximized if the agents were taken before bedtime. They tend only to lower BP in those who are already hypertensive. The hypotensive effect is by blocking α-receptors in peripheral arteries allowing the unopposed vasodilatory effect of β-adrenoreceptors – particularly with exercise or stress. β-blockers exert their antihypertensive effects through central, cardiac and renal mechanisms. Tamsulosin was the first specific α_{1a}-blocker. It is long-acting, does not require dose titration and has a minimal effect on BP. Although theoretically useful, more recent trial data with this group of drugs have called their efficacy into

Box 43.1 Side effects of α-blockers

- Fluid retention
- Asthenia, fatigue*
- Postural hypotension
- Dizziness*
- Somnolence
- Nasal congestion
- Ejaculatory dysfunction

*Not always directly related to BP lowering

question and curtailed their further development. Alfuzosin is a non-subtype specific agent that also does not require dose titration and is less likely to cause ejaculatory problems.

Labetalol and carvedilol are non-selective β-blockers with additional α_1-blocking activity. As with other β-blockers they can provoke asthma and bradycardia. Labetalol can also worsen hyperglycaemia and dyslipidaemia. Unlike other β-blockers, carvedilol may actually have a beneficial effect on insulin resistance and glycaemic control. Because it has been used for many years, labetalol is considered safe in pregnancy and its combined α/β action has also proved useful in the management of hypertensive emergencies. The short half-life is a disadvantage in the management of chronic hypertension. The ratio of α to β blockade with labetalol is about 1:3. It is probably not useful in controlling prostatic symptoms although specific studies have not been conducted. Carvedilol has fewer negative inotropic and chronotropic effects than other β-blockers and is licensed for use in left ventricular dysfunction and chronic circulatory failure as well as in hypertension. The immediate release formulation, given twice daily, has been used since the mid-1990s. An extended release preparation for once-daily administration is now available in some countries. The ratio of α to β blockade with carvedilol is 1:8 and is not, therefore, useful in managing prostatic symptoms. At higher doses, carvedilol also has antioxidant and calcium channel-blocking effects.

Nebivolol is a highly selective β_1-adrenorecptor antagonist with an additional vasodilatory effect mediated by nitric oxide. The latter is achieved by activation of the endothelial nitric oxide synthase enzyme and by decreased nitric oxide breakdown. Additionally, it has beneficial effects on oxidative stress and endothelial function. In uncomplicated hypertension, trial data[2] show that nebivolol is as effective as other β-blockers and other classes. As nebivolol improves both systolic and diastolic function, it is also licensed for use in chronic HF. For example, in the SENIORS (Study of Effects of Nebivolol Intervention on Outcomes and Rehospitalization in Seniors With Heart Failure) study (2005)[2] nebivolol (compared with placebo) decreased mortality and hospital admissions in older patients with HF. In these patients, increased central aortic pressure contributes to left ventricular afterload, leading to myocyte hypertrophy. Decreased aortic diastolic BP impairs coronary perfusion, which contributes to subendocardial ischaemia with consequent fibrosis. Altered myocardial remodelling (myocyte hypertrophy and fibrosis) leads to impaired diastolic function. The combined actions of nebivolol favourably influence both the remodelling process and the underlying mechanical vascular changes that are apparent in many elderly people with hypertension. Nebivolol is at least neutral in relation to total and low-density lipoprotein-cholesterol, blood glucose and body weight. It modestly decreases triglycerides and may have a protective effect against the development of diabetes. Side effects are not usually severe but include headache, tiredness and dizziness. A lower starting dose should be used for the elderly. The dose should be decreased in those with renal impairment and the drug is best avoided with severe hepatic impairment.

Recent Developments

1   In spite of the results of ALLHAT,[1] doxazosin should not be abandoned and is often useful as a third-line agent. In addition to its neutral metabolic profile, it may have an anti-inflammatory action. Its peripheral action is also useful in the elderly, decreasing arterial stiffness and thus making it potentially very useful in isolated systolic hypertension.[3] As for prostatic symptoms, there may be benefits for hypertension with a night-time dose of doxazosin. A decreased morning surge in BP resulting from night-time dosing can contribute to decreasing Left Ventricular Mass Index.[4]

2   Trial data with the controlled release formulation of carvedilol are encouraging[5] – 40 mg of this formulation is equivalent to 12.5 mg BD of the immediate release formulation. BP-lowering effects persist through the 24-hour period with a single daily dose of the controlled release preparation. With the beneficial effects of round the clock BP control and favourable effects on renal and cardiac haemodynamics, carvedilol may have significant antioxidant and anti-inflammatory properties contributing to its ability to modulate atherosclerosis.[6]

3   The metabolism of nebivolol is highly dependent on the cytochrome P450 2D6 enzyme (CYP2D6). Steady-state plasma levels can be up to 15 times higher in patients classified as poor metabolizers. Astonishingly, this wide variation in plasma concentrations does not seem to affect the beneficial BP-lowering properties.[7]

4   A short-term multicentre trial of nebivolol in 909 patients with mild to moderate hypertension[8] confirmed its ability to lower both systolic BP (by 4–10 mmHg) and diastolic BP (by 8–11 mmHg). The relatively higher reduction in diastolic BP has been consistently reported and is greater than that seen, for example, with angiotensin-converting enzyme inhibitors. The effect of nebivolol in reducing brachial systolic BP is similar to that of atenolol, but it has a greater effect in decreasing aortic pulse pressure.[9] It is not clear whether this benefit translates into improved end-point outcomes. Nebivolol may be useful in high-risk groups, including African Americans who typically respond poorly to β-blockers.[10] The drug was also very well tolerated in this group who are often more prone to adverse effects of antihypertensives because they need more therapy.

Conclusions

Adrenergic blockers, which are not classical (first- or second-generation) β-blockers, have an important and emerging place in the management of hypertension (Figure 43.1).

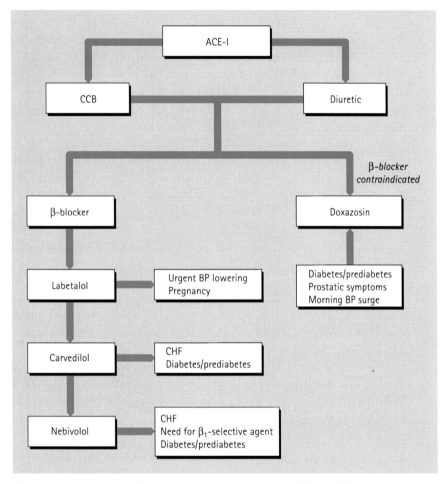

Figure 43.1 Use of drugs. ACE-I, angiotensin-converting enzyme inhibitor; CCB, calcium channel blocker; CHF, congestive heart failure

α-blockers remain important third-line drugs and have often been used in men with prostatic symptoms. They are valuable because of their metabolic neutrality and also because a night-time dose can be useful in patients with a morning BP surge. They should not be used alone because fluid retention and neurohumoral activation may offset the benefit of their BP-lowering effect. Available combined α/β blockers are not useful in the management of prostatic symptoms as they do not have sufficient α-blocking activity. Carvedilol has found a major place in patients with HF. It has additional antioxidant properties, and its controlled release preparation should prove very useful. Nebivolol is a vasodilating cardioselective β-blocker that has considerable support from recent studies showing its utility in patients with hypertension and in those with HF. The decline of β-blockers as first-line agents has coincided with the emergence of newer agents that combine the benefits of β-blockade with other properties.

References

1   ALLHAT Officers and Coordinators. Major cardiovascular events in hypertensive patients randomized to doxazosin vs chlorthalidone. *JAMA* 2000; **283**: 1967–75.

2   Moen MD, Wagstaff AJ. Nebivolol. A review of its use in the management of hypertension and chronic heart failure. *Drugs* 2006; **66**: 1389–409.

3   Wykretowicz A, Guzik P, Krauze T, Adamska K, Milewska A, Wysocki H. Add-on therapy with doxazosin in patients with hypertension influences arterial stiffness and albuterol-mediated arterial vasodilation. *Br J Clin Pharmacol* 2007; **64**: 792–5.

4   Ikeda T, Gomi T, Shibuya Y, Shinozaki S, Suzuki Y, Matsuda N. Add-on effect of bedtime dosing of the alpha(1)-adrenergic receptor antagonist doxazosin on morning hypertension and left ventricular hypertrophy in patients undergoing long-term amlodipine monotherapy.[See comment.] *Hypertens Res* 2007; **30**: 1097–105.

5   Weber MA, Bakris GL, Tarka EA, Iyengar M, Fleck R, Sica DA. Efficacy of a once-daily formulation of carvedilol for the treatment of hypertension. *J Clin Hypertens* 2006; **8**: 840–9.

6   Dandona P, Ghanim H, Brooks DP. Antioxidant activity of carvedilol in cardiovascular disease. *J Hypertens* 2007; **25**: 731–41.

7   Lefebvre J, Poirier L, Poirier P, Turgeon J, Lacourciere Y. The influence of CYP2D6 phenotype on the clinical response of nebivolol in patients with essential hypertension. *Br J Clin Pharmacol* 2007; **63**: 575–82.

8   Weiss RJ, Weber MA, Carr AA, Sullivan WA. A randomized, double-blind, placebo-controlled parallel-group study to assess the efficacy and safety of nebivolol, a novel beta-blocker, in patients with mild to moderate hypertension. *J Clin Hypertens* 2007; **9**: 667–76.

9   Dhakam Z, Yasmin, McEniery CM, Burton T, Brown MJ, Wilkinson IB. A comparison of atenolol and nebivolol in isolated systolic hypertension. *J Hypertens* 2008; **26**: 351–6.

10 Saunders E, Smith WB, DeSalvo KB, Sullivan WA. The efficacy and tolerability of nebivolol in hypertensive African American patients. *J Clin Hypertens* 2007; **9**: 866–75.

44 Angiotensin–converting Enzyme Inhibitors

Case History

John is 48 years old, and has recently been noted to be hypertensive. His parents both had treatment for hypertension, and renal failure contributed to his father's death at the age of 67 years. A urine stick test for protein was recently positive. Subsequent testing was negative but urine sent to the laboratory showed him to have microalbuminuria (confirmed on two occasions). You discuss the options with him and decide that an angiotensin-converting enzyme inhibitor (ACE-I) would be useful, both to control his blood pressure (BP) and to protect his kidneys.

Does it matter which ACE-I is prescribed?

What precautions should be taken when starting an ACE-I?

Are there benefits beyond lowering of BP?

Background

Inhibition of the renin–angiotensin system (RAS) has been one of the major developments in cardiovascular (CV) medicine over the past three decades. RAS is not only involved in regulating BP, but also participates in several key processes that contribute to vascular disease. These include inflammation, cell proliferation and oxidative stress. The system works not only in the systemic circulation but components of RAS are also expressed in many tissues (Figure 44.1). Angiotensinogen is an α_2-globulin that is constitutively secreted by the liver, and is acted upon by renin (secreted by the juxtaglomerular cells apparatus) to produce the decapeptide angiotensin (Ang) I. Renin secretion is stimulated by decreased pressure in the afferent arterioles, decreased sodium delivery or by sympathetic stimulation. By cleavage of the two carboxyterminal amino acids, ACE yields the octapeptide Ang II, which, in turn, binds to the receptors AT_1, AT_2 and AT_4. Other enzymes, including chymases and cathepsins, can also cleave Ang I to Ang II.

The major BP-regulating effects (vasoconstriction, aldosterone secretion and vascular remodelling) are mediated through the AT_1 receptor. The AT_2 receptor is most active during foetal life and antagonizes many of the effects of AT_1, although the two may synergize in regulating inflammatory responses. AT_4 activation leads to vasodilatation, plasminogen activator inhibitor-1 release, and central nervous system responses. β-blockers

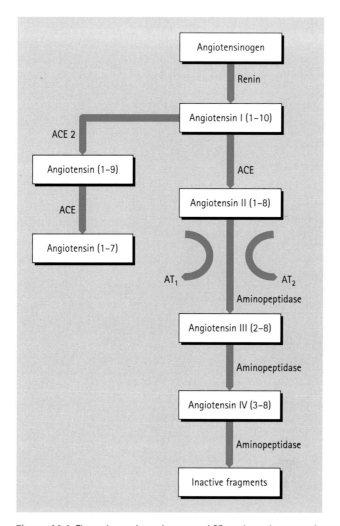

Figure 44.1 The renin–angiotensin system. ACE, angiotensin-converting enzyme

decrease RAS activity by inhibiting renin release. ACE2 is an enzyme with sequence similarity to ACE and which produces angiotensin (1–7), a heptapeptide that produces vasodilatation and levels of which increase with ACE-Is and angiotensin receptor blockers.[1] Increased RAS activity is involved in a variety of types of hypertension – renin-secreting tumours (rare), renovascular (including atherosclerotic and fibromuscular renal artery) stenosis (increased renin release due to decreased renal perfusion), essential hypertension (renin elevated in 15% but inappropriately high in up to 50%), malignant hypertension (renal ischaemia), phaeochromocytoma (catecholamine excess), and states of mineralocorticoid excess.

Studies in the early 1960s showed that the venom of the Brazilian arrowhead viper (*Bothrops jararaca*) inhibited the enzyme that later became known as ACE. Later, peptide and non-peptide inhibitors of this enzyme were shown to decrease BP. This led to the development of the first ACE-I, captopril. Others have largely superseded this drug because of its short half-life and high incidence of taste disturbances and skin rashes. The latter two effects are attributable to the drug's sulphydryl group. This group has been replaced with a carboxyl group in the majority of currently available ACE-Is, except fosinopril, which has a phosphoryl group. ACE-Is have been widely used because of their protective effects on the heart and kidney. Some key early studies were:[1]

- CONSENSUS (Cooperative North Scandinavian Enalapril Survival Study, 1987): showing improved survival in patients with chronic circulatory failure.

- SOLVD (Studies of Left Ventricular Dysfunction, 1991): showing decreased mortality and lower hospitalization rates in patients with heart failure who were treated with enalapril.

- SAVE (Survival and Ventricular Enlargement, 1992): in which captopril improved survival and protected against heart failure in patients with myocardial infarction.

Two meta-analyses have examined more recent trials of ACE-Is in patients who have apparently normal left ventricular function: Dagenais *et al.*[2] analysed outcomes and mortality in the 29 805 patients who participated in the HOPE (Heart Outcomes Prevention Evaluation), EUROPA (EUropean trial on Reduction Of cardiac events with Perindopril) and PEACE (Prevention of Events with ACE inhibition) studies. Combining data from these studies, ACE-Is reduced all-cause mortality, CV mortality, myocardial infarction, stroke and heart failure. In HOPE, the baseline BP was 139/79 and decreased by 3/3 mmHg with ramipril. Baseline BP in EUROPA was 137/82 and decreased by 6/4 mmHg with perindopril, while in PEACE the baseline was 133/78 and decreased by 4/4 mmHg with trandolapril. Clearly, the patient groups in these studies were not particularly hypertensive but the studies do illustrate that the protective effects of ACE-Is are out of proportion to their BP-lowering effect. Al-Mallah *et al.*[3] analysed data from 16 772 patients enrolled in six trials. Again, ACE-I usage was associated with decreased risk of CV events. For a mean treatment of 4.4 years, 100 patients would have to be treated to prevent one event. This argues against the universal use of RAS-blocking drugs in all patients with CV risk factors.

Commonly used ACE-Is are summarized in Table 44.1, and a schema for starting ACE-Is is proposed in Figure 44.2. In terms of efficacy for lowering BP, protecting against CV events and side-effect profile, there seems little to choose between different members of this class. Adverse effects include:

- Cough in 6–8%. This is thought to be due to increased bradykinin, which is normally broken down by ACE. Tachykinins, substance P and prostaglandins may also be involved. Women, black or Asian patients, and those with ACE genotype II are at increased risk. The cough usually resolves within days of stopping the drug, but resolution may take several weeks. The cough has been treated with local anaesthetic agents, theophylline, and non-steroidal anti-inflammatory drugs (particularly sulindac). Cough is the commonest side effect of ACE-Is and occurs uniformly with all members of the class.

- Angio-oedema is a less common but serious and potentially fatal side effect. Increased bradykinin levels may contribute. The patient complains of rapid development of swelling of the lips and tongue, along with constriction of the

Table 44.1 Angiotensin–converting enzyme inhibitors

Drug	Brand names	Half–life (h)	Daily dose (mg)
Captopril	Capoten, Acenorm Capothexal, Topace	2	25–50 TDS
Enalapril	Amprace, Renitec, Enahexal, Alphapril	11	5–40
Fosinopril	Monopril	12	10–40
Lisinopril	Lisodur, Prinivil Liprace, Zestril	12	10–40
Perindopril	Coversyl	25	5–10
Quinapril	Accupril, Asig	2	20–40 BD
Ramipril	Ramace, Tritace	15	5–20
Trandolapril	Gopten, Odrik	18	2–4

The half-lives given are the effective half-life (drug + metabolites). Intermediate duration agents are better divided into two doses when higher doses are used. Combination preparations:

- Accuretic: Quinapril + hydrochlorthiazide
- Coversyl Plus: Perindopril + indapamide
- Monoplus: Fosinopril + hydrochlorthiazide
- Renitec Plus: Enalapril + hydrochlorthiazide
- Tarka: Trandolapril + verapamil
- Zestoretic: Lisinopril + hydrochlorthiazide

upper airways. ACE-Is are the commonest drugs to cause angio-oedema (0.1–0.5% of users). Other drugs include bupropion (Zyban), non-steroidal anti-inflammatory drugs, antidepressants (selective serotonin reuptake inhibitors [SSRIs] and others), and statins. Unlike with cough, patients who develop angio-oedema with ACE-Is may also develop it with angiotensin receptor blockers.

- Hypotension can occur in those who are concurrently using diuretics, or where there is dehydration through poor oral intake, excessive sweating, vomiting or diarrhoea.

- Worsening of renal function – decreased tone in efferent vessels along with lowering of systemic BP both contribute to decreased glomerular filtration pressure. A small increase in creatinine is common – up to 20% is considered reasonable.

- Hyperkalaemia-decreased aldosterone leads to sodium loss but with potassium retention.

Recent Developments

1 In a subgroup analysis of ALLHAT (Antihypertensive and Lipid-Lowering Treatment to Prevent Heart Attack Trial) l,[4] patients with the metabolic syndrome had a 17.1% incidence of diabetes with chlorthalidone, 16.0% with

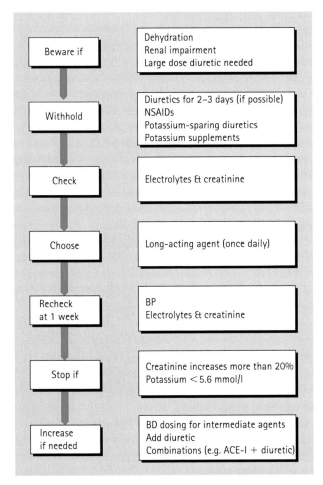

Figure 44.2 Starting an ACE-I. ACE-I, angiotensin-converting enzyme inhibitor; NSAIDs, non-steroidal anti-inflammatory drugs.

amlodipine and only 12.6% with lisinopril. In spite of this statistically significant difference in metabolic outcome, chlorthalidone was superior in terms of preventing heart failure or other CV events. Metabolic variables are only one aspect of CV disease prevention with antihypertensive drugs.

2 Dipeptidyl peptidase IV (DPP IV) inhibitors are being increasingly used as treatments for type 2 diabetes. They inhibit breakdown of glucagon-like peptide-1, which is an incretin, stimulating insulin release in response to food. DPP IV and aminopeptidase P are also involved in the inactivation of bradykinin and substance P. Decreased levels of these enzymes has been reported in patients with ACE-I-related angio-oedema.[5] There is no evidence for an association to date but concurrent use of DPP IV inhibitors and ACE-Is could increase the incidence of angio-oedema.

3 There is a suggestion that ACE-Is may retard cognitive decline in patients prone to Alzheimer's disease.[6] ACE is involved in the cleavage of amyloid-β peptide, deposition of which is increased in the brains of patients with Alzheimer's.[7] The rate of cognitive decline may be slower in patients with the ACE-I polymorphism.

4 A report involving patients from the Rotterdam study[8] showed that patients with the D allele of the insertion/deletion (I/D) polymorphism of the ACE gene had higher mean levels of BP and also higher pulse pressure. The D allele is associated with the higher endogenous activity of ACE. Common polymorphisms exist in the genes for ACE, angiotensinogen and the AT_1 receptor. These may not only help determine the susceptibility to hypertension, but may also determine the response to treatments, including RAS blockade.[9] Vasodilatation mediated by bradykinin also contributes to the BP-lowering effect of ACE-Is. This response may also be partly genetically determined through a common polymorphism in the bradykinin type 2 receptor gene.[10]

5 ACE2 is a highly efficient enzyme, which, by catalysing formation of angiotensin (2–7) diverts substrate away from the formation of Ang II. In the future, gene transfer strategies to increase ACE2 activity or the use of ACE2 activators may provide a novel treatment for hypertension. Initial studies with the latter in animal models have proved encouraging.[11]

Conclusions

ACE-Is and angiotensin receptor blockers block the RAS and are among the most commonly used antihypertensive agents. ACE-Is are safe and generally very well tolerated. The available agents are very similar in terms of efficacy and tolerability. Compliance is likely to be higher with a once-daily agent. For agents that are of intermediate duration of action, twice daily dosing should be considered with higher doses. There is a very useful synergy with diuretics that should be added at an early stage, perhaps even before maximizing the dose of ACE-I. The major risks when starting an ACE-I are hypotension, hyperkalaemia and deteriorating renal function (Figure 44.2). Hyperkalaemia is more likely in old age, where there is pre-existing renal impairment, with diabetes, peripheral vascular disease (increased risk of renal artery stenosis), and with potassium-sparing diuretics. ACE-Is are not the most powerful agents available for lowering BP. However, the many actions of the RAS mean that the benefits of ACE-Is extend way beyond simple BP reduction.

References

1 Schmieder RE, Hilgers KF, Schlaich MP, Schmidt BMW. Renin–angiotensin system and cardiovascular risk. *Lancet* 2007; **369**: 1208–19.

2 Dagenais GR, Pogue J, Fox K, Simoons ML, Yusuf S. Angiotensin-converting-enzyme inhibitors in stable vascular disease without left ventricular systolic dysfunction or heart failure: a combined analysis of three trials. *Lancet* 2006; **368**: 581–8.

3 Al-Mallah M, Tleyjeh IM, Abdel-Latif AA, Weaver WD. Angiotensin-converting enzyme inhibitors in coronary artery disease and preserved left ventricular function. *J Am Coll Cardiol* 2006; **47**: 1576–83.

4   Black HR, Davis B, Barzilay J, Nwachuku C, Baimbridge C, Marginean H, *et al.* Metabolic and clinical outcomes in nondiabetic individuals with the metabolic syndrome assigned to chlorthalidone, amlodipine, or lisinopril as initial treatment for hypertension: a report from the Antihypertensive and Lipid-Lowering Treatment to Prevent Heart Attack Trial (ALLHAT). *Diabetes Care* 2008; **31**: 353–60.

5   Byrd JB, Touzin K, Sile S, Gainer JV, Yu C, Nadeau J, *et al.* Dipeptidyl peptidase IV in angiotensin-converting enzyme inhibitor associated angio-oedema.[See comment.] *Hypertension* 2008; **51**: 141–7.

6   Hajjar IM, Keown M, Lewis P, Almor A. Angiotensin converting enzyme inhibitors and cognitive and functional decline in patients with Alzheimer's disease: an observational study. *Am J Alzheimer's Dis Other Dementias* 2008; **23**: 77–83.

7   Miners JS, Ashby E, Van Helmond Z, Chalmers KA, Palmer LE, Love S, *et al.* Angiotensin-converting enzyme (ACE) levels and activity in Alzheimer's disease, and relationship of perivascular ACE-1 to cerebral amyloid angiopathy. *Neuropathol Appl Neurobiol* 2008; **34**: 181–93.

8   Mattace-Raso FUS, Sie MPS, van der Cammen TJM, Safar ME, Hofman A, van Duijn CM, *et al.* Insertion/deletion gene polymorphism of the angiotensin-converting enzyme and blood pressure changes in older adults. The Rotterdam study. *J Hum Hypertens* 2007; **21**: 736–40.

9   Bhatnagar V, O'Connor DT, Schork NJ, Salem RM, Nievergelt CM, Rana BK, *et al.* Angiotensin-converting enzyme gene polymorphism predicts the time-course of blood pressure response to angiotensin converting enzyme inhibition in the AASK trial. *J Hypertens* 2007; **25**: 2082–92.

10 Van Guilder GP, Pretorius M, Luther JM, Byrd JB, Hill K, Gainer JV, *et al.* Bradykinin type 2 receptor BE1 genotype influences bradykinin-dependent vasodilation during angiotensin-converting enzyme inhibition. *Hypertension* 2008; **51**: 454–9.

11 Hernandez Prada JA, Ferreira AJ, Katovich MJ, Shenoy V, Qi Y, Santos RAS, *et al.* Structure-based identification of small-molecule angiotensin-converting enzyme 2 activators as novel antihypertensive agents. *Hypertension* 2008; **51**: 1312–17.

45 Angiotensin Receptor Blockers and Dual Blockade

Case History

Albert is 62 years old and was recently started on an angiotensin-converting enzyme inhibitor (ACE-I), following which he developed an irritating cough. He also takes hydrochlorthiazide and amlodipine for his blood pressure (BP), which is not perfectly controlled. He suffered a myocardial infarction (MI) 4 years ago, and there is a strong family history of vascular disease. He no longer smokes and is a moderate alcohol drinker. His electrocardiogram (ECG) fulfils criteria for left ventricular hypertrophy. This is confirmed by an echocardiogram but he has good left ventricular function. You decide that an angiotensin receptor blocker (ARB) would be the most logical next step, after stopping his ACE-I.

Is there anything to choose between the available ARBs?

Have ARBs been shown to protect against cardiovascular (CV) events as well as lowering BP?

Is there evidence to support dual renin–angiotensin system (RAS) blockade with ACE-I and ARB?

Background

Losartan and eprosartan were the first drugs of a class that inhibited the angiotensin type 1 receptor. The drugs have found wide usage in the treatment of hypertension as well as in chronic kidney disease (CKD), including diabetic nephropathy and in heart failure. In the early days of these drugs, it was hoped that by inhibiting the binding of angiotensin II to its receptor, these drugs might offer an advantage over ACE-Is. In fact, the efficacy of the two classes appears to be roughly equivalent. Stimulus to the development of RAS-blocking drugs came from evidence that the harmful effects of angiotensin II were not entirely mediated through increased BP. Furthermore, patients with hypertension but low renin levels were at less risk of MI, stroke and renal disease than were those with high renin. RAS-blocking drugs have proved to be protective in high-risk groups, including those with left ventricular failure, CKD and diabetic nephropathy.

ARBs are generally well tolerated with a very low incidence of serious side effects. They can cause hypotension with first dose exposure. As with ACE-Is, patients starting ARBs

Table 45.1 Commonly used angiotensin receptor blockers

Drug	Brand names	Half–life (h)	Daily dose (mg)
Candesartan	Atacand	8	8–16
	Atacand Plus*		16/12.5
Eprosartan	Teveten	7	600–800
	Teveten Plus*		600/12.5
Irbesartan	Avapro, Karvea	13	150–300
	Avapro HCT*		150/12.5
	Karvezide		150/12.5
			300/12.5
Losartan	Cozaar	2	50–100
Olmesartan	Olmetec	13	20–40
	Olmetec Plus*		20/12.5
			40/12.5
			40/25
Telmisartan	Micardis	24	40–80
	Micardis Plus*		40/12.5
			80/12.5
Valsartan	Diovan	6	80–320

*Angiotensin receptor blocker with hydrochlorthiazide (12.5 mg unless otherwise stated).

should be screened for increased creatinine and hyperkalaemia. A marked increase in creatinine suggests renal artery stenosis, and patients should be investigated accordingly. It is not as well documented as for ACE-Is, but can be assumed that an early increase of creatinine of up to 20–30% above baseline is predictive of long-term renal protective effect.[1] The most common side effect of ACE-Is is cough (up to 8% of patients), which does not occur with ARBs. Angio-oedema is a rare but serious side effect of ACE-Is. Angio-oedema has also been reported with ARBs. Other reported side effects include skin rash, dizziness, headache, gastrointestinal disturbances and muscle cramps. The commonly used ARBs are listed in Table 45.1. Losartan, the first to be marketed, has a very short half-life and is better given as a twice-daily dose. Irbesartan, olmesartan and telmisartan have longer half-lives, perhaps explaining why these drugs have found very wide usage. The duration of action of these drugs has also been expressed as the pressor effect 24 hours after they are administered. For most of the drugs used, this is in the range 40–70%. Apart from duration of action, there is little to suggest that there is much difference in the actions of the different drugs in this class. Losartan is somewhat uricosuric, but it is not clear if this is clinically significant.

Kjeldsen and Julius (2004)[2] reviewed the larger ACE-I and the early ARB trials. In all, six ACE-I trials and five ARB trials were reviewed although three of the ARB trials were still in progress at the time. In general, a 6–12 mmHg reduction in systolic BP or a 5–6 mmHg reduction in diastolic BP in these trials equated to a 35–42% reduction in risk of a stroke and 10–16% reduction in risk of MI. The major ACE-I trials reviewed showed the benefits of RAS blockade, but also the difficulty in interpreting the effects of RAS-blocking drugs in combination with other drug classes and in determining whether beneficial effects were related to, or independent of, BP lowering. The major ACE-I trials were:

● CAPPP (Captopril Prevention Project) (1999) followed 10 985 subjects for a mean of 6.1 years, comparing the effects of ACE-I with diuretic and β-blocker. There was no difference in the primary end-point but captopril reduced the risk of CV death and MI (fatal and non-fatal), although it increased the risk of stroke.

● STOP-2 (Swedish Trial in Old Patients with Hypertension) (1999) included 6614 subjects aged 70–84 years and followed them for a mean of 4.5 years. With ACE-I compared with other agents, there was no difference in mortality or major CV event rate, but there were decreased rates of MI and heart failure.

● HOPE (Heart Outcomes Prevention Evaluation) (2000) compared ramipril with placebo and followed 9297 high-risk subjects over 4 years. Ramipril decreased CV morbidity and mortality. The benefits were also seen in patients with diabetes, whether or not they were hypertensive.

● PROGRESS (Perindopril Protection against Recurrent Stroke Study) (2001) followed 6105 subjects with stroke or transient ischaemic accident over 4 years, comparing ACE-I ± diuretic with placebo. In addition to a marked reduction in BP, there was decreased stroke risk during the follow-up period.

● ALLHAT (Antihypertensive and Lipid-Lowering Treatment to Prevent Heart Attack Trial) (2002) recruited over 42 000 subjects with hypertension and at least one other risk factor, and aimed to compare calcium channel blocker, α-blocker, ACE-I and diuretic. The α-blocker wing was stopped early. Otherwise, follow-up was for a mean of 4.9 years. Compared with other agents there was no difference with ACE-I for the primary end-point but there was increased relative risk (RR) for stroke.

● ANBP2 (Second Australian National Blood Pressure Study) followed 6083 hypertensive subjects aged 65–84 years for a mean of 4.1 years. Compared with diuretic, ACE-I treatment was associated with an 11% reduction in risk of CV events, including death. The beneficial effect of ACE-I was primarily in men.

The above studies in the late 1990s and early 2000s showed the potential benefit of RAS blockade in preventing CV events in patients with hypertension. They were followed by studies using the ARBs, the first of which was the LIFE (Losartan Intervention For Endpoint reduction, 2002) study. Here, 9222 patients with hypertension and ECG criteria for left ventricular failure were followed for a mean of 4.8 years, comparing enalapril with atenolol.[2] Despite similar reductions in BP, losartan was associated with a 13% risk reduction for CV events compared with atenolol. The effect of the ACE-I was even more impressive in the substudy involving only patients with diabetes, although there was a 2 mmHg difference in systolic BP (lower for losartan) in this substudy.[2] SCOPE (Study on Cognition and Prognosis in the Elderly, 2003) compared candesartan with placebo (each ± hydrochlorthiazide) in 4937 mildly hypertensive patients followed for 3.7 years.[2] Candesartan decreased risk for stroke by 28% and risk of major CV events by 11%. Not

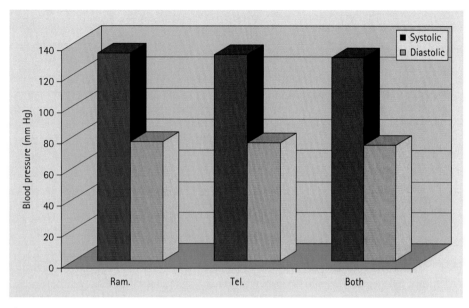

Figure 45.1 Blood pressure control in the ONTARGET study. Data are from the ONTARGET Study[4] comparing ramipril (Ram.), telmisartan (Tel.), or the combination (Both) in high-risk patients. Combined angiotensin-converting enzyme inhibitor and angiotensin receptor blocker treatment did not lower blood pressure any more than either agent used alone

surprisingly, there was also a greater reduction in BP compared with placebo. Finally, VALUE (Valsartan Antihypertensive Long-term Use Evaluation, 2004) recruited 15 314 patients with hypertension and associated risk factors, and followed them for a mean of 4.2 years.[2] Valsartan was compared with amlodipine. There was no difference in hypertension control, and also no difference in the primary end-point.

Is there any evidence that ARBs are superior to ACE-Is? This was addressed in a recent systematic review that included 61 studies where the two classes of drug were directly compared. Many of the studies were of relatively short duration. As expected, cough was consistently found to be more common with ACE-Is. This is probably the reason for the greater persistence rate with ARBs. The two classes had very similar effects on BP. There was no difference in CV events, left ventricular mass or function, renal disease, lipid levels, development of diabetes, need for additional agents, or quality of life.

Recent Developments

1   Some studies have suggested that ACE-I and ARB together may confer additional protection compared with use of either class alone. However, two large studies have documented no benefit of combining the two classes. In the VALIANT (Valsartan in Acute Myocardial Infarction) study,[3] valsartan, ramipril, and the combination of the two were compared in patients with left ventricular dysfunction or failure following MI. The ACE-I and the ARB conferred identical

protective effects and there was no additional benefit from combining the two. Post-treatment BP was comparable in all three wings of the study. The recently published ONTARGET (Ongoing Telmisartan Alone and in Combination with Ramipril Global Endpoint Trial) study[4] compared telmisartan, ramipril, or the combination, in patients with vascular disease or high-risk diabetes. There were no differences in CV outcomes. Adverse effects – hypotension, syncope, cough, diarrhoea and renal impairment – were all more common with the combination compared with either drug alone. There was no advantage of the combination for BP control (Figure 45.1).

2   A meta-analysis of ACE-I or ARBs in high-risk patients included 25 trials with a total of nearly 46 000 patients with CKD and proteinuria,[5] and showed a decreased risk of CV outcomes, MI and heart failure. The benefits of RAS blockade were apparent in patients with non-diabetic nephropathy and also when diabetic patients were included in the analysis. There is evidence that dual blockade, while it does not necessarily markedly improve BP control, might be more protective than either agent class alone for renal and myocardial function. However, the combination of the ACE-I and ARB is associated with a marked increase in adverse events compared with either drug class used alone.[6] There is emerging evidence that the combination of spironolactone with either ACE-I or ARB may be more effective and a safer combination.

3   Aliskiren is a non-peptide inhibitor of renin that is as effective as ACE-Is or ARBs in lowering BP. Unlike the latter two classes it lowers, instead of increasing, circulating renin, and it has no effect on BP in normotensive subjects. It can be used effectively in combination with diuretic.[7] The recent AVOID (Aliskiren in the Evaluation of Proteinuria in Diabetes) study[8] evaluated the drug in combination with losartan. The study demonstrated that aliskiren appeared to have renoprotective effects over and above its ability to lower BP in patients with diabetic nephropathy. Other developments in the pipeline for blocking RAS include dual action angiotensin and endothelin receptor antagonists. Atrial natriuretic peptide is a vasodilator and is degraded by neutral endopeptidase. Compounds are being investigated which are dual ACE/neutral endopeptidase inhibitors. Triple inhibitors are ACE/neutral endopeptidase inhibitors with endothelin converting enzyme inhibitory activity in addition, and are currently being investigated.

4   *In vitro* studies with telmisartan have shown that it has anti-inflammatory and antioxidant effects.[9] Other studies have shown that ARBs can decrease the effect of excess dietary salt on the vasculature, and that they may directly affect endothelial precursor cell function. A better understanding of the role of these processes may lead to design of drugs with multiple therapeutic actions.

Conclusions

Considerations around prescribing ARBs are summarized in Figure 45.2. ACE-I and ARBs have a similar potency for decreasing BP to other major classes of antihypertensive drug. Available evidence suggests, but does not absolutely prove, that the two classes of RAS-blocking drug may have organ-protective effects beyond BP lowering. In some

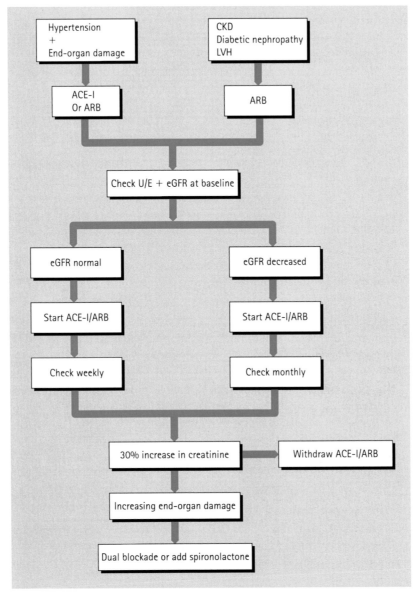

Figure 45.2 Prescription of ARBs. ACE-I, angiotensin-converting enzyme inhibitor; ARB, angiotensin receptor blocker; CKD, chronic kidney disease; eGFR, estimated glomerular filtration rate; LVH, left ventricular hypertrophy

studies where benefit has been attributed to RAS-blocking drugs, slightly better BP reduction could have accounted for some of the differences in outcomes documented. There do not appear to be significant differences in the therapeutic effect of different agents in this class. Those with a longer biological half-life are more likely to provide round the clock BP lowering. ARBs or ACE-Is are particularly indicated where hypertension is accompanied by a high risk of end-organ damage, e.g. in diabetic nephropathy, CKD or with left ventricular failure (Figure 45.2). Dual blockade with ACE-I plus ARB has been widely used in recent years. It does not, however, offer a marked advantage in terms of BP reduction. It may add to end-organ protection compared with either drug alone, and there is a marked increase in adverse events, including hyperkalaemia and worsening of renal function.

References

1   Bakris GL, Weir MR. Angiotensin-converting enzyme inhibitor-associated elevations in serum creatinine. Is this a cause for concern? *Arch Intern Med* 2000; **160**: 683–93.

2   Kjeldsen SE, Julius S. Hypertension mega-trials with cardiovascular endpoints: effect of angiotensin-converting enzyme inhibitors and angiotensin receptor blockers. *Am Heart J* 2004; **148**: 747–54.

3   Pfeffer MA, McMurray JJV, Velazquez EJ, Rouleau JL, Kober L, Maggioni AP, *et al.* Valsartan, captopril, or both in myocardial infarction complicated by heart failure, left ventricular dysfunction or both. *N Engl J Med* 2003; **349**: 1893–906.

4   Yusuf S, Teo KK, Pogue J, Dyal L, Copland I, Schumaker H, *et al.* Telmisartan, ramipril or both in patients at high risk for vascular events. *N Engl J Med* 2008; **358**: 1547–59.

5   Balamuthusamy S, Srinivasan L, Verma M, Adigopula S, Jalandara N, Hathiwala S, Smith E. Renin angiotensin system blockade and cardiovascular outcomes in patients with chronic kidney disease and proteinuria: a meta-analysis. *Am Heart J* 2008; **155**: 791–805.

6   Phillips CO, Kashani A, Ko DK, Francis G, Krumholz HM. Adverse effects of combination of angiotensin II receptor blockers plus angiotensin-converting enzyme inhibitors for left ventricular dysfunction: a quantitative review of data from randomized clinical trials. *Arch Intern Med* 2007; **167**: 1930–6.

7   Gradman AH, Kad R. Renin inhibition in hypertension. *J Am Coll Cardiol* 2008; **51**: 519–28.

8   Parving HH, Persson F, Lewis JB, Lewis EJ, Hollenberg NK. Aliskiren combined with losartan in type 2 diabetes and nephropathy. *N Engl J Med* 2008; **358**: 2433–46.

9   Cianchetti S, Del Fiorentino A, Colognato R, Di Stefano R, Franzoni F, Pedrinelli R. Anti-inflammatory and anti-oxidant properties of telmisartan in cultured human umbilical vein endothelial cells. *Atherosclerosis* 2008; **198**: 22–8.

46 Centrally-acting and vasodilator drugs

Case History

Mrs CS is 59 years old and has tried many antihypertensive drugs, but experienced numerous side effects. Currently, she takes 5 mg amlodipine and 5 mg bendrofluazide. She tolerates this well but her blood pressure (BP) is not well controlled with systolic pressures above 145 mmHg. She has not tolerated higher doses of amlodipine, cannot tolerate β-blocker, and has previously had a cough with angiotensin-converting enzyme inhibitors and possible angio-oedema with candesartan. She is keen to have her BP controlled, as there is a family history of vascular disease.

What is the present place of drugs of the above two classes?

How useful are the centrally acting drugs?

What are the prospects for drugs that are direct vasodilators?

Background

Although drugs of the above classes are not generally used as first- or second-line, their use is still frequently considered. Commonly used agents are summarized in Table 46.1. The centrally acting drugs cross the blood–brain barrier and are agonists at the α_2-adrenergic or imidazoline receptors in the rostral ventrolateral medulla. The effect of their action on these receptors is to decrease peripheral sympathetic tone. Methyldopa was once very commonly used, and is still used by some patients who have been treated for hypertension for many years. Its current use is largely confined to hypertension in pregnancy. Methyldopa is converted to α-methyl-noradrenaline, which acts as a selective α_2-agonist. Side effects include dry mouth, gastrointestinal symptoms and postural hypotension. Haemolytic anaemia and systemic lupus erythematosus-like syndrome are rare side effects. Effects on reproductive function are common – hyperprolactinaemia, decreased libido, menstrual irregularities, gynaecomastia and ejaculatory failure. Side effects are less common if the daily dose is less than 1000 mg. Rebound hypertension can occur if the drug is stopped suddenly.

In addition to its use in hypertension, clonidine is also used for neuropathic pain, opiate withdrawal, migraine, and for vasomotor symptoms related to the menopause. It acts through both α_2-adrenoreceptors and imidazoline I_1 receptors. Most of the side effects are mediated through the α_2 receptors and include dry mouth, drowsiness, postural

Table 46.1 Commonly used agents			
Agent	Brand name	Half-life (h)	Usual daily dose (mg)
1. Centrally acting drugs			
α-methyldopa	Aldomet	2*	500–2000**
Clonidine	Catapres, Dixarit	12–16	0.2–0.6**
Moxonidine	Physiotens	2–3	0.2–0.6**
2. Vasoldilators			
Hydralazine	Apresoline, generic	2	50–200
Minoxidil	Loniten, Rogaine	4	20–40

*Actual duration of hypotensive effect much longer.
**Divided for higher doses.

hypotension and constipation. Sudden withdrawal may cause rebound hypertension and tachycardia. Clonidine is widely used as a diagnostic test for phaeochromocytoma – administration of the drug normally suppresses peripheral catecholamines but fails to do so in patients with phaeochromocytoma. Other centrally acting α_2-agonists include guanabenz (Wytensin) and guanfacine (Tenex, Intuniv).

Moxonidine is a selective imidazoline I_1 receptor agonist with only minor α_2-agonist activity.[1] Cardiac I_1 receptors are involved in increasing atrial natriuretic peptide release but there is no convincing evidence that this mechanism contributes to the therapeutic effect of moxonidine. Decreases in systolic BP and diastolic BP are comparable with those with other agents when moxonidine is used as monotherapy, and the drug can usefully be combined with a variety of other agents. It has no significant negative effect on cardiac haemodynamic parameters. Potentially, a major advantage is that the decreased sympathetic activity with the drug leads to improvements in insulin sensitivity and glucose tolerance. This is especially so in patients with a high baseline sympathetic activity (resting pulse rate >80 beats/min). Both fasting and postprandial glucose levels are decreased. The drug is at least weight neutral and may even promote modest weight loss. Moxonidine has no meaningful effect on lipid profile. Side effects are similar to those of other centrally acting drugs, but usually much milder. Drowsiness may be markedly increased when the drug is taken with alcohol or benzodiazepines. Bradycardia, rebound hypertension and erectile dysfunction do not occur. The dose should be decreased in those with moderate, or worse, renal impairment – as with clonidine. In short-term trials, moxonidine has been shown to be useful in combination with diuretic, angiotensin-converting enzyme inhibitors, or calcium channel blockers. A particularly useful synergy exists with vasodilator drugs as the central sympatholytic effect of moxonidine prevents reflex tachycardia. There are no sizeable long-term outcome studies, although its BP-lowering effect is well documented to be associated with decreased microalbumin.

Moxonidine is contraindicated in patients with heart failure and in those with dysrhythmias. Patients with heart failure poorly tolerate higher doses. The MOXCON (Moxonidine Congestive Heart Failure) study[2] planned to recruit over 4500 patients with New York Heart Association class II–IV cardiac failure from 425 centres in 17 countries. It was terminated early because of an excess of deaths in the moxonidine (compared with placebo) group. Only 1934 patients were actually recruited. There were 54 deaths (5.5%) in the treated group compared with 32 (3.4%, $P = 0.012$) in the placebo arm. There were also more hospital admissions in the moxonidine arm. Thus, in spite of its efficacy, low incidence of side effects, and beneficial metabolic profile, there are concerns in relation to long-term prognosis.

Hydralazine is another drug that has traditionally been widely used but is now rarely used. It is a direct vasodilator that acts by decreasing calcium release from the sarcoplasmic reticulum, and thus relaxing the vascular smooth muscle. Side effects include loss of appetite, nausea and vomiting, reflex tachycardia, palpitation, increased angina, flushing and postural hypotension. Arthralgia and myalgia may occur, and the drug can cause a systemic lupus erythematosus-like syndrome. It is useful in hypertensive emergencies, including those during pregnancy. For pregnancy, it is classified as category C – some suggestion of adverse effects from animal studies, insufficient systematic studies in humans, but suitable for use in pregnancy where benefits are judged to outweigh risks. There has been a recent increase in hydralazine use because of the preparation Bidil (isosorbide dinitrate 20 mg + hydralazine 37.5 mg) – licensed in the USA for the treatment of heart failure in black Americans.

Minoxidil is a powerful vasodilator that probably acts as a nitric oxide donor but also opens potassium channels. It should be reserved for severe hypertension resistant to other agents. It causes reflex tachycardia and sodium/water retention. Because of these effects it is usually prescribed with a β-blocker and a loop diuretic. It can precipitate angina or heart failure. Pericardial effusion, which is sometimes severe enough to cause tamponade, has been described. Hypertrichosis has long been noted as a side effect and the drug is used systemically and topically to reverse baldness.

More recent approaches to development of vasodilator drugs are:

● Fenoldopam (Corlopam) is a very short-acting dopamine D_1 receptor agonist used in emergency treatment of hypertension. Postural hypotension is a well recognized side effect.

● The endothelin receptor antagonist bosentan is efficacious in pulmonary hypertension. There is hope that selective endothelin A receptor antagonists such as darusentan may be useful in patients with systemic hypertension.

● Inhibitors of the enzyme Rho kinase such as fasudil may not only attenuate some of the vasoconstrictor effects of angiotensin II but also have positive effects on insulin sensitivity and vascular remodelling.

Recent Developments

1   While there is doubt as to the place of central sympathetic inhibition, recent data with moxonidine confirm the metabolic benefits of this drug compared with other antihypertensives. Derosa et al.[3] in a study over 6 months involving patients with type 2 diabetes and moderate hypertension showed that, in addition to improved BP, there were improvements in HbA_1c and lipids.

2   Arterial stiffening is the major cause of increased systolic and pulse pressure in older subjects. Brachial BP does not entirely reflect central pressure – the pressure

transmitted to heart, brain and kidneys. Increased central pressure is an important determinant of cardiovascular events. Vasodilator drugs do not affect the underlying arterial stiffness but they do considerably modify pulse wave reflection and are thus most useful in older subjects with hypertension.[4]

3   Darusentan has recently been studied in a group of patients with resistant hypertension.[5] Mean systolic BP decreased by 11.5 mmHg and diastolic BP by about 6.5 mmHg. The drug was very well tolerated with mild oedema and headache being the most frequent side effects. Selective endothelin antagonists show considerable promise, but are a long way from being regarded as first-line agents.

4   Activators of large-conductance calcium-activated potassium (BK) channels are a novel approach to vasodilatation and hypertension management.[6] Increased expression of these channels has been noted in animal models of hypertension and is thought to be a compensatory mechanism. BK channels are activated by certain naturally occurring long-chain polyunsaturated fatty acids. In addition to their antihypertensive effects, BK channel activators also act on the kidney leading to potassium conservation.[7]

5   Some of the benefits of calcium channel blockers on outcomes may relate to effects of vascular remodelling. Rho kinase inhibitors may also have this dual action. Migration and hypertrophy of vascular smooth muscle cells is a normal response to increased BP and is partially mediated by Rho kinase. Inhibitors of the enzyme can alter this process[8] and can also favourably affect the response of the myocardium to increased pressure load.[9]

Conclusions

Mechanistic considerations (Figure 46.1) suggest that central sympatholytic drugs and direct vasodilators should be important agents in managing hypertension. At present, the place of these two classes is somewhat limited. Methyldopa is still widely used in the management of hypertension in pregnancy – this relates to prolonged experience with the drug, which is safe, rather than efficacy considerations. Hydralazine, and occasionally minoxidil, is still used in states of severe or resistant hypertension but other agents have largely superseded them. The favourable metabolic profile of minoxidil is a considerable advantage but studies are needed to resolve questions about its safety in relation to causing or precipitating heart failure. Given recent increases in understanding about the importance of altered physical properties of arteries in older subjects, it is certain that vasodilator drugs will find increased usage in the next few years. Several classes of drug are in advanced stages of development.

References

1   Fenton C, Keating GM, Lyseng-Williamson KA. Moxonidine. A review of its use in essential hypertension. *Drugs* 2006; **66**: 477–96.

2   Cohn JN, Pfeffer MA, Rouleau J, Sharpe N, Swedberg K, Straub M, *et al.* Adverse mortality effect of central sympathetic inhibition with sustained-release moxonidine in patients with heart failure (MOXCON). *Eur J Heart Fail* 2003; **5**: 659–67.

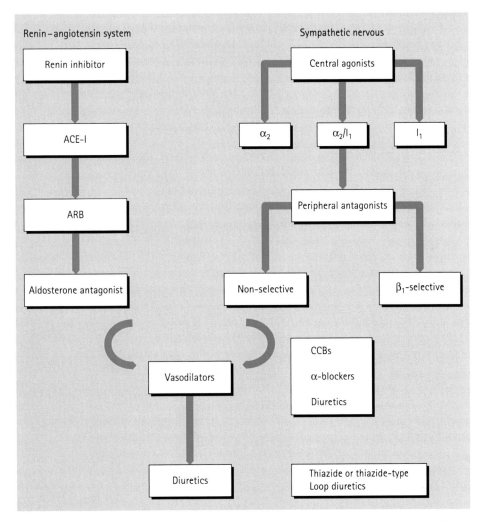

Figure 46.1 Antihypertensive drug mechanisms. ACE-I, angiotensin-converting enzyme inhibitor; ARB, angiotensin receptor blocker; CCB, calcium channel blocker.

3 Derosa G, Cicero AFG, D'Angelo A, Fogari E, Salvadeo S, Gravina A, *et al.* Metabolic and antihypertensive effects of moxonidine and moxonidine plus irbesartan in patients with type 2 diabetes mellitus and mild hypertension: a sequential, randomized, double-blind clinical trial. *Clin Ther* 2007; **29**: 602–10.

4 Nichols WW, Denardo SJ, Wilkinson IB, McEniery CM, Cockcroft J, O'Rourke MF. Effects of arterial stiffness, pulse wave velocity, and wave reflections on the central aortic pressure waveform. *J Clin Hypertens* 2008; **10**: 295–303.

5 Black HR, Bakris GL, Weber MA, Weiss R, Shahawy ME, Marple R, *et al.* Efficacy and safety of darusentan in patients with resistant hypertension: results from a randomized, double-blind, placebo-controlled dose-ranging study. *J Clin Hypertens* 2007; **9**: 760–9.

6   Calderone V, Fiamingo FL, Amato G, Giorgi I, Livi O, Martelli A, *et al.* New amido derivatives as potential BKCa potassium channel activators. XI. *Eur J Med Chem* 2008; **43:** 792–9.

7   Grimm PR, Sansom SC. BK channels in the kidney. *Curr Opin Nephrol Hypertens* 2007; **16:** 430–6.

8   Onoue N, Nawata J, Tada T, Zhulanqiqige D, Wang H, Sugimura K, *et al.* Increased static pressure promotes migration of vascular smooth muscle cells: involvement of the Rho-kinase pathway. *J Cardiovasc Pharmacol* 2008; **51:** 55–61.

9   Phrommintikul A, Tran L, Kompa A, Wang B, Adrahtas A, Cantwell D, *et al.* Effects of a Rho kinase inhibitor on pressure overload induced cardiac hypertrophy and associated diastolic dysfunction. *Am J Physiol* 2008; **294:** H1804–14.

Index

Page numbers in italics refer to figures or tables.